RADIOLOGY 101
The Basics and Fundamentals
of Imaging

D1472739

Radiology 101

The Basics and Fundamentals of Imaging

Editor

William E. Erkonen, M.D.
Associate Professor
Department of Radiology
University of Iowa College of Medicine
University of Iowa Hospitals and Clinics
Iowa City, Iowa

Associate Editor

Wilbur L. Smith, M.D.
Professor
Department of Radiology and Pediatrics
University of Iowa College of Medicine
University of Iowa Hospitals and Clinics
Iowa City, Iowa

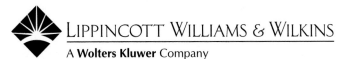

LIPPINCOTT WILLIAMS & WILKINS
A **Wolters Kluwer** Company

Philadelphia • Baltimore • New York • London
Buenos Aires • Hong Kong • Sydney • Tokyo

Acquisitions Editor: James Ryan
Developmental Editor: Brian Brown
Manufacturing Manager: Dennis Teston
Production Manager: Jodi Borgenicht
Production Editor: Karen G. Edmonson
Cover Designer: Diana Andrews
Indexer: Gloria Hamilton
Compositor: Bi-Comp, Inc.
Printer: Courier Westford

Printed in the United States of America

9 8 7 6 5 4 3 2

Library of Congress Cataloging-in-Publication Data
Radiology 101: The Basics and Fundamentals of Imaging / editor, William E.
Erkonen; associate editor, Wilbur L. Smith.
     p.   cm.
   Includes bibliographical references and index.
   ISBN 0-397-51499-9
   1. Radiography, Medical.   2. Diagnosis, Radioscopic.   I. Erkonen,
William E.   II. Smith, Wilbur L.   III: Title: Radiology one hundred one.
IV. Title: Radiology one hundred and one.
   [DNLM: 1. Radiology. 2. Diagnostic Imaging.   WN 100 R1285 1998]
RC78.R242   1998
616.07′54—dc21
DNLM/DLC   98-2597
for Library of Congress   CIP

To Beth Vandermyde Erkonen

Contents

Section I: Basic Principles

Section II: Diagnostic Radiology

Contributing Authors

David Bushnell, M.D. *Chief of Diagnostic Imaging, Veterans Administration Hospital, Iowa City, Iowa; Associate Professor, Department of Radiology, University of Iowa College of Medicine, University of Iowa Hospitals and Clinics, 200 Hawkins Road, Iowa City, Iowa 52247-1077*

Paul J. Chang, M.D. *Associate Professor of Radiology, Director, Division of Radiology Informatics, Department of Radiology, University of Pittsburgh Medical Center, 200 Lothrop Street, Pittsburgh, Pennsylvania 15213*

William E. Erkonen, M.D. *Associate Professor, Department of Radiology, University of Iowa College of Medicine, University of Iowa Hospitals and Clinics, 200 Hawkins Road, Iowa City, Iowa 52247-1077*

Thomas A. Farrell, M.B. *Assistant Professor, Department of Radiology, University of Chicago, 5841 S. Maryland Avenue, Chicago, Illinois 60637*

Wilbur L. Smith, M.D. *Professor of Radiology and Pediatrics, Department of Radiology, University of Iowa College of Medicine, University of Iowa Hospitals and Clinics, 200 Hawkins Road, Iowa City, Iowa 52242-1077*

Preface

In 1995, we celebrated the centennial of Roentgen's discovery of x-rays. This discovery marked the birth of radiology. During the last twenty years, radiology has played a critical role in patient diagnosis and care on the wings of extraordinary technologic advances. As one develops a better understanding of radiology, improved patient diagnosis and care are likely to follow.

The basics of radiologic imaging can be understood by most students, and recent research documented that first year medical students enrolled in a gross anatomy course recognized anatomic structures on images at an 88% correct response rate immediately following instruction. The same group had a long-term retention rate at 1 year post-instruction of 74% (Chapter 1) (1). This supported previously held views that visual instruction is generally superior to verbal instruction (Chapter 1) (2). Thus, this book places heavy emphasis on images of both normal anatomy and commonly encountered pathology.

Anatomy is, after all, the language of radiology; a sound foundation in old-fashioned radiologic anatomy is essential to understand the manifestations of disease on radiologic images. We have presented clearly labeled images of the normal anatomy of the major organ systems in the human body to facilitate this understanding, and have presented this anatomy from a variety of angles. More importantly, we present normal anatomy not only on radiographs, but also on magnetic resonance images and CT scans, which are currently so commonly used as to be routine.

The first section of this book presents basic, easily understandable discussions of how the major imaging modalities are used and operated. These discussions are important because understanding how radiologic images are produced is vital to understanding what the images portray. The strengths and weaknesses of the various modalities are described in clinical tips within the text (e.g., "What are the basic differences between T-1 and T-2 images and what are the clinical indications for each?"). We have included a substantial chapter on interventional radiology, which is of increasing importance. Section One concludes with a pragmatic assessment of radiologic decision-making. The information in this chapter properly places the interpretation of radiologic studies in the clinical context of day-to-day practice, including important reminders about the limits of what imaging studies can portray and, with what degree of certitude.

The second section systematically examines the imaging of anatomic areas and major organ systems and contains, as stated above, extensive presentations of normal anatomy, normal anatomic variants, and commonly encountered pathology. Each chapter begins with a chapter outline to make topics easier to find and with the exception of chapter 5, concludes with a summary list of key points. We have attempted to make each chapter in the book user-friendly. The writing tends to be informal and dispenses common-sense tips and pointers freely (e.g., how to systematically examine a PA chest radiograph, including how to be sure that the film is positioned correctly on the view box).

Although this book is not intended to transform the reader into a radiologist or a radiologist look-a-like, it could well serve as a general field guide. The true purpose of this book is to give the reader a "feel" for radiologic anatomy and the radiologic manifestations of some common disease processes. This "feel" for radiology will enable you to request radiologic consultations in an intelligent manner and to approach image viewing without feeling intimidated. This book will give the reader the basic foundation for further study on the subject.

William E. Erkonen
Wilbur L. Smith

Acknowledgments

A deep debt of gratitude is owed to the entire Radiology faculty and resident staff at the University of Iowa for providing images and advice for this book. Special thanks to Doctors Monzer Abu-Yousef, Thomas Barloon, Eric Brandser, Bruce Brown, Daniel Crosby, William Daniel, J. G. Fletcher, Jeffrey Galvin, Elvira Lang, Charles Lu, Brian Mullan, Hoang Nyguyen, Retta Pelsang, Patrick Rheingans, Parvez Shirazi, William Sickels, William Stanford, Brad Thompson, and Donald C. Young. We are also indebted to technologists Stephanie Ellingson, Mary Burr, Scot Heery, Deborah Troyer, and Heidi Berns.

A special thanks to Dr. George El-Khoury, Dr. Ronald Bergman, and Kathy Martensen, RTR, for their encouragement, suggestions, and general advice.

The skillful illustrations of Shirley Taylor and the late Frank J. Sindelar are greatly appreciated. Brian Clarke provided the original drawings for Figures 3-1, 3-2, 3-18, 3-21, and 3-23.

SECTION I

Basic Principles

CHAPTER 1

Radiography, Computed Tomography, Magnetic Resonance Imaging, and Ultrasonography

Principles and Indications

William E. Erkonen

Very few of us take the time to study, let alone enjoy, the physics of the technology that we use in our everyday lives. Almost everybody drives an automobile, for instance, but only a few of us have working knowledge about what goes on under our car hoods. The medical technology that produces imaging studies is often met with a similar reception: we all want to drive the car, so to speak, but we don't necessarily want to understand the principles underlying the computed tomograms or magnetic resonance images we study. Yet a basic understanding of imaging modalities is extremely important because you will most likely be reviewing images with a radiologist during radiologic consultations for the rest of your professional life, and the results of these consultations will at times profoundly affect your clinical decision making. Add to this the fact that the interpretation of imaging studies is to a considerable degree dependent on understanding how the images are produced. Here is where our analogy breaks down: one doesn't necessarily have to be a mechanic to be a skilled driver, but reaching a basic understanding of how imaging studies are produced is a necessary first step to viewing the studies themselves. This chapter is designed to demonstrate the elementary physics of radiologic diagnostic imaging.

RADIOGRAPHY

Radiographs are the most common imaging consultations requested by clinicians. So let's set off on the right foot by referring to radiologic images as *radiographs, images, or films,* but not *x-rays.* After all, x-rays are electromagnetic waves produced in an x-ray tube. It is acceptable for a layperson to refer to a radiograph as an x-ray, but the knowledgeable clinician and health care worker should avoid the term. Your usage of appropriate terminology demonstrates *savoir-faire* (the ability to say and do the right thing) to your colleagues and patients.

Whenever possible, radiographs are accomplished in the radiology department. The number of views obtained during a standard or routine study depends

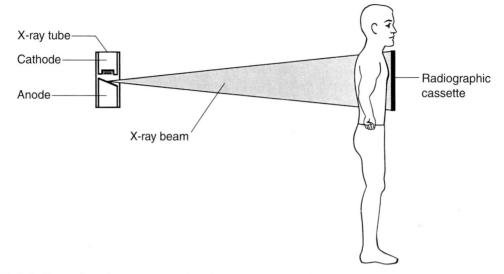

X-ray tube

Cathode

Anode

Radiographic
cassette

X-ray beam

FIG. 1-1. Illustration of a posteroanterior chest radiograph. The patient's chest is pressed against the cassette with hands on the hips. The x-ray beam emanating from the x-ray tube passes through the patient's chest in a posterior-to-anterior or back-to-front direction. The x-rays that pass completely through the patient eventually strike the radiographic film and screens inside the radiographic cassette.

on the anatomic site being imaged. The common radiographic views obtained are named posteroanterior (PA), anteroposterior (AP), oblique, and lateral views.

The chest will be used to illustrate these basic radiographic terms, but this terminology applies to almost all anatomic sites. PA indicates that the central x-ray beam travels from posterior to anterior or back to front as it traverses the chest or any other anatomic site (Fig. 1-1). Lateral indicates that the x-ray beam travels through the patient from side to side (Fig. 1-2). When the patient is unable to cooperate for these routine views, a single AP upright or supine view is obtained. AP means that the x-ray beam passes through the chest or other anatomic site from anterior to posterior or front to back (Fig. 1-3). PA and AP radiographs have similar appear-

ances. When the patient cannot tolerate a transfer to the radiology facility, a portable study is obtained, which means that a portable x-ray machine is brought to the patient wherever he or she is located. AP is the standard portable technique with the patient sitting or supine (Fig. 1-4).

Radiographs have traditionally been described as shades of black, white, and gray. What causes a structure to appear black, white, or gray on a radiograph? Actually, it is the density of the object being imaged that determines how much of the x-ray beam will be absorbed or attenuated (Fig. 1-5). In other words, as the density of an object increases, fewer x-rays pass through it. It is the variable density of structures that results in the four basic radiographic densities: air (black), fat (black), water (gray), and metallic or bone (white)

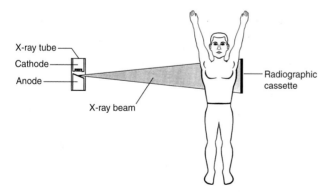

X-ray tube

Cathode

Anode

Radiographic
cassette

X-ray beam

FIG. 1-2. Illustration of a lateral chest radiograph. The x-ray beam passes through the patient's chest from side to side. The x-rays that pass completely through the patient eventually strike the radiographic film and screens. Note that the patient's arms are positioned as to not project over the chest.

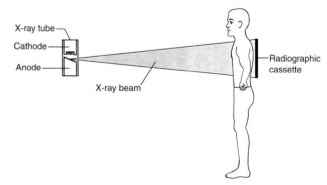

X-ray tube

Cathode

Anode

Radiographic
cassette

X-ray beam

FIG. 1-3. An anteroposterior chest radiograph. The x-ray beam passes through the patient's chest in an anterior-to-posterior or front-to-back direction. Note that the hands are on the hips.

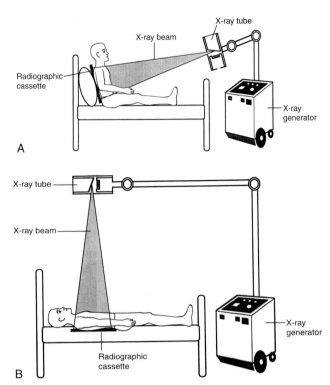

FIG. 1-4. An anteroposterior portable chest radiograph with the patient either sitting **(A)** or supine **(B)**. The x-ray beam passes through the patient's chest in an anterior-to-posterior direction. The x-ray machine has wheels and that allows it to be used wherever needed throughout the hospital.

(Table 1-1). For example, the lungs primarily consist of low-density air, which absorbs very little of the x-ray beam. Thus, air allows a large amount of the x-ray beam to strike or expose the radiographic film. As a result, air in the lungs will appear black on a radiograph. Similarly, fat has a low density but its density is slightly greater than air. Fat will appear black on a radiograph but slightly less black than air. High-density objects such as bones, teeth, calcium deposits in tumors, metallic foreign bodies, R and L lead film markers, and intravascularly injected contrast media absorb all or nearly all of the x-ray beam. As a result, the radiographic film receives little or no x-ray exposure, and these dense structures appear white. Muscles, organs (heart, liver, spleen), and soft tissues are shades of gray, and the shades of gray range

TABLE 1-1. *Basic radiograph film densities or appearances*

Object	Film density
Air	Black
Fat	Black
Bone	White
Metal	White
Calcium	White
Organs, muscles, soft tissues	Shades of gray

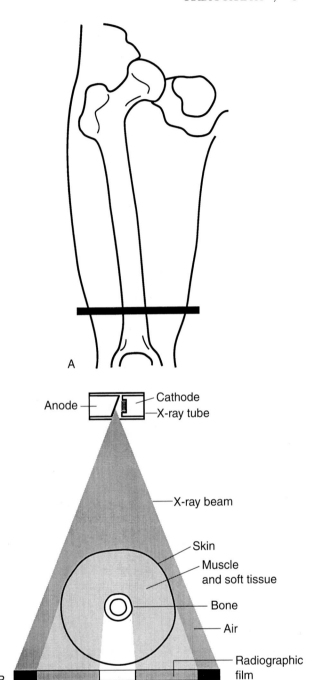

FIG. 1-5. A: The level in the distal thigh through which the x-ray beam is passing in B. **B:** Cross-section of the distal thigh at the level indicated in A. Notice that when the x-ray beam passes through air, the result is a black area on the radiograph. When the x-ray beam strikes bone, the result is a white area on the radiograph. If the x-ray beam passes through soft tissues, the result is a gray appearance on the film.

somewhere between white and black depending on the structure's density. These shades of gray are referred to as *water density*.

Radiographic screens are positioned on either side of the radiographic film inside the light-tight cassette

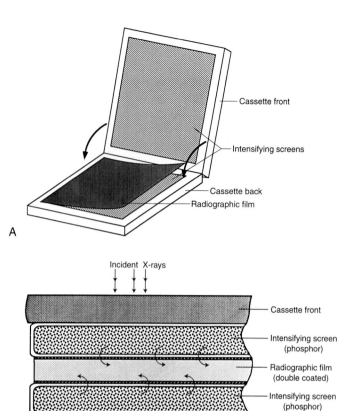

FIG. 1-6. A: An open radiographic cassette containing one sheet of radiographic film and two intensifying screens. A radiographic screen is positioned on each side of the film, and the screens will emit a light flash (fluoresce) when struck by an x-ray. Also, some x-rays directly strike the radiographic film. It is this combination of light flashes from the screens as well as x-rays directly striking the film that causes the radiographic film to be exposed. This is similar to photographic film. **B:** Cross-section illustration of a radiographic cassette. Note the lead foil in the back of the cassette that is designed to stop any x-rays that have penetrated the full thickness of the cassette. The curved arrows represent light flashes that are created when x-rays strike the screens.

or film holder (Fig. 1-6A). The chemical structure of the screens causes them to emit light flashes or to fluoresce when struck by x-rays (Fig. 1-6B). Roentgen's famous discovery of the x-ray was based on his observation that certain chemicals on a laboratory bench across the room actually fluoresced when a cathode ray tube was activated. Later he found that the fluorescence occurred when wood and other materials were placed between the cathode ray tube and the chemicals. He did not know what these highly penetrating invisible rays were, so he called them x-rays. Actually, it is the fluoresced light from the screens on both sides of the film that accounts for the major exposure of the radiographic film. The direct incident x-rays striking the radiographic film account for a small proportion of the film exposure. The use of screens decreases the amount of radiation required to produce a radiograph, and this in turn decreases the patient exposure to radiation.

It is important to remember that both radiographic and photographic film respond in a similar manner to light and x-rays.

Contrast Media

Because soft tissues (muscles, blood vessels, organs) appear approximately the same on a radiograph, we often need a way to distinguish between these structures and their surroundings. Thus, high-density contrast agents are injected intravenously to enhance organs and other soft tissues. It is this enhancement (which increases their density or makes them whiter) that enables the viewer to detect subtle differences between normal and abnormal soft tissues and between an organ and the surrounding tissues on a radiograph. Contrast media usage varies from a simple injection into a fistulous tract to an invasive procedure such as an angiogram, and this will be discussed in greater detail in Chapter 2.

Another type of contrast media employed is that for the gastrointestinal (GI) tract. To accomplish a GI contrast examination, barium sulfate suspension is introduced into the GI tract either by oral ingestion (upper GI series), or through an intestinal tube (small bowel series), or as an enema (barium enema). When air is introduced into the GI tract along with the barium, the result is called a double-contrast study. Barium studies are safer, better tolerated by patients, and relatively inexpensive than the more invasive GI endoscopic studies. Barium studies can be effective in diagnosing a wide variety of GI pathology, as they are quite sensitive and specific.

When the integrity of the GI tract is in question there exists a potential for catastrophic extravasation of the barium into the mediastinum or peritoneum. In these situations barium studies are contraindicated, and a water-soluble iodinated compound should be employed. As a general rule, images produced with water-soluble contrast agents are less informative than barium studies because the water soluble agents are less dense than barium and result in poorer contrast.

Oral ingested tablets containing iodinated compounds can be used to visualize the gallbladder (oral cholecystogram). These compounds are removed from the blood by the hepatic cells and excreted into the biliary tree and concentrated in the gallbladder. This study provides information about gallbladder function and the presence or absence of filling defects such as calculi and tumors.

Often it is necessary to visualize the urinary tract *(excretory urogram)* when searching for a wide variety of pathologic conditions and when seeking anatomic and physiologic information. This study uses intravenously injected ionic high and low osmolar iodinated compounds that are excreted by the kidneys. These same compounds are used in angiography, arthrography, and computed tomography (CT).

Angiography is merely the injection of contrast media directly into a vein or artery via a needle and/or catheter (see Chapter 2).

Arthrography is the injection of contrast media and/or air into a joint. Air may be used alone or in combinations with these compounds to improve contrast. Arthrography has been used to image multiple joints such as rotator cuff injuries of the shoulder and to assess meniscus injuries in the knee. Since the advent of CT and magnetic resonance imaging (MRI), the arthrogram has become less important.

Myelography is the placement of contrast media in the spinal subarachnoid space, usually via a lumbar puncture. This procedure is useful for diagnosing diseases in and around the spinal canal and cord. Due to the advent of the less invasive CT and MRI modalities, the use of myelogram studies has been decreasing.

COMPUTED TOMOGRAPHY

Now is the appropriate time to discuss sectional anatomy imaging, or anatomy in the coronal, sagittal, and axial (cross-section, transverse) planes. These terms, which can be confusing, are clearly illustrated in Fig. 1-7. Sectional anatomy has always been important to the physician and health care worker, but the newer imaging modalities of computed tomography (CT), magnetic resonance imaging (MRI), and ultrasonography (US) demand an in-depth understanding of anatomy displayed in this manner.

Computed tomography (CT or CAT scan) technology was developed in the 1970s, and the rock group The Beatles gave a big boost to CT development when they

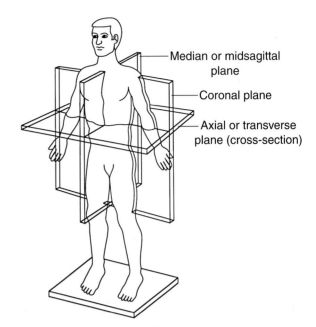

FIG. 1-7. Sagittal, coronal, and axial anatomic planes.

invested a significant amount of money in a business called Electric Musical Instruments Limited (EMI). It was EMI engineers who subsequently developed CT technology. Initially, EMI scanners were utilized exclusively for brain imaging, but this technology was rapidly extended to the abdomen, thorax, spine, and extremities.

CT imaging is best understood if the anatomic site to be examined is thought of as a loaf of sliced bread, and an image of each slice of bread is created without imaging the other slices (Fig. 1-8). This is in contradistinction to a radiograph, which captures the whole loaf of bread, as in a photograph.

The external appearance of a typical CT unit or machine is illustrated in Fig. 1-9. CT images are produced by a combination of x-rays, computers, and detectors. A computer-controlled couch transfers the patient in short increments through the hole or opening in the scanner housing. In the standard CT unit the x-ray tube located in the housing (gantry) rotates around the patient, and each anatomic slice to be imaged is exposed to a pencil-thin x-ray beam (Fig. 1-10). Each image or slice requires only a few seconds; therefore breath holding is usually not an issue. The thickness of these axial images or slices can be varied from 1 to 10 mm depending on the indications for the study. For example, in the abdomen and lungs we commonly use a 10-mm slice thickness because the structures are large. A slice thickness of only a few millimeters is used to image small structures like those found in the middle and inner ear. An average CT study takes approximately 10–20 minutes depending on the circumstances.

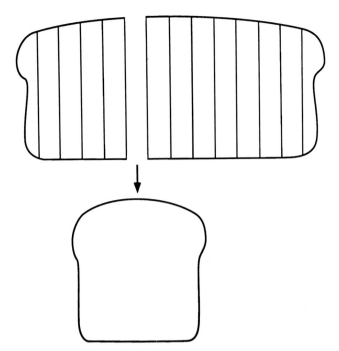

FIG. 1-8. Illustration of how CT technology creates an image of a single slice of bread from a loaf of sliced bread without imaging the other slices.

As in a radiograph, the amount of the x-ray beam that passes through each slice or section of the patient will be inversely proportional to the density of the traversed tissues. The x-rays that pass completely through the patient eventually strike detectors (not film), and the detectors subsequently convert these incident x-rays to an electron stream. This electron stream is digitized or converted to numbers called Hounsfield units (HU); then computer software converts these numbers to corresponding shades of black, white, and gray. A dense structure, such as bone, will absorb most of the x-ray

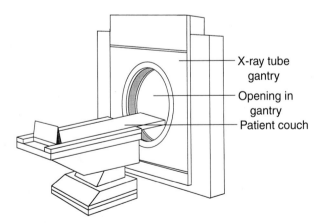

FIG. 1-9. A standard CT scanner or machine. The patient couch or cradle is fed through the opening in the x-ray tube gantry or housing, and the anatomic part to be imaged is centered in this opening. The x-ray tube is located inside the gantry and moves around the patient to create an image.

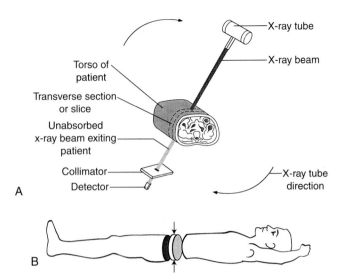

FIG. 1-10. A: Illustration of how the x-ray tube circles the patient's abdomen to produce an image (slice) as shown in B. **B:** Demonstration of how a CT scan creates a thin slice axial image of the abdomen *(arrows)* without imaging the remainder of the abdomen.

beam and allow only a small amount of x-rays to strike the detectors. The result is a −1000 Hounsfield value and a white density on the film. On the other hand, air will absorb little of the x-ray beam, allowing a large number of x-rays to strike the detectors. The result is a −1000 Hounsfield value and a black density on the image. Water density is assigned a Hounsfield value of zero and is gray on an image.

This CT digital information can be displayed on a video monitor, stored on magnetic tape, transmitted across computer networks, or printed on radiographic film via a format camera.

Because CT technology utilizes x-rays, the densities of the anatomic structures being imaged are the same on both CT and radiograph images. In other words, air appears black on both a CT image and a radiograph, and bone appears white on both modalities. One major difference between a radiograph and a CT image is that a radiograph displays the entire anatomic structure, whereas a CT image allows us to visualize the same structure in slices. Another major difference is that in radiography the x-rays that pass through an object are recorded on film, whereas in CT the x-rays are recorded by devices called detectors and converted to digital data.

CT imaging is accomplished with and/or without intravenously injected contrast media. The intravenous contrast media enhance or increase the density of blood vessels, vascular soft tissues, organs, and tumors, as in a radiograph. This enhancement assists in distinguishing between normal tissue and a pathologic process. Contrast media is not needed when searching for intracerebral hemorrhage, for a suspected fracture, or

TABLE 1-2. *Some common indications for CT imaging*

Trauma
Intracranial hemorrhage (suspected or known)
Abdominal injury, especially to organs
Fracture detection and evaluation
Spine alignment
Detect foreign bodies (especially in joints)
Diagnosis of primary and secondary neoplasms
   liver, renal, brain, lung, and bone
Tumor staging

evaluating a fracture fragment within a joint. However, contrast is used when evaluating the liver, kidney, and brain for primary and secondary neoplasms. A few of the common indications for CT imaging are listed in Table 1-2.

Whenever possible, oral GI contrast agents are administered prior to an abdominal CT to delineate the contrast-filled GI tract from other abdominal structures.

High-Resolution Computed Tomography

High-resolution computed tomography (HRCT) refers to CT studies that use thin slices that are approximately 1.5–2.0 mm thick. This technology has become very useful in the diagnosis of parenchymal lung diseases.

Helical or Spiral Computed Tomography

Helical or spiral CT imaging is a recent development. This technology is similar to standard CT but with a few new twists. In helical or spiral CT the patient continuously moves through the gantry while the x-ray tube is continuously circling the patient (Fig. 1-11A). This combination of the patient and x-ray tube continuously moving results in a spiral configuration. This technology can produce 1 slice per second, and the slice can vary

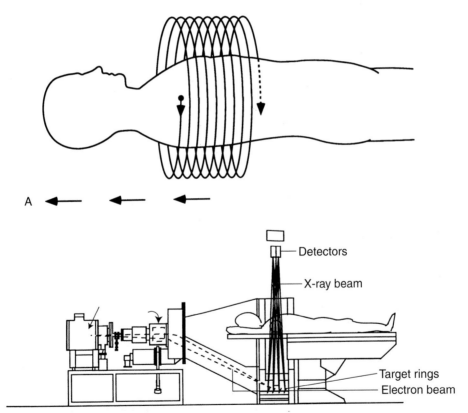

FIG. 1-11. A: A helical or spiral CT scanner. The x-ray tube continuously circles the patient while the patient couch moves continuously through the opening in the x-ray tube gantry. The combination of continuous patient and x-ray tube movement results in a spiral configuration; hence the name "helical." In a standard CT or nonhelical scanner, the patient couch moves in short increments toward the gantry opening and stops intermittently to allow the x-ray tube to move around the patient. Thus, the x-ray tube only moves around the patient when the couch is stationary. **B:** An ultrafast CT scanner or electron beam CT scanner. An electron beam is produced by an electron gun *(straight arrow)*, and the deflection coil *(curved arrow)* causes the electron beam to strike multiple fixed targets that in turn deflect multiple central x-ray beams through the patient. Some x-rays pass through the patient and strike a detector and are processed into an image in much the same manner as in any other CT scanner. (Courtesy of Immatron, Inc., South, San Francisco, CA)

TABLE 1-3. *Advantages and disadvantages of Ultrafast CT (UFCT)*

Advantages
Static and cine or movie images
Noninvasive
Rapid filming results in decreased motion artefact
Good spatial resolution
Disadvantages
Expensive
Limited availability

in thickness from 1 to 10 mm. The resolution and contrast of these images are better than on standard CT images resulting in improved images in areas such the thorax and abdomen.

Ultrafast Computed Tomography

Ultrafast CT (UFCT®) (Immatron, Inc., South, San Francisco, CA) or electron beam computed tomography (EBCT) has been around for a number of years. This technology produces an image in milliseconds or up to 17 images per second (Fig. 1-11B), whereas a conventional CT study requires at least 1–2 seconds to produce one image. The ability to produce multiple images per second results in a cine or movie of moving objects such as contracting cardiac chambers and moving valves. UFCT is used to evaluate a number of cardiac and vascular problems including congenital defects, coronary artery calcifications, and possible aortic dissections. Some of the advantages and disadvantages of UFCT are listed in Table 1-3.

Computed Tomographic Angiography

This term refers to noninvasive angiography using either an UFCT or helical CT scanner. The procedure produces 3-mm slices during the rapid injection of contrast media. This information can be used to create three-dimensional reconstructions.

TABLE 1-4. *Advantages and disadvantages of MRI*

Advantages
Static and cine or movie images
Multiple plane images
Good contrast
No known health hazards
Good for soft tissue injuries of the knee, ankle, and shoulder joints
Disadvantages
More expensive than CT
Long scan times can cause claustrophobia and motion artefacts
Limited availability

TABLE 1-5. *Contraindications for MRI studies*

Pregnancy unless an emergency
Cerebral aneurysms clipped by ferromagnetic clips
Cardiac pacemakers
Inner ear implants
Metallic foreign bodies in and around the eyes

MAGNETIC RESONANCE IMAGING

Magnetic resonance imaging (MRI or MR) is another method for displaying anatomy in the axial, sagittal, and coronal planes, and the slice thicknesses vary between 1 and 10 mm. MRI is especially good for coronal and sagittal imaging, whereas axial imaging is the forte of CT. One of the real strengths of MRI is its ability to detect small changes (contrast) within soft tissues, and MRI soft tissue contrast is better than that found on CT images and radiographs.

CT and MR imaging modalities are digital-based technologies that require computers to convert digital information to shades of black, white, and gray. The major difference in the two technologies is that in MRI the patient is exposed to external magnetic fields and radiofrequency waves, whereas the patient is exposed to x-rays during a CT study. The magnetic fields used in MRI are believed to be harmless. MR scanning can be a problem for people who are prone to develop claustrophobia because they are surrounded by a tunnel-like structure for approximately 30–45 minutes. Some of the advantages and disadvantages of MRI are summarized in Table 1-4. There are a few contraindications for an MRI study, and these are listed in Table 1-5.

The external appearance of an MRI scanner or machine is similar to a CT scanner with the exception that the opening in the MR gantry is more tunnel-like (Fig. 1-12). As in CT, the patient is comfortably positioned

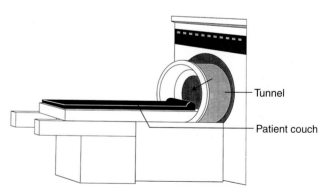

FIG. 1-12. Illustration of an MRI scanner. Notice that its external appearance is similar to a that of CT scanner. The major difference, of course, is that there is a magnetic field around the gantry opening and not an x-ray tube.

supine, prone, or decubitus on a couch. Unlike CT, the couch does not move during the exam, and the patient hears and feels a jackhammer-like thumping while the study is in progress.

The underlying physics of MRI is complicated, and strange-sounding terms proliferate. Let's keep it simple: *MRI is essentially the imaging of protons.* The most commonly imaged proton is hydrogen, as it is abundant in the human body and is easily manipulated by a magnetic field. However, other nuclei can be imaged. Because the hydrogen proton has a positive charge and is constantly spinning at a fixed frequency, called the *spin frequency,* a small magnetic field with a north and south pole surrounds the proton. Remember that a moving charged particle creates a surrounding magnetic field. Thus, these hydrogen protons act like magnets and align themselves within an external magnetic field much like nails in a magnetic field or the needle of a compass.

While in the MR scanner, or magnet, short bursts of radio-frequency waves are broadcast into the patient from radio transmitters. The broadcast radio wave frequency is the same as the spin frequency of the proton being imaged (hydrogen in this case). The hydrogen protons absorb the broadcast radio wave energy and become energized, or resonate. Hence the term *magnetic resonance.* Once the radiofrequency wave broadcast is discontinued, the protons revert or decay back to their normal or steady state that existed prior to the radio wave broadcast. As the hydrogen protons decay back to their normal state or relax, they continue to resonate and broadcast radio waves that can be detected by a radio wave receiver set to the same frequency as the broadcast radio waves and the hydrogen proton spin frequency (Fig. 1-13). The intensity of the radio wave signal detected by the receiver coil indicates the numbers and locations of the resonating hydrogen protons. For example, there are many hydrogen atoms and protons present in fat, and the received radio wave signal will be intense or very bright. However, there is much

less hydrogen in bone cortex, and the received radio wave signal is of low intensity or black. The overall result is a three-dimensional proton density plot or map of the anatomic slice being examined. This analog (wave) data received by the receiver coil is subsequently converted to numbers (digitized), and the numbers are converted to shades of black, white, and gray by computers.

Now comes the complicated part. The received radio wave signal intensity from the patient is determined not only by the number of hydrogen atoms but by the T1 and T2 relaxation times. If the radio receivers listen early during the decay following the discontinuance of the radio wave broadcast, it is called a T1-weighted sequence. In a T1 image the fat is white, and the gray soft tissue detail is excellent. If the radio receivers listen late during the decay, it is called a T2-weighted sequence wherein the water in soft tissues is now a lighter gray and fat appears gray. The simplest way to think of T1 and T2 is as two different technical ways to look at the same structure. This is analogous to the PA and lateral radiographs being two different ways to view a bone or the chest. We tend to use T1 imaging when seeking anatomic information. T2 imaging is helpful when searching for pathology because most pathology tends to contain considerable amounts of water or hydrogen, and T2 causes water to light up like a lightbulb. In general, T1 images have good resolution and T2 images have better contrast than T1 images.

Although human anatomy is always the same no matter what the imaging modality, the appearances of anatomic structures are very different on MR and CT images. Sometimes it is difficult for the beginner to differentiate between a CT and an MR image. The secret is to *look to the fat.* If the subcutaneous fat is black, it is a CT image as fat appears black on studies that use x-rays. If the subcutaneous fat is white (high-intensity signal), then it has to be an MR. Next, *look to the bones.* Bones should have a gray medullary canal and a white cortex on radiographs and CT images. The medullary

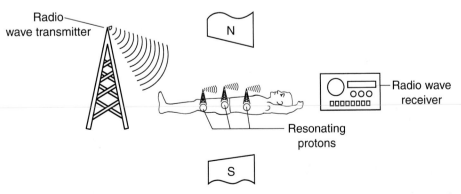

FIG. 1-13. The general principles of MRI physics. The frequencies of the radio wave transmitter, the radio wave receiver, and the spin frequency of hydrogen atom protons are the same.

canal contains bone marrow and the gray is due to the large amount of fat in bone marrow. On a T1 MR image, nearly all of the bone appears homogeneously white as the bone marrow is fat that emits a high-intensity signal and appears white. Also, on MR the cortex of the bone will appear black (dark or low-intensity signal), whereas on CT images the cortex is white. Soft tissues and organs appear as shades of gray on CT and MR. Air appears black on CT and has a low-intensity signal (black or dark) on MR. Table 1-6 compares the appearances of various structures on MR and CT images. Don't fight it; just learn it.

Standard iodinated contrast agents are of no use in MRI. Instead, we use magnetically active substances (paramagnetic) such as gadolinium to enhance certain disease processes. Gadolinium does not produce an MR signal, but it shortens the T1 relaxation time in tissues where it has localized. Gadolinium creates improved contrast between tissues especially on T1 images, and it is useful for imaging tumors, infections, and acute stroke. Gadolinium is safer than the iodinated contrast media.

Magnetic resonance angiography (MRA) is a special

TABLE 1-6. *A comparison of structure appearances on images*

Object	CT and radiographs	MRI T1	MRI T2
Air	Black	Dark	Dark
Fat	Black	Very bright	Intermediate-dark
Muscles	Gray	Dark	Dark
Bone cortex	White	Dark	Dark
Bone marrow	Gray	Bright	Intermediate-dark
Gadolinium		Very bright	Bright

Remember: On MR images the words *dark, low-intensity signal,* and *black* are synonymous; *bright, high-intensity signal,* and *white* are synonymous, and *intermediate intensity signal* and *gray* are synonymous.

noninterventional study that can specifically image cerebral and carotid vessels without using needles, catheters, or iodinated contrast media. As a general rule, flowing blood appears black on most MR images, but by using a special imaging technique (gradient-echo pulse sequence) the arterial and venous blood appears as a high-intensity signal, or bright (Fig. 1-14).

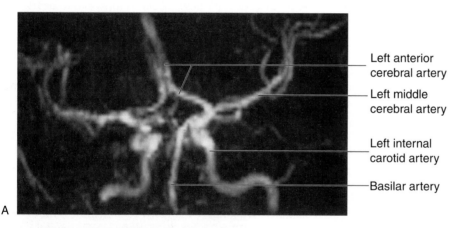

Left anterior cerebral artery

Left middle cerebral artery

Left internal carotid artery

Basilar artery

A

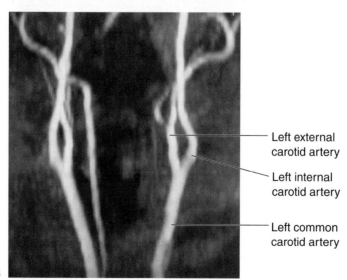

Left external carotid artery

Left internal carotid artery

Left common carotid artery

B

FIG. 1-14. A: Magnetic resonance angiography axial image of the circle of Willis arteries: normal. **B:** MRA coronal image of the carotid arteries: normal.

TABLE 1-7. *Some common imaging applications for diagnostic ultrasound*

Obstetrics
Pediatric brain
Testicle and prostate
Female pelvis
Chest for pleural effusion drainage
Abdomen(kidney, pancreas, liver, and gallbladder)
Vascular disease

This procedure takes approximately 10 minutes, and three-dimensional images of the vasculature can be reconstructed with the digital information. MRA has not been as effective for imaging the arteries and veins in the extremities, abdomen, and chest, as in the carotid and cerebral vessels.

ULTRASONOGRAPHY

Ultrasonography (US) is another useful diagnostic imaging tool that is noninvasive and does not employ x-rays or radiation. US has significantly improved the diagnosis, treatment, and management of a number of diseases. Some common imaging applications of US are listed in Table 1-7. It has achieved excellent patient acceptance because it is safe, fast, painless, and inexpensive when compared to the other imaging modalities. A complete CT of the abdomen costs approximately $750, abdominal MRI approximately $1200, and US approximately $300. The advantages and disadvantages of US are listed in Table 1-8.

Ultrasound technology produces sectional anatomy images or slices in multiple planes much like CT and MRI. An US machine consists of an US wave source, a computer, and a transducer (Fig. 1-15). The US machine emits high-frequency sound waves, ranging from 1 to 10 MHz, that are considerably above the human ear's audible range of 20 to 20,000 Hz. Short bursts of these high-frequency sound waves are alternately broadcast into the patient by a transducer, and some of the reflected sound waves from body tissues are intermittently

TABLE 1-8. *Advantages and disadvantages of ultrasound diagnostic imaging*

Advantages
Multiple plane imaging including obliques
Safe—no known biological harm at diagnostic sound frequency levels
Painless (noninvasive)
Less expensive than CT and MRI
Equipment cost is less than that of CT and MRI
Real-time or cine is possible
Very portable

Disadvantages
Requires technical skill or is operator-dependent
Not good for bone and lung imaging

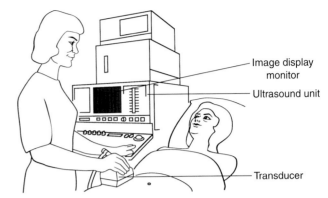

FIG. 1-15. An ultrasound unit, an ultrasonographer, and the patient. The transducer is centered over the abdomen. The ultrasonographer moves the transducer with the right hand while making technical adjustments on the ultrasound unit with the left hand.

received by the transducer (Fig. 1-16). The acoustic impedance *(Z)* of a structure determines the amount of sound energy transmitted and reflected at its boundary (*Z* = tissue density × sound velocity). When a sound wave encounters an acoustic interface or the boundary between two media of different acoustic impedance, the sound waves may be absorbed, deflected, or reflected (Fig. 1-17).

The analog sound waves that are reflected directly back to the transducer are subsequently digitized. Next, a computer converts this digital information to an image with shades of black, white, and gray. US, like MRI and CT, depends on computer technology to store digital information and subsequently convert it to an image.

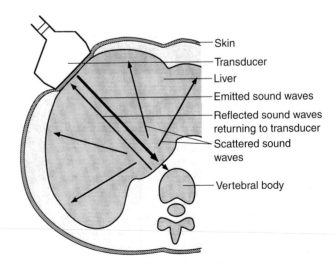

FIG. 1-16. A transducer placed on the skin overlying the liver. The transducer broadcasts short bursts of high-frequency sound waves into the liver and deeper structures. Reflected sound waves are intermittently received by the transducer when it is not broadcasting sound waves. Note that some of the sound waves are deflected away from the transducer and are of no use for imaging.

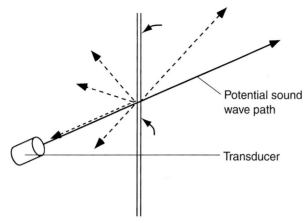

FIG. 1-17. Illustration of what can happen to sound waves when they encounter an acoustic interface. An acoustic interface represents the intersection of two structures that possess different acoustic impedances or densities. When the sound waves are broadcast from the transducer *(solid black line)* and strike an acoustic interface *(curved arrows)*, a number of things can happen to them such as the following: they can be reflected back to the transducer, deflected away from the transducer, pass through the interface, or absorbed at the interface.

Each organ and tissue has its own characteristic echo pattern. Solid organs have a homogeneous echo pattern, whereas fluid-filled organs and masses such as the urinary bladder, cysts, and the gall-bladder have relatively fewer internal echoes.

The terminology employed to describe the US image planes is slightly different from that used in describing CT and MR image planes. In US an axial view may be referred to as a *transverse* scan, and a sagittal view may be associated with a *longitudinal* scan or view (Fig. 1-18).

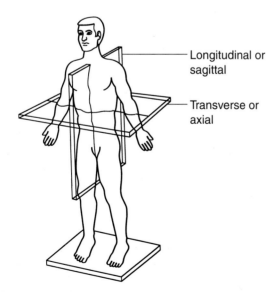

FIG. 1-18. Clarification of some of the terminology used to describe sectional anatomy planes on US images.

As previously noted, a significant part of medicine is just learning the lingo.

While an US study is in progress, the images are viewed on a monitor. The monitor is analogous to a movie screen or television, and this viewing mode is called *real time.* This allows onlookers to observe a beating heart or the movements of an intrauterine fetus. Also, static images may be reproduced on film by a format camera.

NUCLEAR MEDICINE

Various organs and organ systems can be imaged by administering small amounts of radionuclides tagged to compounds that are selectively taken up by a target organ or system such as the heart, the lungs, or the bones. The radioactive emissions from the radionuclides are detected and recorded by a special camera with a sodium iodide crystal, and this information is converted to a diagnostic image. The detailed basics of this important imaging modality are discussed in Chapter 3.

INTERVENTIONAL RADIOLOGY

This radiology subspecialty includes a wide range of important invasive procedures that utilize needles, catheters, radiography, CT, and MRI. This area of radiology is expanding rapidly and becoming more and more important in the diagnosis, treatment, and management of disease processes (see Chapter 2).

TELERADIOLOGY

This is simply the transmission of images from one site to another across telephone lines. This technology allows an image to be transferred to a radiologist's office or home for instant interpretation. Thus, a distant site without a radiologist present can transfer images to a radiologist at another site.

COMPUTED RADIOGRAPHY

This is the process of producing a digital radiographic image. A cassette containing a phosphor plate (instead of photographic film) is exposed to the x-ray beam. The phosphor plate is scanned by a laser beam, and the digital data are subsequently converted to an image by computer. The subsequent image can be viewed on a monitor or transferred to radiographic film. The beauty of this system is that the digital image can be transferred via networks to multiple sites in or out of the hospital, and the digital images

Key Points

- There are four basic densities or appearances to observe on radiographs and CT images: *air,* which appears black; *fat,* which also appears black; *soft tissues and organs,* which appear gray; and *metal, calcium, and bone,* which appear white.
- Plain radiography images are produced by x-rays and radiographic film. CT images are produced by x-rays, detectors and computers. MR images are produced by magnetic fields, radiofrequency waves, and computers. Ultrasound images are produced by high-frequency sound waves, transducers, and computers.
- Sectional anatomy is the imaging of anatomy in multiple planes, including the axial plane (transverse or cross-section), the sagittal plane, and the coronal plane.
- A key to distinguishing an MRI from a CT image is that the fat in an MRI appears white.
- T1 MR images tend to have excellent resolution and are therefore used to procure anatomic information. T2 MR images have better contrast than T1 images and cause water to light up; they are therefore frequently used when searching for pathology, which tends to contain a lot of water.
- The high resolution of CT makes it effective for imaging anatomy. MRI has high soft tissue contrast that makes it especially useful for soft tissue imaging.
- Commonly used contrast agents include barium sulfate, high and low osmolar iodinated compounds, ionic iodinated and nonionic (low osmolar) contrast media, air, and gadolinium. Images produced with water-soluble iodinated agents are generally less informative than barium studies because they are less dense and result in poorer contrast.

are easily stored in a computer or server. For example, a digital chest radiograph obtained in an intensive care unit (ICU) can be transmitted to the radiology department for consultation and interpretation in a matter of minutes. Then, the radiologist could send this image via a network back to the ICU or to the referring physician's office. Of course, this digital information would be stored in a computer (server) for future recall. As this technology improves, it will become more and more important to the routine practice of medicine.

REFERENCES

1. Erkonen WE, Albanese MA, Smith WL, Pantazis NJ. Effectiveness of teaching radiologic interpretation in gross anatomy: a long-term follow-up. *Invest Radiol* 1992;27:264.
2. Paivio A. Imagery and long-term memory. In: Dennedy A, Wildes AJ, eds. *Studies in Long-term Memory.* London: John Wiley and Sons; 1975:57.

BIBLIOGRAPHY

1. Hashemi RH, Bradley WG. *MRI: The Basics.* Baltimore: Williams and Wilkins, 1997.

CHAPTER 2

Interventional Radiology

Thomas A. Farrell

Interventional radiology (IR) is a specialty in which radiologists diagnose and treat disease nonoperatively. The interventional radiologist uses catheters, guidewires, needles, balloons, stents, and other devices with radiologic imaging to perform procedures that are often alternatives to surgery. These procedures, which may be categorized as vascular (i.e., angiography) and nonvascular (e.g., decompression and drainage of obstructed kidneys and bile ducts), are performed in an interventional radiology suite and are often done on an outpatient basis. Many procedures that were previously performed surgically are now accomplished by an interventional radiologist with less morbidity and a shorter hospital stay.

Interventional radiology is constantly evolving as new techniques and technologies are developed and applied to enhance patient care. Because of the invasive nature of many of the procedures performed, interventional radiologists tend to be more involved in patient care. Patients undergoing procedures are routinely worked up by the IR service and are subsequently followed up postprocedure. The preprocedure workup consists of

patient assessment as well as evaluation of previous imaging studies (Table 2-1). Postprocedure follow-up is essential to determine if the procedure has been successful and free of complications. This all-inclusive type of clinical service underlines that there is more to IR than simply doing procedures.

Because most procedures performed by interventional radiologists are invasive, a certain amount of risk for developing complications exists. It is important that the patient be aware of this risk so that an informed decision can be made by weighing the possible risks of a procedure against its benefits. A physician should never place a patient in a position of risk unless this has been discussed, understood, and consented to before the procedure. It is in the physician's best interest to be honest and forthright when dealing with patients and their expectations about the outcomes of a procedure, partly because such a rapport may reduce risk of litigation in the event of complication.

The aim of this chapter is to explain the background, indications, and basic techniques of commonly used pro-

TABLE 2-1. *Interventional radiology preprocedure checklist*

Indication for procedure/question(s) to be answered from procedure
Contraindications for procedure
Review prior imaging and noninvasive studies
Check for contrast allergy
Written informed consent
Check coagulation parameters and serum creatinine
Need for prophylactic antibiotics
Patient should be fasting and well hydrated
Discontinue heparin infusion

cedures so that the reader will gain an understanding of how IR can contribute to patient care.

ANGIOGRAPHY

Angiography is a technique of imaging blood vessels, usually by injecting contrast material via an intraluminally placed catheter. Blood vessels may also be visualized noninvasively by magnetic resonance angiography (MRA), which takes advantage of the inherent contrast between flowing blood and stationary tissue (see Fig. 1-14).

The Seldinger technique (Fig. 2-1) is a method of gaining vascular access using a needle, guidewire, and catheter. It has also been used to gain access to the stomach, renal pelvis, biliary tract, etc. The Seldinger technique can be summarized in as follows: Needle in, wire in, needle out, catheter in, wire out. Once the catheter tip is in a satisfactory position, it is aspirated and flushed with saline and a test injection of contrast is given to confirm the position of the catheter.

PERIPHERAL VASCULAR DISEASE

Generally, the diagnosis of peripheral vascular disease (PVD) has already been made by the time a lower limb angiogram is requested. The referring physician should have assessed the patient's symptoms and reviewed the noninvasive imaging tests such as segmental limb pressures before proceeding to angiography. Rather than being an endpoint, the angiogram helps formulate a comprehensive plan in the patient's subsequent treatment as it evaluates the extent and severity of disease and provides a road map for future intervention (balloon angioplasty, stenting, surgery, etc.). Diabetic patients may present with a more advanced stage of ischemia as they are prone to developing peripheral neuropathy that may mask the above symptoms. Diabetics also tend to have a greater prevalence of small vessel disease, which is more difficult to treat surgically and contributes to a less favorable long-term prognosis compared to nondiabetics with PVD.

Arteriographic evaluation of patients with PVD may be divided into three anatomic regions: the abdominal aorta, the pelvic arteries, and the arteries below the inguinal ligament. Aortic aneurysms occur most commonly below the level of the renal arteries. The number of renal arteries should also be noted as should the presence of stenoses in these vessels. Bilateral oblique views of the pelvic arterial system should be obtained as hemodynamically significant stenoses can be missed if only a frontal view is performed. After injection of contrast, the angiographic table moves at a predetermined speed, following the bolus of contrast down to the feet. This initial angiogram should be reviewed and supplemented with further views if necessary.

In general, arterial stenoses are not regarded as significant unless they reduce the lumen diameter by 70% angiographically. The significance of a stenosis can be more accurately assessed by measuring a pressure gradient across it. The presence of a 10 mm Hg gradient or greater across a stenosis is regarded as significant and

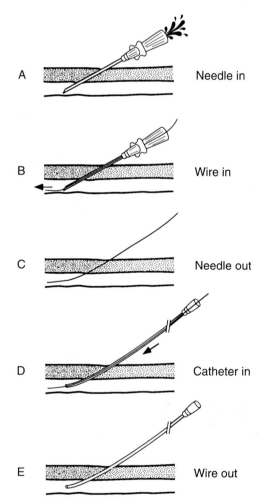

FIG. 2-1. Seldinger technique. **A:** The vessel is punctured with the needle. **B:** A guidewire is advanced through the needle into the vessel. **C:** The needle is removed leaving the guidewire in place. **D:** A catheter is advanced over the guidewire into the vessel. **E:** The guidewire is removed and the catheter flushed.

TABLE 2-2. *Complications of angiography*

Systemic
Allergic contrast reaction
Renal failure
Local
Puncture site:
    Hematoma
    Pseudoaneurysm
    Arteriovenous fistula
Intraluminal:
    Subintimal dissection
    Thrombosis
    Distal embolization

worthy of further treatment such as angioplasty or stenting. If the gradient is less than 10 mm Hg, a vasodilator such as nitroglycerin may be given intraarterially to simulate exercise and possibly unmask a significant stenosis.

An antegrade common femoral artery puncture is useful if angioplasty below the knee is contemplated as it provides a more direct route. In the absence of satisfactory femoral pulses bilaterally, either the brachial or axillary arteries can be punctured.

COMPLICATIONS OF ANGIOGRAPHY

Complications of angiography may be divided into those that are systemic and those that are related to the vessel puncture (Table 2-2).

Systemic Complications

The frequency and severity of allergic or idiosyncratic reactions to contrast media depends on the type, dose, route, and rate of delivery. Reactions may be categorized as mild, moderate, or severe (Table 2-3). The prevalence of most reactions is greater with the intravenous route. Severe contrast reactions resulting in cardiac arrest and convulsions are rare, with an incidence of less than 1 per 1000 examinations. Many studies suggest a lower incidence of severe reactions when nonionic iodinated contrast is used. The mortality rate, which is equivalent for high and lower osmolar contrast agents, is approximately 1 per 45,000 examinations. Moderate contrast reactions characterized by hypertension, hypotension, wheezing, and laryngospasm occur in 1% to 2% of examinations. Mild reactions (nausea, cough, hives, and flushing) are even more common and can be treated symptomatically. Premedication with steroids for 24 hours prior to angiography has reduced the incidence of idiosyncratic contrast reactions.

Contrast-Induced Renal Failure

Contrast induced renal failure is usually mild and self-limiting, with serum creatinine levels peaking by 3–5 days and returning to normal within 2 weeks. The pathophysiology of this complication is thought to be due to a combination of vasoconstriction and direct toxicity of contrast on the renal tubules. Diabetics and patients with preexisting renal impairment (serum creatinine greater than 2 mg %) are at increased risk for developing contrast-induced renal failure. Some studies suggest that nonionic contrast is less nephrotoxic than ionic contrast. Adequate hydration prior to angiography is a key element in minimizing the deleterious effects of iodinated contrast. An alternative to iodinated contrast is carbon dioxide gas, which is nontoxic and inexpensive. However, meticulous technique is necessary for the visualization of smaller vessels.

Puncture Site Complications

A hematoma may occur at the puncture site during the procedure or following removal of the catheter. The risk factors for this complication include hypertension and obesity. Prevention involves meticulous technique including vessel puncture over the femoral head and constant manual pressure directly over the puncture site after removal of the catheter until hemostasis is achieved. The hematoma may extend into the retroperitoneum when the puncture site is above the inguinal ligament. Incomplete or intermittent compression over the puncture site may also result in the formation of a pseudoaneurysm.

TABLE 2-3. *Allergic contrast reactions*

Type:	Mild	Moderate	Severe
Incidence (%)	5–15	1–2	0.1
Clinical features	Nausea	Bronchospasm	Laryngospasm
	Vomiting	Dyspnea	Facial edema
	Urticaria	Vasovagal reaction	Cardiorespiratory arrest
		Hypertension	Seizures
Treatment	Monitor vital signs	Oxygen	Oxygen/IV fluids
	Observe for clinical deterioration	β_2 agonist	Epinephrine SC or IV
			β_2 agonist
			Diazepam
			Cardiopulmonary resuscitation

The arterial wall may be dissected inadvertently by passage of a guidewire between the intimal and muscle layers, a complication that may be avoided by use of a floppy tipped or J-tipped guidewire rather than a straight guidewire. Complications following brachial or axillary arterial puncture are more common than with femoral artery puncture because of the smaller vessel size and the close proximity of the vessels to nerves within a common sheath in the arm.

VASCULAR INTERVENTIONS

Thrombolysis

Thrombolysis is a technique whereby blood clot is dissolved by injecting a drug such as urokinase or tissue plasminogen activator directly into it. Urokinase converts plasminogen to plasmin, which in turn degrades fibrin. Thrombolytic drugs are infused via multiple-side-hole catheters and wires placed directly into the thrombosed grafts and vessels to ensure a very high local concentration of the drug. Active internal bleeding or recent intracranial hemorrhage or surgery are absolute contraindications for thrombolysis (Table 2-4). Arterial thrombolysis should not be undertaken in a limb which has become so ischemic that it is not viable because systemic acidemia, hyperkalemia, and myoglobinuria may result when reperfusion of necrotic tissue occurs.

Thrombolysis is not without potential complications such as bleeding and embolization of thrombus distally. The cumulative probability of major complications increases with duration of infusion, rising from less than 10% after 16 hours to more than 30% at 40 hours. Once thrombolysis is complete balloon angioplasty or surgery can be used to treat any underlying vessel stenoses that contributed to the occlusion.

Balloon Angioplasty

Percutaneous transluminal balloon angioplasty (PTA) has become an established technique in the treatment of vascular stenoses due to atherosclerotic plaque and fibromuscular dysplasia. The precise pathophysiologic mechanism of PTA in atherosclerotic plaque is controversial. However, most agree that PTA results in a con-

TABLE 2-4. *Contraindications for arterial thrombolysis*

Absolute
Active GI *or* GU bleeding
Recent (<2 months) cerebral hemorrhage/infarct/surgery
Irreversible limb ischemia
Relative
History of GI *or* GU bleeding
Recent thoracic/abdominal surgery
Recent trauma
Severe uncontrolled hypertension

trolled plaque and intimal fracture with localized dissection into the underlying media thereby increasing the intraluminal diameter. The plaque, intima, and media are subsequently remodeled to give a smoother endoluminal surface. The appropriate angioplasty balloon catheter should be chosen so that its inflated diameter is the same size or slightly larger than the nondiseased vessel. Initially, the stenosis is crossed with a guidewire that is left across the lesion until the procedure is finished. Heparin and nitroglycerin may be given intraarterially to prevent thrombosis and vessel spasm, respectively. The angioplasty balloon is advanced across the stenosis and is inflated and deflated slowly under fluoroscopic guidance. Repeat angiography and pressure measurements should be obtained to evaluate the results of angioplasty.

Iliac artery angioplasty improves inflow to the lower limb and requires balloons that are 7–10 mm in diameter. Again, a guidewire is left across the stenosis during the procedure, the success of which is judged on angiographic and hemodynamic criteria. Stent placement should be considered if the postangioplasty pressure gradient is greater than 10 mm Hg or if a flow-limiting dissection is present (Fig. 2-2). Simultaneous PTA of both common iliac arteries—known as the kissing-balloons technique—is effective in treating bilateral proximal common iliac artery stenoses.

Renal artery angioplasty is usually performed with a 5- to 7-mm-diameter balloon. Atheromatous disease usually involves the proximal or ostial portion of the vessel in contrast to fibromuscular dysplasia which usually affects the midportion of the vessel. The improvement in renal function and hypertension following renal artery angioplasty is equivalent to that obtained after surgical revascularization (Fig. 2-3). Renal artery stenting is performed if there is a residual stenosis or significant dissection postangioplasty (Fig. 2-4).

Infrageniculate angioplasty (anterior/posterior tibial and peroneal artery angioplasty) is usually done for limb salvage or to reduce the extent of an impending below-the-knee or forefoot amputation for ischemia. This technique requires a fine guidewire (010–018) and angioplasty balloon (2–3 mm in diameter) because of the smaller vessel size. An antegrade common femoral arterial approach where the artery is punctured in a downstream direction is helpful as are higher doses of heparin and nitroglycerin to prevent vessel thrombosis and spasm.

Endovascular Stents

There are two main indications for endovascular stent placement: (a) a residual pressure gradient of more than 10 mm Hg postangioplasty, which is regarded as an indication for either repeat angioplasty or stent place-

text continues on page 23

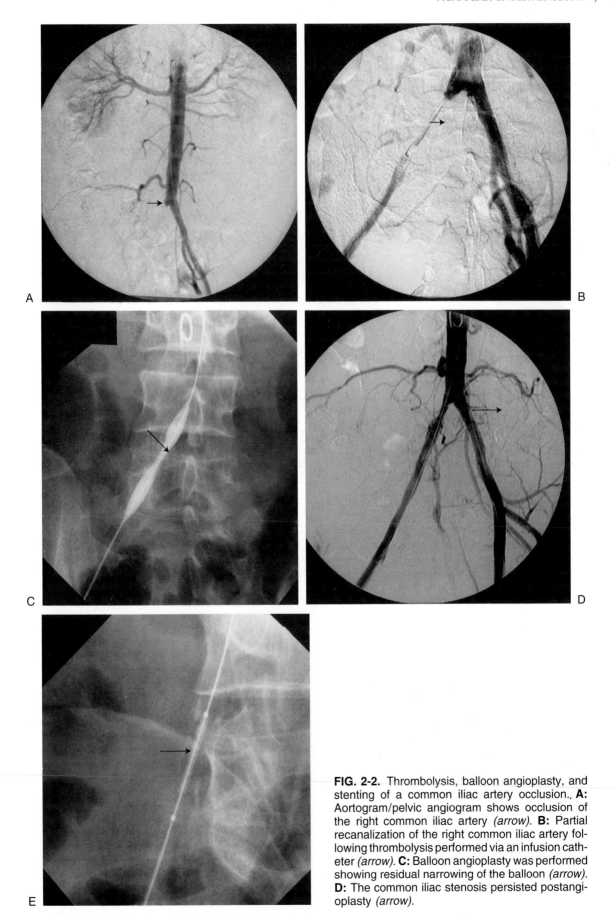

FIG. 2-2. Thrombolysis, balloon angioplasty, and stenting of a common iliac artery occlusion., **A:** Aortogram/pelvic angiogram shows occlusion of the right common iliac artery *(arrow)*. **B:** Partial recanalization of the right common iliac artery following thrombolysis performed via an infusion catheter *(arrow)*. **C:** Balloon angioplasty was performed showing residual narrowing of the balloon *(arrow)*. **D:** The common iliac stenosis persisted postangioplasty *(arrow)*.

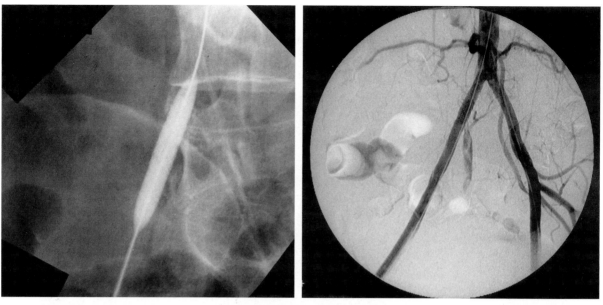

FIG. 2-2. *Continued.* **E, F:** A balloon expandable stent was deployed across the stenosis. The undeployed stent *(arrow)* can be seen on the distal portion of the angioplasty balloon. **G:** Poststenting, no residual stenosis is present.

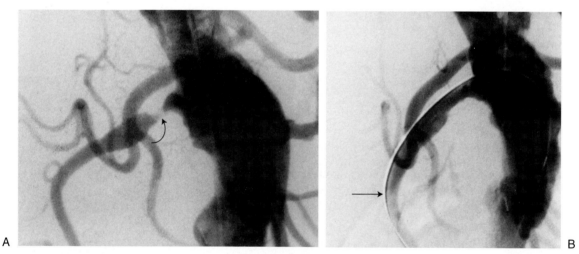

FIG. 2-3. Renal artery angioplasty. **A:** Flush aortogram with a pigtail catheter *(arrow)* showing right renal artery stenosis *(curved arrow).* **B:** Residual stenosis persists post–balloon angioplasty. Note that the guidewire *(arrow)* is left across the stenosis.

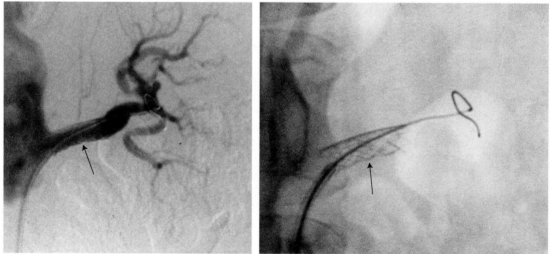

FIG. 2-4. Renal artery stenting. A Palmaz stent *(arrow)* has been placed across a left renal artery stenosis.

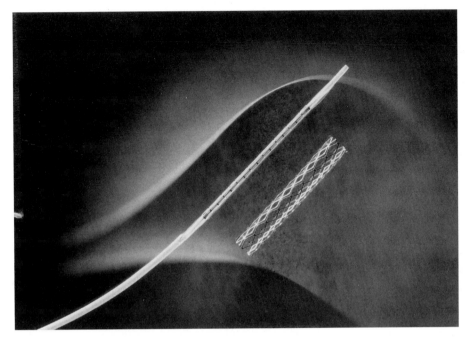

FIG. 2-5. Palmaz stent mounted on an angioplasty balloon and in its expanded form. (Photograph courtesy of Cordis Corporation.)

ment; (b) dissection postangioplasty where the aim of stent placement is to appose the dissected flap against the wall and improve flow. Currently, two metallic stents are approved by the U.S. Food and Drug Administration for intravascular use: the Palmaz stent (Johnson and Johnson, Warren, NJ). This stent is hand-mounted on an angioplasty balloon. The balloon–stent combination is placed across the stenosis and the balloon is inflated, thus opening and deploying the stent. The balloon is then deflated and removed (Fig. 2-5). On the other hand, the Wallstent (Schneider, Minneapolis,

MN) is self-expanding and does not require mounting on an angioplasty balloon. Deployment involves withdrawal of a covering sheath, after which the stent expands. The Wallstent is more flexible than the Palmaz stent, which is an advantage when stenting tortuous vessels (Fig. 2-6).

TRAUMA

The interventional radiologist has an important role in the management of trauma patients. In general, imaging does not cure trauma patients, so that the number of radiographs allowed in the emergency room should be inversely proportional to the severity of injury. The seriously injured patient needs only three radiographs: a lateral cervical spine, a frontal chest, and a pelvis. Although it is tempting to further evaluate trauma patients by obtaining extra views and by doing more studies, these should be deferred until the patient's condition has stabilized. Remember, perfect is the enemy of good.

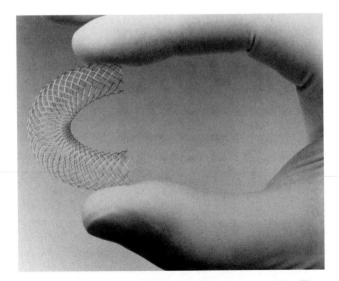

FIG. 2-6. The Wallstent is self-expanding and flexible. (Photograph courtesy of Schneider, Inc.)

Aortic Transection

Eighty percent of those who sustain a laceration to the thoracic aorta following blunt trauma die at the scene of the accident, en route to the hospital, or shortly after arriving in hospital. The cause of death in most cases is exsanguination from aortic transection. The precise mechanism of aortic transection is uncertain. It may be due to sudden deceleration where the mobile descending aorta shears from the relatively fixed aortic arch, as the most common site for aortic transection is just distal to the origin of the left subclavian artery. As in all trauma patients, clinical evaluation is important, but up to 50% of patients surviving accidents with blunt aortic injuries have no external physical signs of injury. There is much debate as to the optimal imaging algorithm of patients with suspected aortic transection. One school of thought is that a normal-appearing mediastinum on chest radiography and computed tomography (CT) virtually excludes transection and that these two modalities should be used for screening patients prior to arch aortography. Others argue that as well as being time consuming, chest radiography and CT in trauma patients have limitations and that aortography, with its low morbidity, is the gold standard for diagnosing vascular injury and should be performed when there is the slightest suspicion of aortic transection. An arch aortogram is performed by advancing a 6- or 7F pigtail catheter carefully through the common femoral artery over the aortic arch so that the catheter tip lies just above the aortic valve. The left anterior oblique (LAO) projection provides an optimal view of the aortic arch. A second view in an orthogonal plane, right anterior oblique (RAO), should detect an injury in the posteromedial wall not seen on the initial LAO projection. One should be aware of a normal anatomic variant in the aortic arch that may be misdiagnosed as transection—the so-called ductus bump, which lies proximally on the inferior surface of the aortic arch and represents the site of attachment of the ductus arteriosus (Fig. 2-7).

Hemorrhage Associated with Pelvic Fracture

Prior to the introduction of external fixation devices, much of the early mortality associated with pelvic fractures was due to hemorrhage. Presently, up to 20% of patients with pelvic fractures require the services of interventional radiology for the diagnosis and treatment of hemorrhage. In general, surgery is not a satisfactory treatment option for this problem as exploration will decompress the pelvic hematoma, reduce the tamponade effect, and lead to further blood loss.

A diagnostic pelvic angiogram is performed with a pigtail catheter placed above the aortic bifurcation and active hemorrhage is diagnosed by extravasation of contrast. The bleeding vessel may then be embolized with either a stainless steel Gianturco coil or pledgets of gelatin sponge, both of which can be placed through a selective 5F angiographic catheter. Gelatin sponge results in temporary vascular occlusion that recanalizes within 2–3 weeks, whereas a Gianturco coil might result in a permanent occlusion. Pelvic ischemia following selective arterial embolization is unusual due to the extensive collateral blood supply.

Gastrointestinal Hemorrhage

Selective angiography and therapeutic embolization have become important techniques in the management of patients with gastrointestinal (GI) bleeding. Initially, a nuclear medicine study using radiolabeled red cells should be done to confirm the presence and anatomic location of the bleeding vessel. Selective angiography of either the celiac, superior mesenteric, or inferior mesenteric arteries is then performed. Once a bleeding site has been demonstrated, the catheter can be used to control bleeding either by selectively infusing vasopressin to constricts the vessel or by deploying embolic materials such as gelatin sponge pledgets or coils to mechanically occlude flow. The specific treatment depends on the nature and location of the hemorrhage. Upper GI bleeding is more commonly treated by embolization because of the richer collateral arterial supply, whereas selective vasopressin infusion is preferred in the lower GI tract, which is more prone to ischemia.

Pulmonary Arteriography

Pulmonary arteriography is regarded as the gold standard in the diagnosis of pulmonary embolism (PE) (Fig. 2-8). This procedure has a low morbidity and is usually performed in patients who have already had a ventilation-perfusion (V/Q) scan of the lungs (see Chapter 3). However, a V/Q scan is reported in terms of probability of PE (high, intermediate, low probability, and normal) and when taken on its own this examination has limitations. It is just as important to avoid overdiagnosing PE as it is to avoid underdiagnosing it because the treatment includes anticoagulation with heparin and warfarin (Coumadin), which is associated with a significant morbidity. The Prospective Investigation of Pulmonary Embolism Disease (PIOPED) study (1) reviewed the role of pulmonary arteriography and V/Q scanning in patients with suspected PE. Among its conclusions were the following: (a) a normal V/Q scan virtually excludes a PE. (b) A high-probability V/Q scan has a positive predictive value for PE in the region of 90%. However, this pattern occurs in only 40% of patients with PE. (c) The incidence of PE in patients with a low-probability V/Q scan but with high clinical suspicion of PE is about 40%.

Depending on the clinical circumstances, V/Q scanning will yield an accurate diagnosis in over one-third of cases with suspected PE: those with high-probability scans and those with normal scans. In the remainder of patients, pulmonary arteriography must be undertaken for a definitive diagnosis (Table 2-5). Pulmonary arteriography is also helpful in the diagnosis of pulmonary arteriovenous fistulas and pulmonary hypertension.

Pulmonary angiography is performed with a pigtail catheter which is manipulated through the right side of the heart to the pulmonary artery. Pressure readings

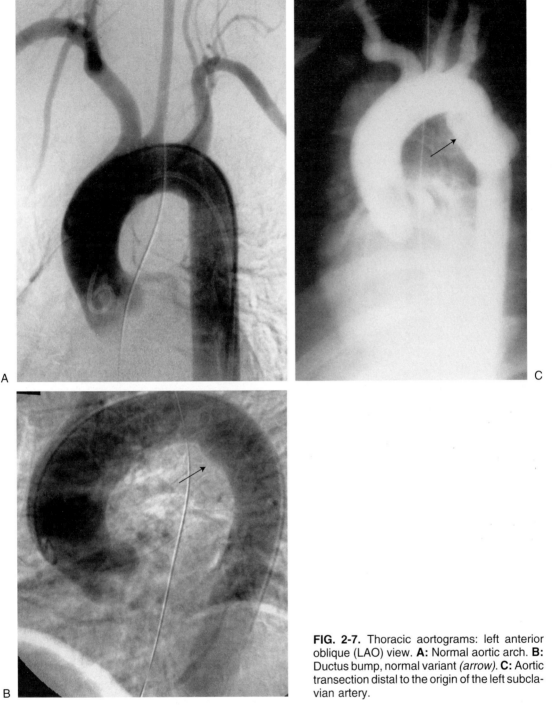

FIG. 2-7. Thoracic aortograms: left anterior oblique (LAO) view. **A:** Normal aortic arch. **B:** Ductus bump, normal variant *(arrow)*. **C:** Aortic transection distal to the origin of the left subclavian artery.

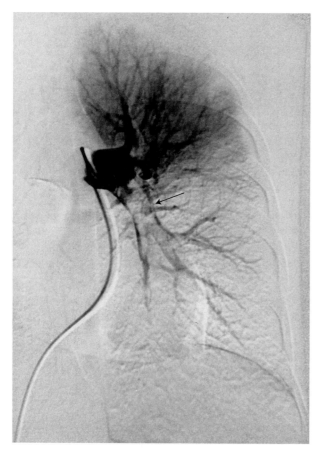

FIG. 2-8. Pulmonary angiogram showing an embolism *(arrow)* in the left lower lobe pulmonary artery. Note the normal appearance of the left upper lobe.

are recorded to detect pulmonary arterial hypertension. ECG monitoring is essential as left bundle branch block may be converted to complete heart block during passage of the catheter through the right heart. As most of the blood flow is to the lower lobes, these are the most common sites for PE. If PE is diagnosed and anticoagulation is contraindicated, an inferior vena cava filter can be placed using the same venous access site through which the pulmonary arteriogram was performed.

TABLE 2-5. *Indications for pulmonary angiography*

Low-probability V/Q scan and high clinical suspicion for PE
Intermediate or indeterminate V/Q scan
High-probability V/Q scan and low clinical suspicion for PE in a patient in whom anticoagulation or thrombolysis carries a high risk.
Evaluation of chronic pulmonary thromboembolic disease prior to thromboembolectomy
Evaluation of congenital malformations, e.g., arteriovenous fistula

PE, pulmonary embolism

Inferior Vena Cava Filters

The purpose of an inferior vena cava (IVC) filter is to prevent pulmonary embolism by trapping a clot before it gets to the lungs. The filter is usually placed in patients in whom anticoagulation is contraindicated or ineffective. Currently, there are several types of permanent filters available (Fig. 2-9). Three filters are made from stainless steel alloys and the fourth, the Simon Nitinol filter, is made from an alloy of nickel and titanium. The bird's nest filter is the device of choice when the IVC diameter exceeds 28 mm. It is composed of four lengths of five wire that coil and form a mesh within the IVC to trap clot. The other three filter types depend primarily on their legs to trap clot. All filters may be placed percutaneously via a common femoral or internal jugular vein approach. A transbrachial or subclavian vein approach is also possible for placement of the Simon Nitinol filter because of its smaller (9F) size. Filters should be placed in the infrarenal IVC to reduce risk of renal vein thrombosis. One disadvantage of the currently available filters is that they are designed for permanent placement as their retaining hooks become incorporated into the IVC wall within a few weeks.

Central Venous Access

Central venous catheters are placed for a variety of indications including administration of antibiotics, chemotherapy, and hemodialysis. There are essentially two types of catheters: tunneled and nontunneled. Tunneling refers to the creation of a subcutaneous tract in which the catheter lies before it enters the vein. The tunnel acts as a physical barrier reducing the incidence of catheter related infection and also enhances catheter security. A Dacron cuff is present on some catheters causing a localized fibrotic reaction, stabilizing it within the subcutaneous tissues. Most long-term catheters are made of Silastic, a biocompatible material. The optimal position for placement of the catheter tip is at the junction of the superior vena cava and the right atrium. The right internal jugular vein or the right subclavian vein is commonly used for the placement for these catheters. Another type of tunneled venous access is a port device consisting of a subcutaneously implanted reservoir in the chest wall or upper arm to which the catheter is connected. Ports can be accessed percutaneously with a noncoring needle.

For short-term venous access (less than 90 days) nontunneled catheters, such as a Hohn, or peripherally inserted central catheters (PICCs) are appropriate. Hohn catheters are usually placed via a subclavian vein and PICCs are inserted by direct percutaneous puncture of either arm or forearm veins. The catheter is then advanced until the tip lies in the SVC.

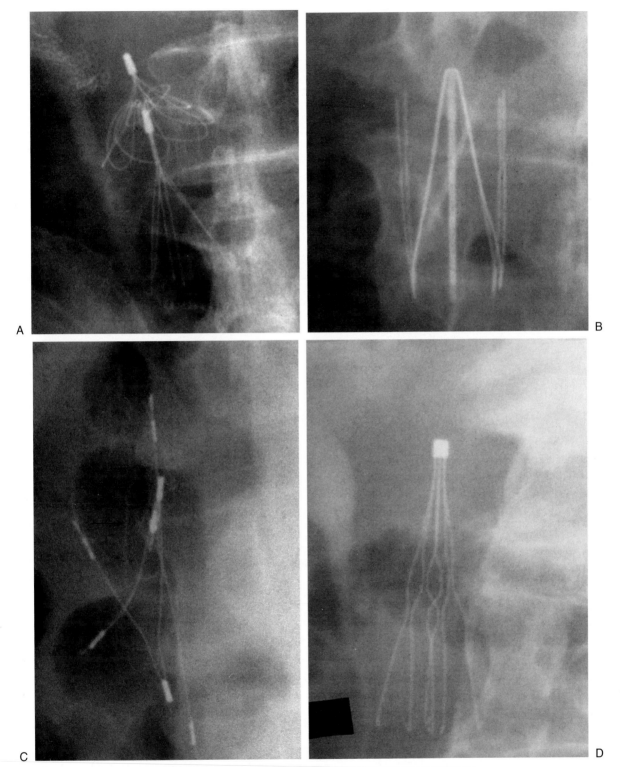

FIG. 2-9. Intravenous catheter filters. **A:** Simon Nitinol filter. **B:** Braun Venatech filter. **C:** Bird's nest filter (arrow represents wire mesh). **D:** Greenfield filter.

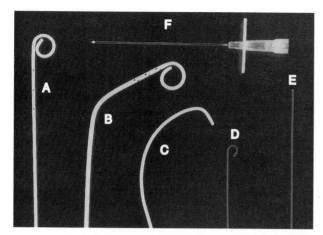

FIG. 2-10. Tools of the trade. **A:** Pigtail catheter. **B:** Angled pigtail catheter. **C:** Cobra catheter. **D:** J-tipped guidewire. **E:** Straight (Bentson) guidewire. **F:** An 18-gauge needle for vessel puncture.

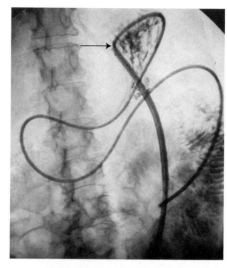

FIG. 2-11. Double-lumen gastrojejunostomy tube allows delivery of enteral nutrition through the distal tip of the catheter into small bowel while the gastric contents are drained through the proximal portion *(arrow)* preventing aspiration of gastric contents into the lungs.

Tools of the Trade: Catheters, Guidewires, and Needles

There are numerous preformed shapes and types of angiographic catheters, most of which are made from flexible plastic material such as polyethylene or polyurethane. Wire braiding may be incorporated into the catheter shaft to increase stiffness and improve its torque. Catheter diameters are measured in French (F) size, where 3F = 1.0 mm (outside diameter). Most angiographic catheters are in the 4F to 7F range. Aortic angiography is performed with pigtail catheters that have several side holes proximal to the tip allowing rapid flow of a contrast bolus while the pigtail loop stabilizes the catheter preventing recoil (Fig. 2-10A). Pulmonary angiography is also performed with a pigtail catheter. However, this catheter has a curve near its tip that facilitates its passage through the right atrium and ventricle and then selectively into either pulmonary artery (Fig. 2-10B). Selective angiography (renal, celiac and superior mesenteric arteries) is performed with a curved end-hole catheter such as a Cobra C2 (Fig. 2-10C). A variety of catheters and guidewires may be necessary during a procedure, and placement of a vascular sheath with a hemostatic valve at the site of access reduces vessel trauma and facilitates rapid catheter and guidewire exchange.

Catheters used in the drainage of abscesses, obstructed kidneys (percutaneous nephrostomy), and bile ducts are made of polyurethane and are of greater diameter than angiographic catheters (8–12F). These drainage catheters are usually placed using the Seldinger technique after which they are secured in position by deploying a locking pigtail mechanism formed by pulling on a suture that runs in most of the catheter shaft and is attached to its tip. The pigtail loop itself contains large side holes for drainage. The smaller diameter catheters occlude more easily with debris and should be routinely changed over a guidewire every 6–8 weeks when continued drainage is required.

Guidewires increase the ease and safety of catheter placement. The outer shell of a guidewire consists of a very tightly wound but flexible metal spring coil. A stiff central core provides rigidity over a variable length of the guidewire. The balance between these two components dictates the handling characteristics of the guidewire. For example, the distal 15 cm of a Bentson guidewire is floppy, allowing easy coiling (Fig. 2-10E). A J-tipped guidewire reduces the risk of damaging the vessel wall because of its blunt tip (Fig. 2-10D). Guidewires usually range in diameter from 18 thousandths of an inch (0.018 in.) to 38 thousandths of an inch (0.038 in.). The standard length for most wires is 145 cm, whereas longer guidewires (260 cm) are available to facilitate catheter exchange.

Needles used in arteriography range in size from a 21-gauge needle through which an 0.018-in. guidewire will pass to an 18-gauge needle that accepts an 0.035-in. guidewire (Fig. 2-10F).

NONVASCULAR INTERVENTIONS

Percutaneous Feeding Tubes

Radiologically guided placement of percutaneous gastrostomy and gastrojejunostomy tubes for enteral nutrition has gained widespread acceptance in the management of patients who cannot eat or swallow because of stroke, head injury, head and neck tumors, and so

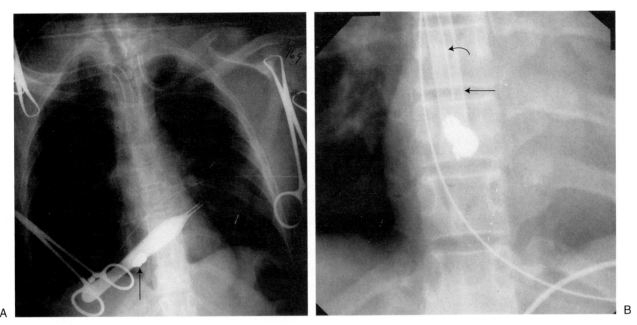

FIG. 2-12. A bullet is lodged deep in the subcutaneous tissue below the right clavicle after deflecting off the patient's chin. Attempted removal of the bullet in the emergency room pushed it deeper into the subcutaneous tissue. A chest radiograph **(A)** showed that the bullet *(arrow)* had migrated to the right atrium. A 24F (8-mm diameter) vascular sheath *(arrow)* was advanced into the right atrium via the right internal jugular vein and a loop snare *(curved arrow)* was placed through this to retrieve the slug **(B)**. This case demonstrates the usefulness of interventional radiology in a situation that would otherwise have required cardiac surgery.

forth. The stomach is accessed percutaneously under fluoroscopic guidance using the Seldinger technique and the tract dilated over a guidewire. A 12- or 14F self-retaining pigtail feeding tube is placed over a guidewire and secured within the stomach. If delivery of liquid feeds directly into the small bowel rather than the stomach is preferred, then a gastrojejunostomy tube can be placed in a transgastric fashion as described above and the tip directed through the pylorus to the distal duodenum (Fig. 2-11). The jejunum may also be punctured percutaneously directly and a feeding tube placed within its lumen for feeding.

VASCULAR INTERVENTION

Example of cardiac intervention (see Fig. 2-12).

Renal Interventions

Percutaneous nephrostomy has become a valuable tool in the treatment of urinary obstruction, which is most commonly caused by calculi, neoplasms, and benign strictures. With the patient in the prone position, the obstructed renal pelvis is accessed using the Seldinger technique during which an 8- or 10F pigtail drainage catheter is passed over a guidewire and the loop formed and secured in the renal pelvis. Further

intervention such as ureteral stenting or stone removal (nephrolithotomy) may be performed through this renal access. Mild hematuria is not uncommon after percutaneous nephrostomy and usually resolves within 72 hours.

Percutaneous Biliary Drainage and Stenting

Obstructive jaundice may be further evaluated by a percutaneous transhepatic cholangiogram (PTC) in whereby a long 22-gauge needle is advanced through the liver parenchyma from a site in the eleventh intercostal space in the right midaxillary line. The needle is then slowly withdrawn while injecting it with contrast to opacify any bile ducts that may have been traversed. Successful PTC is more likely if the ductal system is dilated. Once a duct is opacified a larger (21- or 18-gauge) needle is then used to percutaneously access one of the opacified ducts peripherally. The tract is dilated over a guidewire and an attempt to traverse the biliary obstruction is made followed by an internal-external biliary catheter to decompress the ductal system. Permanent self-expanding metallic stents may be placed percutaneously or endoscopically when internalized biliary drainage is desired, as in the case of a malignant obstruction. Alternatively, temporary short plastic stents may be placed in the common duct when surgery is planned or in patients with benign strictures.

Key Points

- Written informed consent is necessary for most angiographic and interventional procedures. The benefits, risks, and possible complications must be discussed with the patient.
- The Seldinger technique describes a method for gaining vascular or visceral access using a needle, a guidewire, and a catheter.
- Most arteriograms are performed via the common femoral artery, which should be punctured over the femoral head.
- Iodinated contrast is nephrotoxic, particularly in diabetics and patients with preexisting renal impairment.
- Pulmonary angiography has a low morbidity and mortality.
- Most currently available IVC filters are permanent and are placed below the renal veins.
- A positive nuclear medicine scan is helpful in patients with GI bleeding because it not only confirms the diagnosis but also directs the angiographer to the site of bleeding.

REFERENCE

1. The PIOPED investigators: Value of ventilation/perfusion scan in acute pulmonary embolism: results the prospective investigation of pulmonary embolism diagnosis (PIOPED). *JAMA* 1990;263:2753.

BIBLIOGRAPHY

Ansell G, Bettman M, Kaufmann J, Wilkins RA. *Complications in Diagnostic Imaging and Interventional Radiology*, 3rd ed. Boston: Blackwell Scientific, 1996.

Baum S, Pentecost MHJ, eds. *Abrams Angiography*, 3rd ed. Boston: Little, Brown, 1997.

Cope C, Burke D, Meranze S. *Atlas of Interventional Radiology*. Philadelphia: JB Lippincott, 1990.

Kadir S. *Atlas of Normal and Variant Angiographic Anatomy*. Philadelphia: WB Saunders, 1991.

Kandarpa K, Aruny JE. *Handbook of Interventional Radiologic Procedures*, 2nd ed. Boston: Little, Brown, 1996.

CHAPTER 3

Nuclear Imaging

David L. Bushnell

Nuclear medicine is an important medical specialty that utilizes measurements of radioactive tracer behavior in the body to detect and assess various types of diseases. The "physiologic" images generated by nuclear imaging procedures reveal less anatomic detail than radiologic studies. It is therefore often necessary to correlate the nuclear images with the corresponding radiologic images. Although there are also several therapeutic applications for radioactive agents, the primary emphasis of this chapter will be on diagnostic nuclear imaging.

TECHNICAL ASPECTS OF NUCLEAR IMAGING

When molecules with radionuclide components are prepared for administration to human beings, they are called radiopharmaceuticals. The radionuclide portion of the radiopharmaceutical typically emits radiation in the form of gamma rays and/or x-rays that can be detected and used to create the scintigraphic images (often loosely referred to as scans). Radiopharmaceuticals participate in, but do not alter, various physiologic processes. Specific radiopharmaceuticals with particular physiochemical properties are utilized to study an organ or organ system. Although radiopharmaceuticals can be introduced into the body in several different ways, the most common mode of administration is intravenously through a peripheral vein.

Side effects from the administration of radiopharmaceuticals for diagnostic imaging are extremely rare. The probability of an adverse reaction from the radiation exposure received by a patient or technologist during a diagnostic nuclear medicine procedure is so small that it has not been measurable to date.

Gamma ray imaging systems are used to detect the radiation emitted from the patient and to create images that depict the regional distribution of the radiopharmaceutical within the body. The most common of these imaging systems is the gamma camera. Gamma cameras use a sodium iodide crystal to "detect" the gamma rays and x-rays. Photons striking the crystal produce light scintillations that are converted to a digital signal. This digital information is stored in a computer and can be transferred to film or interpreted directly from the computer screen (Fig. 3-1). The resultant "picture" is often referred to as a scan or more appropriately a scintigraphic image. The image is essentially a "physiologic map" of the radiopharmaceutical distribution within the body.

Table 3-1 presents the radiopharmaceuticals and the corresponding imaging procedures that are discussed in this chapter.

VENTILATION AND PERFUSION LUNG IMAGING FOR DIAGNOSIS OF PULMONARY EMBOLISM

Pulmonary thromboembolism (PTE) is a common disorder associated with significant mortality rates, which can be reduced with the appropriate detection and treatment. Establishing the diagnosis of PTE is often very difficult. While dyspnea, tachypnea, and sinus

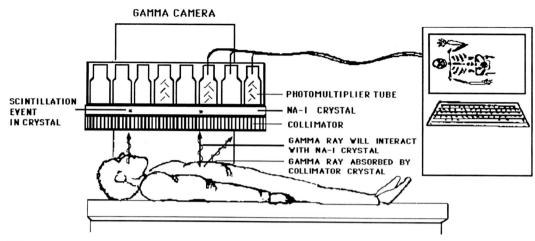

GAMMA CAMERA

SCINTILLATION
EVENT
IN CRYSTAL

PHOTOMULTIPLIER TUBE
NA-I CRYSTAL
COLLIMATOR
GAMMA RAY WILL INTERACT
WITH NA-I CRYSTAL
GAMMA RAY ABSORBED BY
COLLIMATOR CRYSTAL

FIG. 3-1. The basic gamma camera imaging system. The gamma rays that exit the patient perpendicular to the surface of the camera are not absorbed by the collimator and reach the scintillation crystal where they are "detected." The pattern of the gamma ray photons striking the crystal is used to create a digital image on the computer. Na-I indicates sodium iodide.

tachycardia are present in the large majority of individuals with acute PTE, these symptoms and signs may result from any number of cardiopulmonary disorders. *The diagnosis of pulmonary embolism cannot be made with a high degree of reliability based on clinical findings alone.*

A chest radiograph should be obtained in all patients suspected of having pulmonary embolism. The chest x-ray is needed to rule out other causes of the patient's symptoms such as pneumonia, pneumothorax, heart failure, etc. However, the radiograph may appear entirely normal even when PTE is present. Even if the chest radiograph is abnormal and consistent with PTE, the results are never adequately predictive to form the basis of a therapeutic decision. Consequently, more specific diagnostic procedures are necessary for the workup of individuals who fall into this category.

Perfusion lung imaging is an invaluable tool in the workup of PTE and should be obtained in almost all suspected cases of PTE. Scintigraphic perfusion lung imaging has a very high sensitivity for detecting PTE. Although certain image patterns are highly predictive of PTE, many patterns do not yield a definitive result and must be followed by angiography or other diagnostic studies.

TABLE 3-1. *Radiopharmaceuticals discussed in this chapter*

Radiopharmaceutical	Imaging procedure
Tc-99m macroaggregated albumin	Lung perfusion
Xenon-133	Lung ventilation
Tc-99m iminodiacetic acid	Hepatobiliary
Tc-99m diphosphonate	Skeletal
Tc-99m DTPA	Renal GFR
Thallium-201 or Tc-99m sestamibi	Myocardial perfusion

GFR, glomerular filtration rate; DTPA, dethylenetriamine-pentaacetic acid

Pulmonary angiography is currently the most accurate method available for establishing the diagnosis of PTE. However, angiography is costly and associated with side effects that occasionally are severe.

Images of regional pulmonary perfusion are obtained by intravenously injecting several hundred thousand tiny particles of macroaggregated human albumin that are radiolabeled with technetium-99m (Tc-99m). These particles have diameters of 10–40 μm. Because the diameter of pulmonary capillaries and precapillary arterioles is less than 10 μm, the radioactive particles lodge in these vessels throughout the lung fields in concentrations that are directly proportional to the regional pulmonary perfusion (Fig. 3-2). Because less

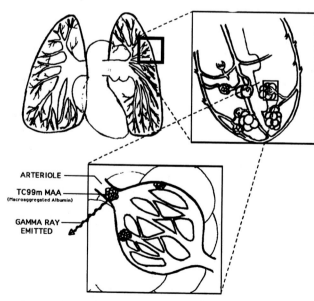

ARTERIOLE
TC99m MAA
(Macroaggregated Albumin)
GAMMA RAY
EMITTED

FIG. 3-2. A Tc-99m MAA particle as it becomes trapped in the pulmonary capillaries and emits gamma rays.

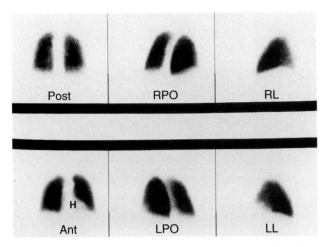

FIG. 3-3. Normal perfusion lung images in six projections. Ant, anterior; Post, posterior; LPO, left posterior oblique; RPO, right posterior oblique; LL, left lateral; RL, right lateral. "H" designates area of absent activity due to the heart.

than 0.1% of the total cross-section of pulmonary vasculature is occluded by the particles, the only potential risk from this procedure is in patients with severe underlying cardiopulmonary disease who have pulmonary hypertension. However, even in these individuals, perfusion scanning can be done safely by reducing the number of particles injected into the patient.

Figure 3-3 shows an example of the normal pulmonary blood flow pattern. Patients with PTE often display diminished or absent blood flow to one or more lung segments (Fig. 3-4A). The emboli are often large enough to occlude the segmental pulmonary arteries and hence the flow defects on the images will often appear "segmental" in configuration. However, thromboembolic occlusion of smaller arteries may occur, and the perfusion pattern may therefore reveal defects that are somewhat smaller.

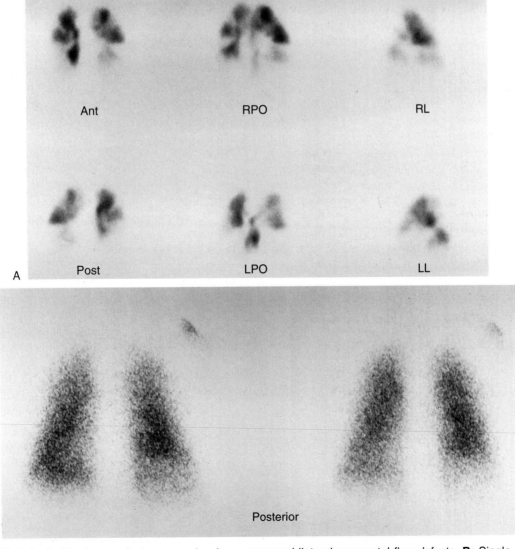

FIG. 3-4. A: Six-view perfusion scan showing numerous bilateral segmental flow defects. **B:** Single-breath ventilation images showing normal ventilation. This pattern is essentially diagnostic for PTE.

TABLE 3-2. *Pulmonary diseases that cause decreased regional lung perfusion with corresponding abnormal ventilation*

Pneumonia
Chronic obstructive lung disease
Atelectasis
Asthma

Lung pathology other than thromboemboli may cause alterations in the regional pulmonary blood flow pattern. Disorders of the lung parenchyma such as pneumonia, chronic obstructive lung disease, and regional atelectasis may lead to abnormalities of lung perfusion due to reflex vasoconstriction in the region of the pathology. As a result, the presence of one or more focal blood flow abnormalities is not necessarily specific for the presence of pulmonary thromboemboli. It is for this reason that scintigraphic ventilation imaging of the lungs is typically combined with the perfusion study in the evaluation of PTE. Determination of the ventilation status of a lung region that shows abnormal perfusion improves the specificity of the test for the diagnosis PTE. Diseases of the lungs that lead to abnormal regional perfusion and corresponding abnormal regional ventilation are summarized in Table 3-2.

Images of regional pulmonary ventilation are obtained using radioactive xenon. The patient inhales the xenon from a device that lets him or her breathe the radioactive gas without allowing the xenon to leak into the room. Images of the initial inhaled distribution of xenon are made along with images depicting the washout or clearance of the xenon from the lungs as the individual begins to breathe room air. A normal ventilation pattern is shown in Fig. 3-5.

Areas of the lung with diminished perfusion secondary to nonembolic lung pathology are associated with "matching" ventilation defects (Fig. 3-6). In contrast, ventilation usually appears normal in regions of the lung that show perfusion defects caused by thromboemboli (Figs. 3-4 and 3-7).

The intrinsic fibrinolytic system will lyse thromboemboli and often restore the pulmonary circulation within

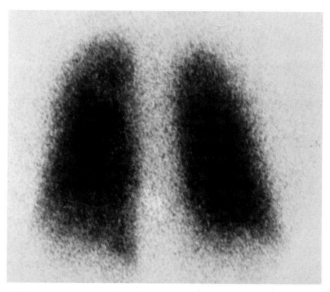

FIG. 3-5. Normal xenon ventilation study. Posterior view of the initial breath hold image.

weeks and even days in some patients (Fig. 3-8). It is therefore important to obtain the ventilation-perfusion (V/P) examination early in the evaluation of the patient with PTE while the flow defects are still present.

Typically, results from the V/P study are used to estimate the probability that acute PTE has occurred. An entirely normal perfusion pattern indicates virtually no chance that the patient has emboli, and the clinician should then focus on a search for other causes of the patient's symptoms. A finding of multiple (two or more) segmental perfusion defects with a correspondingly normal ventilation pattern indicates a very high probability that the patient has PTE. A variety of ventilation-perfusion patterns exist, however, wherein the probability for PTE lies somewhere in between.

If the diagnosis remains uncertain after lung scintigraphy, a noninvasive test for deep vein thrombosis of the lower extremity can be considered because this is where the vast majority of thromboemboli arise. Both ultrasound/Doppler and impedance plethysmography have been used successfully in this capacity. Finally, if

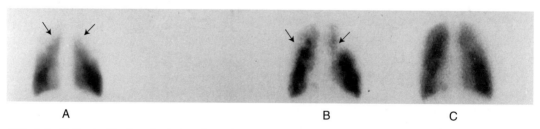

A   B   C

FIG. 3-6. Patient with chronic obstructive pulmonary disease showing "matching" ventilation and perfusion defects in upper lobes *(arrows)*. **A:** Posterior perfusion image. **B:** Posterior initial breath hold ventilation image. **C:** Later "equilibrium" ventilation image showing eventual filling in of defects seen on the initial ventilation image.

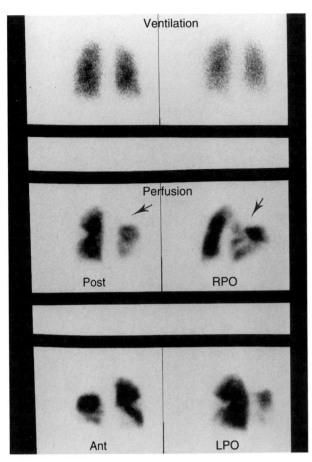

FIG. 3-7. Top two images are posterior ventilation images with xenon-133 showing uniform ventilation to both lungs. Bottom four images are from the perfusion study showing multiple segmental defects. Arrow points to region of absent perfusion in what is probably all three segments of the right upper lobe. Note that the lung regions with flow defects have normal ventilation. This pattern indicates a very high probability for PTE.

a decision is made to perform pulmonary angiography, the perfusion imaging results should serve as a guide to the angiographer for directing the angiography catheter placement to the region of the lung which shows the perfusion defect. Figure 3-9 shows a decision analysis flow chart recommended for the workup of patients with suspected PTE.

HEPATOBILIARY IMAGING

Patients with acute cholecystitis classically present with right upper quadrant pain/tenderness, fever, and leukocytosis. However, the signs and symptoms of acute cholecystitis often vary, and there are a number of pathologic conditions that occasionally present in a similar fashion. Consequently, the provisional diagnosis of acute cholecystitis typically requires confirmatory testing with ultrasound and/or hepatobiliary scintigraphy.

Hepatobiliary scintigraphic imaging is performed us-

ing a Tc-99m-labeled iminodiacetic acid derivative that is an analog of bilirubin. This radiopharmaceutical is actively transported into hepatocytes by the same system which transports bilirubin and is excreted unchanged into the biliary tract.

In normal individuals the hepatobiliary radiotracer will flow into the gallbladder within the first hour after intravenous administration (Fig. 3-10). However, in acute cholecystitis the gallbladder fails to fill with the radiotracer due to cystic duct obstruction by a stone. This test is extremely sensitive and a normal result (i.e., visualization of the gallbladder) virtually excludes the possibility of acute cholecystitis. The possible exception to this occurs in patients who have acalculous cholecystitis (approximately 5% of all cases of cholecystitis). In 10% to 20% of individuals with acute acalculous disease, the gallbladder will be visualized on the hepatobiliary exam.

It is important to note that there are certain conditions that predispose to false-positive results. The most common false-positive result occurs in prolonged fasting of more than 2–3 days. Under this condition, the gallbladder rarely contracts and its contents begin to partially solidify into a gelatinous material that can impede or block the entry of the radioactive bile into the gallbladder. The result is gallbladder nonvisualization. The gallbladder also fails to visualize in many patients who have ingested food within 2 hours of the hepatobiliary study as a result of the high level of circulating cholecystokinin causing gallbladder contraction, which limits entry of the radioactive bile. For this reason, scintigraphic hepatobiliary imaging should not be performed within 2 hours of a meal. Conditions that lead to false-positive (gallbladder nonvisualization) results are summarized in Table 3-3.

The use of morphine with hepatobiliary imaging has been found to be helpful in reducing the number of false-positive results, thereby improving the specificity of the test. Morphine causes constriction of the sphincter of Odi and leads to a rise in biliary system pressure. This augments bile movement through the cystic duct improving gallbladder visualization. For this reason, the use of morphine has become standard practice with this procedure. Figure 3-11 shows a case in which a normal gallbladder became visible only after administration of morphine. Figure 3-12 shows a patient with acute chole-

text continues on page 38

TABLE 3-3. *Conditions that may yield false-positive results with hepatobiliary imaging in the evaluation of acute cholecystitis*

Prolonged fasting (>3 days)
Ingestion of food within 2 hours of the study
Chronic cholecystitis
Chronic alcohol abuse
Pancreatitis

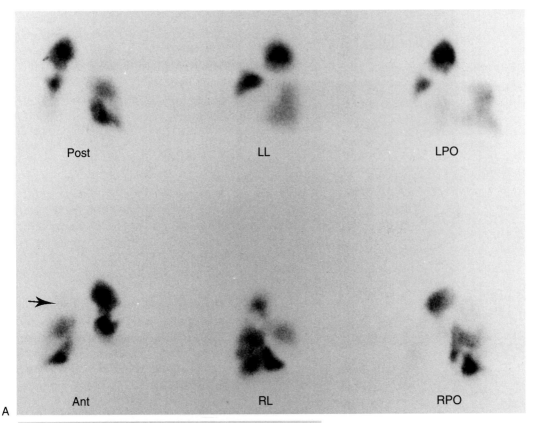

Post   LL   LPO

Ant   RL   RPO

A

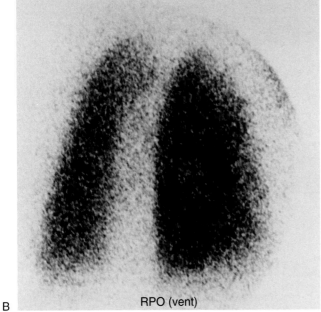

RPO (vent)

B

FIG. 3-8. Patient with PTE showing resolution of flow defects over time. **A:** Lung perfusion study shortly after onset of patients respiratory symptoms. Chest x-ray and ventilation study **(B)** were essentially normal. The diagnosis of PTE was established from these images and the patient was placed on heparin. Ten days later the patient had additional respiratory symptoms and the lung scan was repeated.

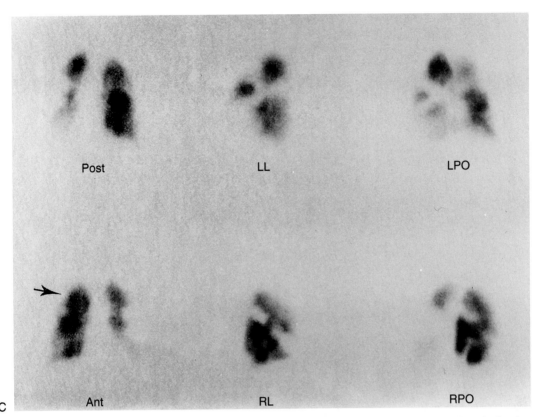

Post   LL   LPO

C   Ant   RL   RPO

FIG. 3-8. *Continued.* The repeat study **(C)** again showed multiple segmental defects of perfusion in the same locations as seen on the first exam. However, blood flow was almost completely restored to at least one large area (right upper lobe indicated by arrow).

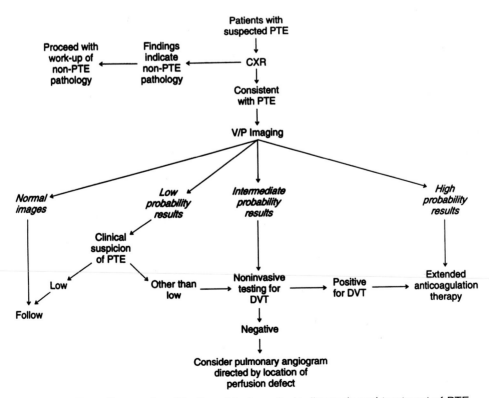

FIG. 3-9. Flow diagram for utilization of test results in diagnosis and treatment of PTE.

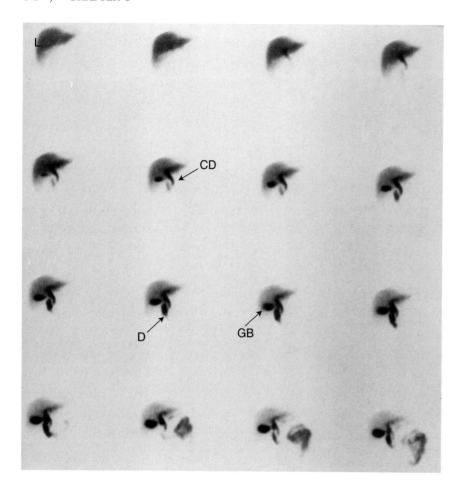

FIG. 3-10. Normal hepatobiliary study. Images obtained in the anterior view every 2 minutes (moving from left to right and top to bottom) following injection of the hepatobiliary radiotracer show good extraction of the agent by the liver (L). The common bile duct *(arrow CD)* is seen along with the duodenum *(arrow D)* and gallbladder *(arrow GB)*.

cystitis and gallbladder nonvisualization both before and after administration of morphine.

Hepatobiliary imaging can be used in infants to help distinguish biliary atresia from neonatal hepatitis, and it is a very sensitive test for detecting acute common bile duct obstruction in adults. The study has also been used successfully to identify biliary leaks due to trauma, surgery, or acute cholecystitis.

SKELETAL IMAGING

Skeletal scintigraphic imaging, more commonly referred to as the bone scan, is a valuable tool for investigation of a number of disorders of the skeletal system. A Tc-99m-labeled diphosphonate derivative is used to perform skeletal scintigraphy because this radiolabeled agent is adsorbed onto the surface of newly forming hydroxyapatite crystal in the bone. New bone formation occurs in response to the presence of almost all skeletal pathology. Consequently, scintigraphic images will demonstrate increased gamma ray emissions localized to the site of bone abnormality.

It is important for clinicians to know whether skeletal metastases are present in patients with malignant tumors. Evaluation of patients for possible metastases is carried out predominantly in those individuals who have tumors that tend to metastasize to the bone, such as breast, lung, prostate, and renal carcinomas. Well-differentiated thyroid cancer is also prone to disseminate to sites in bone but these lesions are probably better detected with iodine-131 imaging.

The normal bone scan appearance is shown in Fig. 3-13. The bone scan in a patient with skeletal metastases typically reveals numerous foci of excessive tracer accumulation, most commonly in the axial skeleton, but also to a lesser extent present in the appendicular skeleton (Fig. 3-14). Skeletal metastases usually arise as a result of hematogenous seeding of tumor cells in the bone marrow. Because most of the adult marrow resides in the axial skeleton, it makes sense that *the large majority of metastatic lesions are detected in the axial skeleton.*

The bone scan is very sensitive for detecting metastatic lesions and in general will identify a metastasis before it can be detected by a conventional radiograph. However, it is often not possible to ascertain whether

text continues on page 41

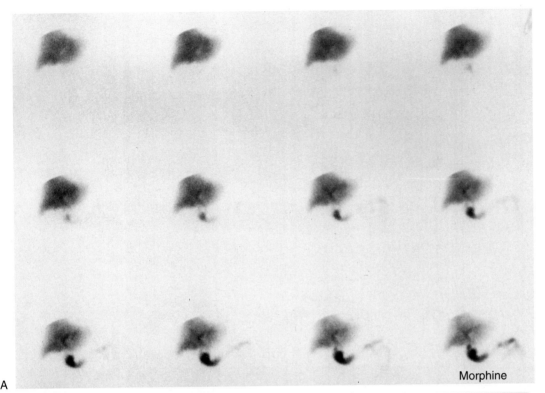

A

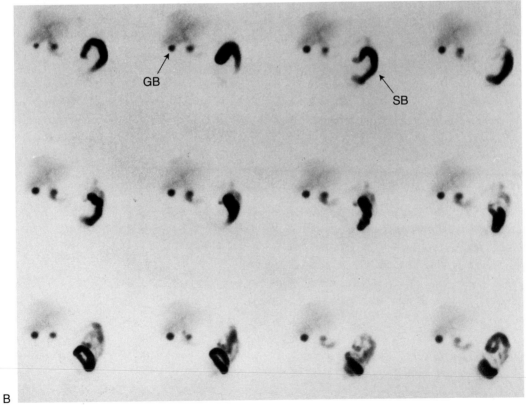

B

FIG. 3-11. Hepatobiliary examination in a patient with right upper quadrant pain. **A:** Initial set of images show normal uptake and excretion by the liver but over time the gallbladder is not visualized and consequently morphine is given at approximately 40 minutes into the study. **B:** Images obtained immediately following administration of morphine show the gallbladder visualization *(arrow GB)* which effectively rules out acute cholecystitis. Note activity in the small bowel *(arrow SB)*.

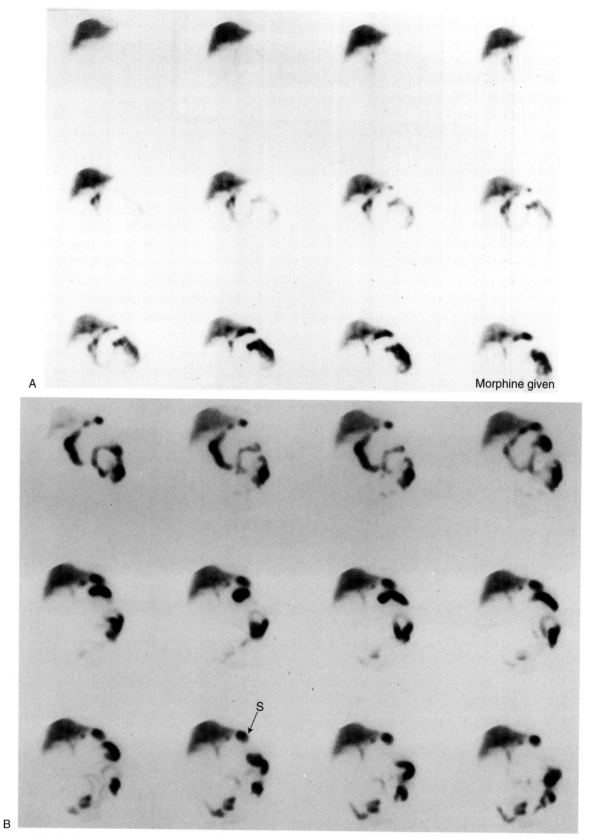

FIG. 3-12. Hepatobiliary study in patient with fever and right upper quadrant pain. **A:** Initial set of images show normal uptake and excretion by the liver but the gallbladder is not visualized and consequently morphine is given at approximately the time of the image at bottom right. **B:** Images obtained immediately following injection of morphine continue to show absence of gallbladder activity indicating cystic duct obstruction and very probably acute cholecystitis. Note the reflux of radioactive bile into the stomach *(arrow S)*. The patient was taken to surgery and found to have acute cholecystitis.

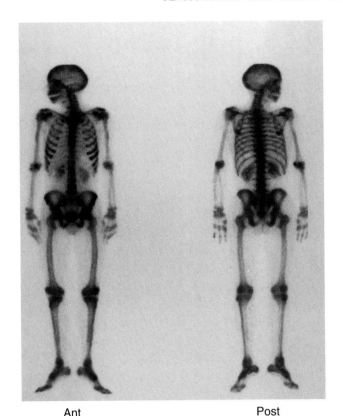

Ant   Post

FIG. 3-13. Anterior and posterior whole-body images of a normal bone scan.

lesions seen on a bone scan are malignant or benign, and this is particularly true for a single lesion, which often is caused by a benign process. *Numerous focal lesions are much more often due to metastatic disease.* In a patient with a single vertebral lesion on bone scan and a normal radiograph, it is often prudent to obtain an MRI study to better determine if a marrow metastasis is present.

Like metastases, osteomyelitis can be detected much earlier with a bone scan than with a radiograph (Fig. 3-15). The bone scan is particularly useful in childhood osteomyelitis where early treatment is very important. The bone scan may also be useful to detect a nondisplaced fracture or traumatic lesion of a type not easily seen on radiographs. For example, lesions that originate from intense physical activity, such as stress fractures (Fig. 3-16) and shin splints (Fig. 3-17), are readily detected on a bone scan and may not be seen on a radiograph. In most cases, fractures through the full thickness of the bone cortex are readily detected by a plain radiograph. Some full-thickness fractures, such as those in the sacrum, scapula, femoral neck, and small bones of the wrist and ankle, are occasionally difficult to visualize on a radiograph, but are detectable by a bone scan.

ANGIOTENSIN-CONVERTING ENZYME INHIBITOR RENAL SCINTIGRAPHIC IMAGING

Scintigraphic imaging procedures can be used to evaluate renal perfusion and various aspects of renal function. Technetium-99m-labeled molecules that are filtered by the renal glomerulus can be used to assess glomerular filtration rate (GFR). Scintigraphic imaging of GFR combined with administration of an angiotensin-converting enzyme (ACE) inhibitor, such as captopril, is used to identify patients with hypertension caused by renal artery stenosis.

In patients with renal vascular hypertension (RVH), renin secretion is enhanced secondary to the hemodynamic effects of a functionally significant stenosis in the renal artery (Fig. 3-18). Decreased perfusion pressure as a result of the stenosis causes the juxtaglomerular cells to increase secretion of renin. Renin acts on angiotensinogen to form angiotensin I. Angiotensin I is con-

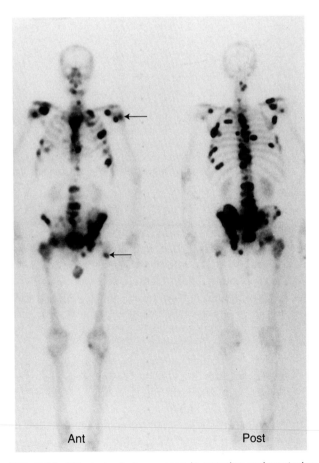

Ant   Post

FIG. 3-14. Whole-body bone scan in anterior and posterior projections of a 65-year-old man with diffuse skeletal metastases from prostate carcinoma. Images reveal numerous metastatic lesions (black foci), primarily in the axial skeleton on both anterior and posterior views. However, lesions are also seen in the proximal femurs and humeri *(arrows)*.

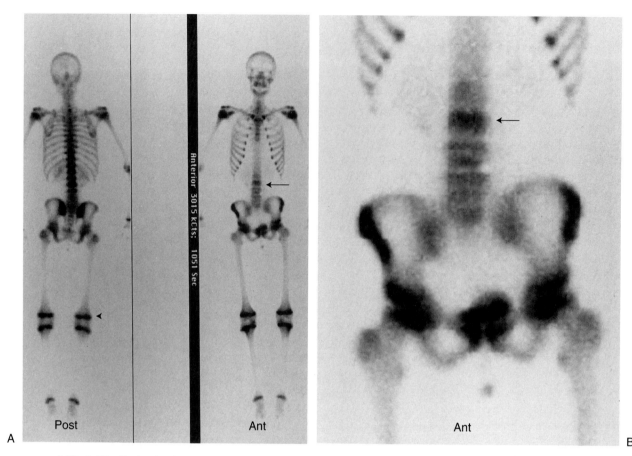

FIG. 3-15. Skeletal scintigraphic images (whole body, **A**; regional view, **B**) from an 18-year-old girl with diabetes who presented with 3–4 weeks of low-back pain. Radiographs of the vertebra were unremarkable. The images show abnormally increased technetium-99m MDP activity in the L-3 vertebral body *(arrow)*. Biopsy of the site confirmed osteomyelitis. Notice the normal intense uptake of Tc-99m MDP at the growth plates in the lower extremities *(arrowhead)* on the whole-body images.

verted to angiotensin II by ACE. Angiotensin II stimulates release of aldosterone, and also acts as a potent vasoconstrictor of the peripheral vasculature and also including vasoconstriction of the efferent renal arterioles distal to the glomerulus in the under perfused kidney with the stenosis. The efferent vasoconstriction acts to preserve the transglomerular pressure gradient and therefore helps to preserve the GFR in the affected kidney. If an ACE inhibitor such as captopril is administered in this setting, angiotensin II levels will drop and the efferent arterioles will dilate, leading to a fall in GFR in the stenotic kidney.

In patients with RVH, scintigraphic images of the kidneys obtained during ACE inhibition demonstrate this deterioration in GFR in the stenotic kidney (Fig. 3-19). In contrast, patients with essential hypertension will have no effect from captopril on the renal scintigraphic images (Fig. 3-20).

What is most important is the ability of this scintigraphic procedure to predict which patients with renal artery stenosis will have their hypertension controlled or cured by a revascularization procedure designed to correct the stenosis. Specifically, patients with a strongly positive scintigraphic ACE inhibitor study are very likely to experience improvement or cure in their hypertension if the stenosis is repaired. Conversely, patients with a completely normal result are very unlikely to respond to repair of the renal artery stenosis.

MYOCARDIAL PERFUSION IMAGING

Perfusion imaging of the myocardium can be performed using intravenous injected thallium-201 chloride or a Tc-99m-labeled agent known as sestamibi. These substances accumulate in the myocardium in direct proportion to the regional myocardial blood flow and the number of viable myocytes. Most imaging centers use SPECT (single-photon emission computed tomography) to obtain perfusion images of the heart in three

text continues on page 45

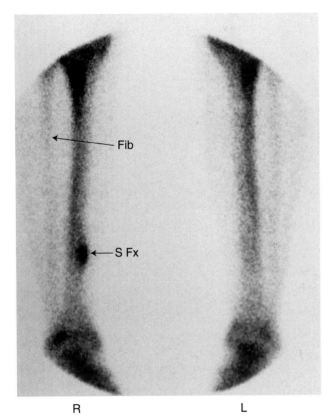

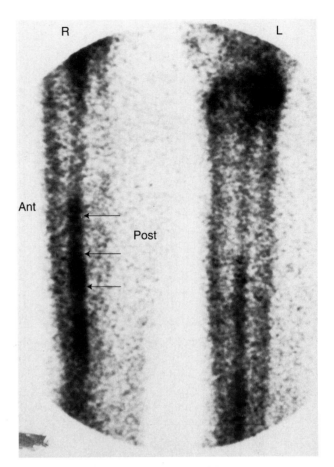

FIG. 3-16. A 20-year-old woman with pain in the right distal lower extremity. Patient was an athlete in training with an extensive running regimen. Radiographs shortly after the onset of pain were normal. Scintigraphic images of the distal lower extremities show focal lesion in the posterior medial aspect of the right distal tibia consistent with a stress fracture *(see arrow)*. Notice that the lesion does not involve the full thickness of the tibia. Fibula indicated by long arrow.

FIG. 3-17. Bone scan in a patient with shin splints showing linear pattern of increased radiopharmaceutical concentration *(arrows)* along the posterior aspect of the tibia.

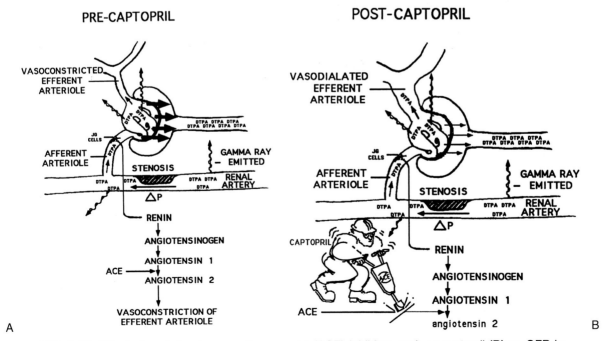

FIG. 3-18. Effect of angiotensin-converting enzyme (ACE) inhibitor, such as captopril **(B)** on GFR in the setting of renal artery stenosis and renal vascular hypertension. **(A)** Without ACE inhibitor.

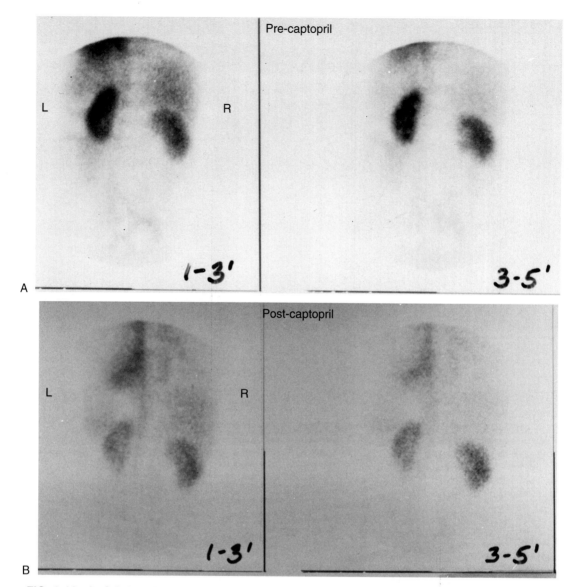

Pre-captopril

L   R

1-3'   3-5'

A

Post-captopril

L   R

1-3'   3-5'

B

FIG. 3-19. A: Scintigraphic images of the kidneys in the posterior projection, 1–3 minutes and 3–5 minutes following IV injection of a Tc-99m-labeled agent that is filtered by the glomerulus. **B:** Repeat images following administration of captopril show a significant decrease in the concentration of this agent (and therefore decrease in GFR) in the left kidney compared to the precaptopril study. This finding indicates renal artery stenosis causing renal vascular hypertension.

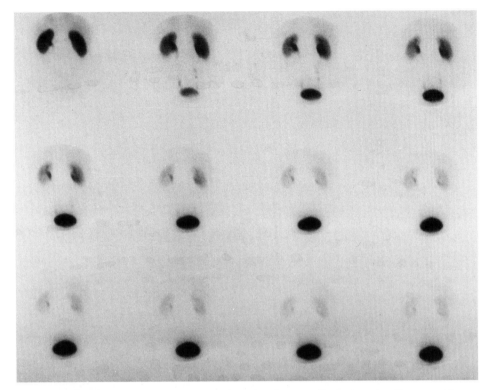

FIG. 3-20. Patient with essential hypertension showing no effect of captopril on renal images.

dimensions (Fig. 3-21). SPECT is a technique that yields a three-dimensional pattern of radiopharmaceutical distribution in the body with images displayed in cross-section much like CT or MRI. A normal cardiac SPECT thallium-201 study shows uniform perfusion throughout the myocardium (Fig. 3-22).

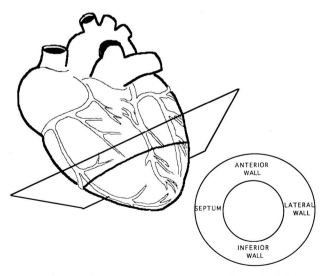

FIG. 3-21. SPECT short-axis cross-section from the left ventricle. The short-axis cross-sectional view is obtained by "slicing" the three-dimensional image of the heart muscle in planes perpendicular to the long dimension of the heart.

Myocardial perfusion "stress" imaging can be performed with either exercise or a pharmacologic agent such as adenosine. Application of the cardiac stress improves the sensitivity of myocardial perfusion imaging for detecting coronary artery disease. Arterioles distal to a normal coronary artery will dilate substantially in response to either exercise or pharmacologic stimulation. As a result, perfusion (and therefore radiotracer concentration) will increase considerably in the myocardium distal to a normal vessel, whereas myocardial perfusion will change little if at all distal to a significant stenosis (Fig. 3-23). Therefore significant coronary artery disease will result in a perfusion "defect" on the cardiac images immediately following the stress (Fig. 3-24).

Perfusion defects seen on the stress images that become less severe or normalize on delayed images are referred to as "reversible" and almost always contain viable myocardium (Fig. 3-24). Defects that do not change from stress to the delayed images (termed "fixed") usually contain scar tissue. However, in some instances fixed defects might still contain viable tissue. This information is very important for making decisions about possible coronary bypass surgery. Figure 3-25 shows an example of a "fixed" thallium defect representing scar tissue from previous infarction.

Myocardial stress imaging can be used to select appropriate candidates with suspected coronary artery disease

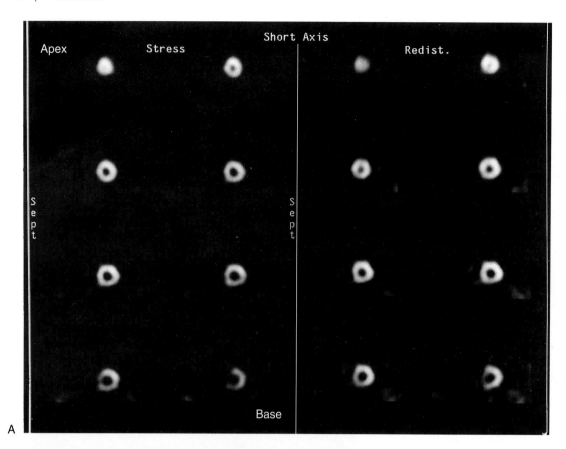

Short Axis

Apex   Stress   Redist.

Sept

Sept

Base

A

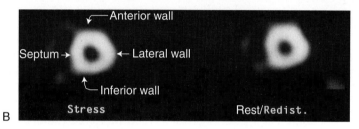

┌─ Anterior wall

Septum →   ← Lateral wall

┌─ Inferior wall

Stress   Rest/Redist.

B

FIG. 3-22. Stress (dipyridamole) and delayed SPECT thallium images showing normal distribution of thallium-201 in the left ventricular myocardium. **A:** All short-axis images from the apex of the heart to the base of the heart. **B:** Selected short-axis images from the mid region of the heart.

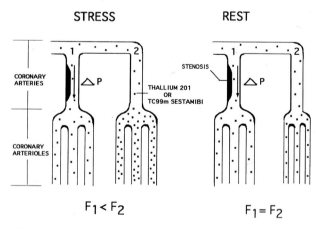

STRESS   REST

CORONARY
ARTERIES

STENOSIS

THALLIUM 201
OR
TC99m SESTAMIBI

ΔP   ΔP

CORONARY
ARTERIOLES

$F_1 < F_2$ $F_1 = F_2$

FIG. 3-23. Diagram showing the effects on the caliber of coronary arterioles from a pressure gradient. Blood flow through the stenosed artery, F1, is essentially the same as flow through the normal artery, F2, at rest due to arteriolar vasodilatation. However, in the presence of a "stress" (exercise or pharmacologic) F2 increases to a greater extent than does F1, creating a discrepancy in regional myocardial perfusion.

TABLE 3-4. *Some radioisotopes used in therapeutic applications*

Radioisotope	Treatment
Iodine-131	Thyroid disorders
Strontium-89	Skeletal metastases
Samarium-153	Skeletal metastases
Phosphorus-32	Polycythemia vera
Iodine-131, yttrium-90-labeled monoclonal antibodies	Lymphoma

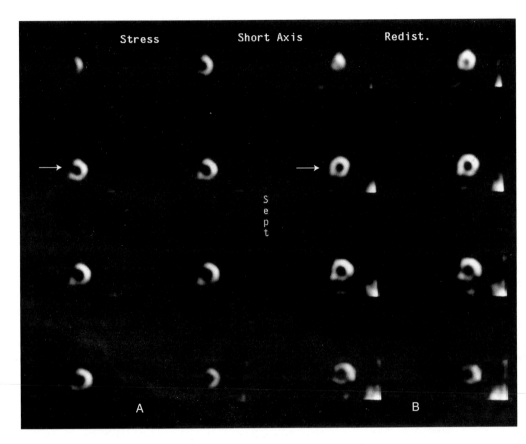

FIG. 3-24. Thallium images from a patient with tight stenosis of the left anterior descending coronary artery; short-axis "stress" images **(A)** showing a severe perfusion defect in the septum which is reversible on rest/redistribution images **(B)**.

for coronary arteriography. In addition, this technique can provide information on the hemodynamic severity of coronary lesions already seen on the angiogram and thus assist in selecting patients for coronary revascularization procedures.

RADIONUCLIDE THERAPY

Although a detailed discussion of the therapeutic applications of internally administered radionuclides is beyond the scope of this chapter, it is important to recognize this aspect of nuclear medicine. Generally, the radioactive isotopes being used now for therapy emit beta particles and in the future alpha particle emitters may also be employed. Currently the most common radioisotope used in therapy is I-131. In its elemental form this agent is used to treat thyroid disorders such as Graves disease and thyroid cancer. Because the iodine is trapped by the abnormal thyroid cells the radiation effect is concentrated at the desired site. A relatively new

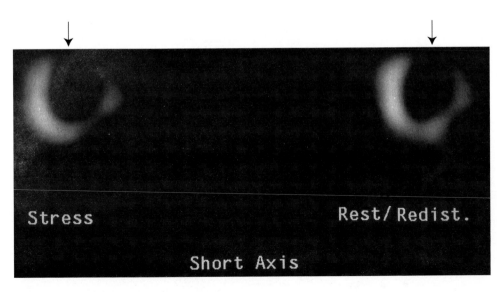

FIG. 3-25. Thallium images from a patient with past infarction of the anterior wall of the heart. Short-axis images show a severe defects in the anterior wall *(arrows)* and lateral wall both of which are fixed (unchanged from stress to rest/redistribution images). These findings are consistent with scarring in the anterior and lateral walls.

Key Points

- Nuclear imaging is performed using radiolabeled molecules injected into the body to create images of organ physiology.
- Ventilation-perfusion lung imaging plays an important role in the workup of patients with suspected PTE.
- Normal pulmonary perfusion essentially rules out the diagnosis of PTE.
- Visualization of the gallbladder with hepatobiliary scintigraphy almost always rules out the diagnosis of acute cholecystis.
- Bone pathology (e.g., metastases) causes increased bone hydroxyapatite formation, leading to increased uptake of the bone scan radiopharmaceutical.
- Bone scintigraphy is a sensitive test for detecting skeletal metastases, osteomyelitis, and fractures.
- Captopril renal imaging accurately detects hemodynamically significant renal artery stenosis in patients with renovascular hypertension.
- Myocardial stress perfusion imaging is an accurate technique for detecting coronary artery disease.

---

way of delivering a radioisotope to a selected target in the body is through the use of radiolabeled monoclonal antibodies (MoAb). The MoAb "carrying" the radio-emitter will bind to a particular tumor cell surface antigen and thus deliver the radioisotope and its radioactive emissions directly to the tumor site. Table 3-4 lists some of the therapeutic uses of internally administered radioisotopes.

ACKNOWLEDGMENTS

The author thanks Brian Clarke CNMT, for his original drawings of Figs. 3-1, 3-2, 3-18, 3-21, and 3-23; Dr. Parvez Shirazi for suppling the images for Fig. 3-17; and Ms. Maryann O'Brien, MA, CNMT, for her assistance in preparing this manuscript.

SUGGESTED READINGS

Henkin RE, Boles MA, Dillehay GL, Halama JR, Karesh SM, Wagner RH, Zimmer AM, eds. *Nuclear Medicine.* St. Louis: CV Mosby, 1996.

Wagner HN, Szabo Z, Buchanan JW, eds. *Principles of Nuclear Medicine.* Philadelphia: WB Saunders, 1995.

CHAPTER 4

Mammography

William E. Erkonen

This chapter is short, but its importance is unrelated to its length. There are a number of good textbooks on this subject that are more encyclopedic, and you can and should refer to these (e.g., 1). The purpose of this chapter is to stress the importance of mammography in the management of breast disease and the screening for early cancer detection.

Approximately one in eight females in the United States will develop cancer of the breast during her lifetime, and this incidence appears to be increasing. Breast cancer currently involves over 180,000 women per year in the United States, and it causes approximately 44,000 deaths per year. An effective strategy to decrease the mortality associated with this disease is to find the lesions at an early and curable stage. Mammography can detect breast lesions before they become symptomatic and/or are palpable, as they can detect early invasive lesions or carcinomas in situ that measure only a few millimeters. It is generally believed that the earlier the disease is diagnosed, the smaller the chance of metastases occurring. Consequently, mammography is widely employed as a routine screening tool to detect occult breast cancer in the general asymptomatic female population. *However, screening mammography must always be used in conjunction with monthly breast self-examination and an annual breast examination performed by a physician.* A recent National Cancer Institute review showed that this approach significantly reduces breast cancer deaths for women of all ages.

Mammography is also a key tool in the evaluation of known and suspected breast disease in both males and females.

There is little doubt that mammograms must be interpreted by qualified radiologists, and the radiologist's role in this disease continues to increase. Radiologists are more frequently being called on to perform breast procedures such as percutaneous breast biopsy and cyst drainage, but all doctors should be aware of the basics of breast imaging due to the prevalence of pathology in this area.

GUIDELINES FOR MAMMOGRAPHY

Some generally accepted guidelines for mammography are listed in Table 4-1. These guidelines provide you with something on which you can hang your hat, but there isn't a unanimous agreement about them. Un-

TABLE 4-1. *General mammography guidelines*

1. Baseline between 35 and 40 years for future comparison.
   a. Baseline before age 35, if mother or sister had premenopausal breast cancer.
2. Every 1–2 years between ages 40 and 49 depending on risk factors. See Table 4-2.
3. Annual mammograms for all women over 50.
4. At any age when there are symptoms or clinical findings suspicious for malignancy.

TABLE 4-2. *Risk factors that can influence the timing for mammography*

1. Prior personal history of breast cancer
2. Family history of premenopausal breast cancer in mother or sister
3. Presence of BRCA-1 and BRCA-2 genes
4. Previous biopsy findings: ductal carcinoma in situ, atypia, juvenile papillomatosis, lobular neoplasia [1]
5. Age (incidence increases with age)
6. Years of menstruation: early age menarche, late age menopause
7. Nulliparous, late age first birth
8. Never breast-fed
9. Postmenopausal obesity
10. Others [1]

TABLE 4-3. *Some attitudinal barriers to mammography*

1. Expense
2. Fear of radiation exposure
3. Fear of causing cancer
4. Fear of pain
5. Fear of overdiagnosis and unnecessary biopsy
6. Denial

fortunately, only about 15% of women over the age of 50 have annual mammograms, and only 10% of physicians use these guidelines for asymptomatic women. As indicated in the guidelines in Table 4-1, risk factors are important and influence the timing for mammography. Some of the common risk factors are listed in Table 4-2. Depending on the risk factors, the time tables may be advanced to younger ages by approximately 5–10 years. Unfortunately, attitudinal barriers to mammography still exist among some patients and doctors, and they are listed in Table 4-3.

TECHNIQUE

The importance of a well-performed mammogram cannot be overemphasized. A standard mammogram consists of a *mediolateral oblique* view with the central x-ray beam traversing the breast obliquely in a medial to lateral direction (Fig. 4-1A), and a *craniocaudal* view (Fig. 4-1B) with the central x-ray beam traversing the breast in a head-to-foot direction. It is usually necessary to compress the breast during the examination to better visualize all the breast tissue, and this may cause a tolerable mild to moderate discomfort. The technical aspects of mammography are very complicated, and it is extremely important that the mammographer be properly trained and qualified. Image quality controls are mandatory.

Normal mediolateral oblique and craniocaudal breast images are shown in Fig. 4-2. Notice that breast images are a combination of fat (black) and water density soft tissues (gray). This background of black and gray, especially the black, enhances visualization of the white calcifications. The major portion of the breast tissue is connective tissue and fat. Breast tissue is predominately connective tissue in the young, and with aging this is gradually replaced by adipose tissue. Only a very small amount of the breast volume is made up of epithelial tissues (lobules and ducts).

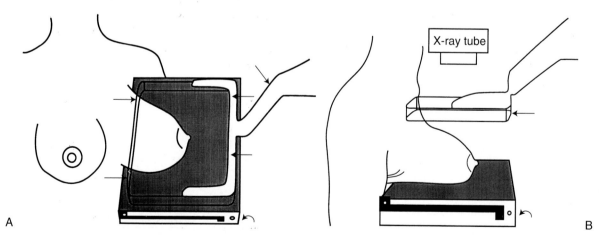

FIG. 4-1. A: Illustration of how the patient is positioned for a mediolateral oblique (MLO) mammogram. The x-ray beam passes obliquely through the breast in a medial to lateral direction. The breast is routinely compressed between the compression device *(straight arrows)* and the radiographic cassette *(curved arrow)*. The cassette contains a radiographic film on which the image will be recorded. Compression improves the diagnostic quality of the images by making the breast a more homogeneous thickness. **B:** Illustration of how the patient is positioned for a craniocaudal (CC) mammogram. The x-ray beam passes through the breast in a head-to-foot or cephalad to caudad direction. The compression device *(straight arrow)* is more easily visualized in this illustration. Again, the image will be recorded on the film in the radiographic cassette *(curved arrow)*.

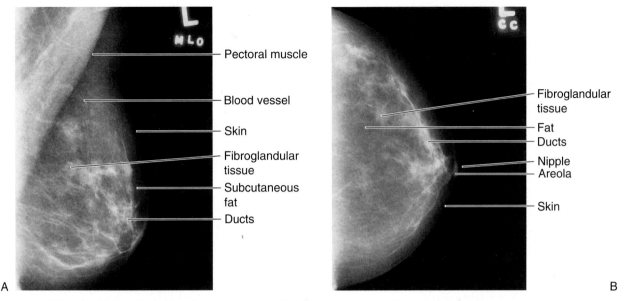

FIG. 4-2. A: Left breast mediolateral oblique (MLO) mammogram. Normal. **B:** Left breast craniocaudal (CC) mammogram. Normal.

MASSES

Benign

Benign disease (Table 4-4) may or may not be symptomatic and may or may not have associated masses. Fibroadenoma (Fig. 4-3) is a benign lesion that must be differentiated from a malignant mass. It generally occurs in young women and may be multiple or single and unilateral or bilateral. On physical examination, fibroadenomas are hard and often movable. The mammographic appearance is a mass with coarse calcifications that may have a popcorn or punctate appearance. On sonograms, these lesions will usually appear hypoechoic.

Another common clinical problem is benign cystic disease, and this problem occurs at all ages. These patients may present with a mass that may or may not be tender, or they may be an asymptomatic incidental mammographic finding. The mammographic appearances are variable, but often there is a water density mass with well-defined sharp borders (Fig. 4-4A). Occasionally there may be mural calcification. Ultrasonography (Fig. 4-4B) usually shows a well-defined anechoic mass with posterior acoustic enhancement. Cysts may or may not require aspiration depending on the clinical

situation, and aspiration under ultrasound control is quite effective.

Breast augmentation implants (Fig. 4-5) are relatively common; over 2 million women now have them (1). The augmentations may be for cosmetic reasons or for postsurgical reconstruction. Special technical views are required to visualize the breast tissue surrounding the implant and to evaluate for implant rupture. Special care must be taken during mammography to avoid rupture of the implant. Mammographic implant appearances vary from water density saline to silicone metallic densities, and they may be discrete surgically implanted masses or multiple masses secondary to silicone injections.

Malignant

Some of the mammographic findings suspicious for malignancy are listed in Table 4-5. Calcifications are very important as they may represent the first sign of

TABLE 4-4. *Partial list of benign breast disease etiologies*

1. Cystic disease
2. Sclerosing adenosis
3. Fibroadenoma
4. Lipoma
5. Foreign body reaction to augmentation

TABLE 4-5. *Mammographic findings suspect for malignancy*

1. Mass on mammogram with:
   a. ill-defined or spiculated borders
   b. malignant calcifications
   c. skin retraction or thickening
2. Microcalcifications with or without a mass
   a. linear or branching
   b. clusters
   c. punctate
3. Mammographic architectural distortion (asymmetry)
4. Hypoechoic solid mass on ultrasound

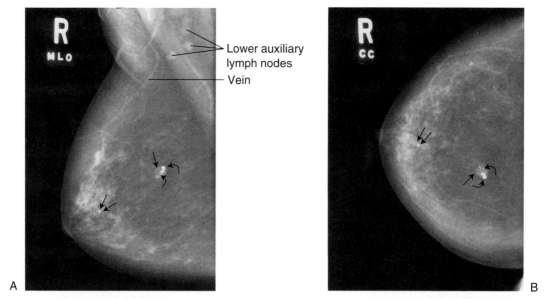

FIG. 4-3. Right breast mediolateral oblique **(A)** and craniocaudal **(B)** mammograms. Calcified benign fibroadenoma. The fibroadenoma mass is only faintly visible *(single straight arrows)*. The benign calcifications within the fibroadenoma are typically globular, coarse, and variable in size *(curved arrows)*. Note the single, benign globular calcification incidentally found without a mass associated *(double straight arrows)*.

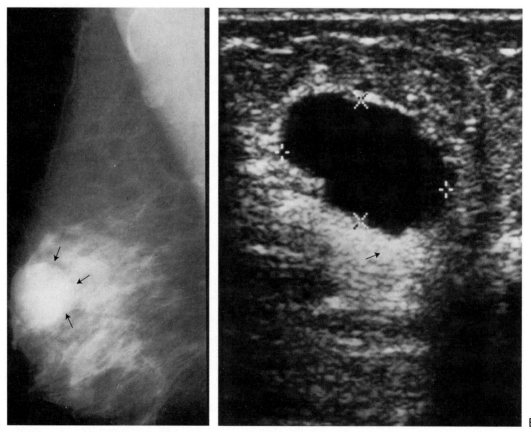

FIG. 4-4. A: Right breast mediolateral oblique mammogram. Benign cyst. The water density cyst *(straight arrows)* has sharp borders and no calcifications. Note the difference between the smooth sharp borders of this benign cyst compared to the irregular and poorly defined borders of the carcinoma in Fig. 4-6. **B:** Right breast sonogram of the lesion in A. This is the classic appearance of a benign breast cyst. The cystic fluid is the anechoic or black area, the hyperechoic or white areas are the cyst wall. The x's and crosses are electronic caliper marks on the cyst's wall that are used in measuring the dimensions of the cyst. Posterior acoustic enhancement *(straight arrow)* is commonly found immediately posterior to a cyst.

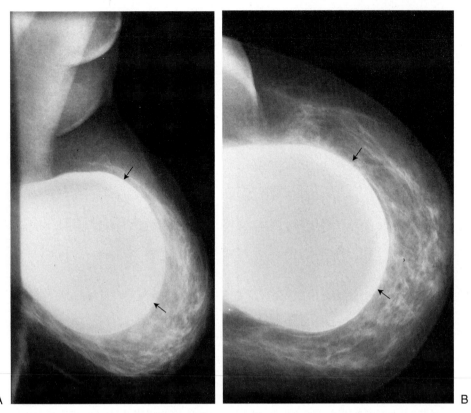

A   B

FIG. 4-5. Left breast mediolateral oblique **(A)** and craniocaudal **(B)** mammograms. Bilateral breast augmentations. The bright white areas represent the surgically implanted silicone augmentations *(straight arrows)*.

malignancy, especially if they are new, punctate (small spots), or branching (Fig. 4-6). It should be emphasized that most calcifications are benign. Therefore, it is essential that the radiologist distinguish between benign and malignant calcifications. Some calcifications are so small that a magnifying glass is mandatory when viewing mammograms. Once suspicious calcifications have been biopsied, the specimen can be radiographed to make sure that the calcifications have been completely removed.

Asymmetric water density masses and asymmetric architectural changes are very suspect for malignancy, especially if they have appeared recently.

MALE BREAST

All of the diseases that occur in the female breast can potentially occur in the male breast. The incidence of male breast carcinoma is approximately 900 cases per year in the United States, and this, of course, is in dramatic contrast to the female population. The indications for male mammography and the image obtained are similar to those for females.

One male breast clinical situation that can be confusing is gynecomastia (Fig. 4-7). The etiologies for male gynecomastia are listed in Table 4-6. It can occur in

neonate males secondary to the maternal estrogen, the majority of pubertal males, and adult men. Usually, adult men present with a tender subareolar breast mass, and it is generally unilateral. On mammography, there is increased soft tissue in the subareolar zone that may or may not be calcified. The need for biopsy will be determined by a combination of symptoms, physical findings, and mammographic findings. There is probably no correlation between gynecomastia and carcinoma.

Male breast carcinomas are similar in appearance and histology to female breast carcinomas.

OTHER TECHNOLOGIES

Computed tomography is rarely used for breast imaging, and magnetic resonance is occasionally used to

---

TABLE 4-6. *Some causes of male gynecomastia*

1. Common in the neonatal male
2. Common in pubertal males
3. Adult men
   a. Any underlying disease causing hormone imbalance (e.g., liver cirrhosis)
   b. Drugs (digitalis, steroids)
   c. Androgen deficiency as in aging

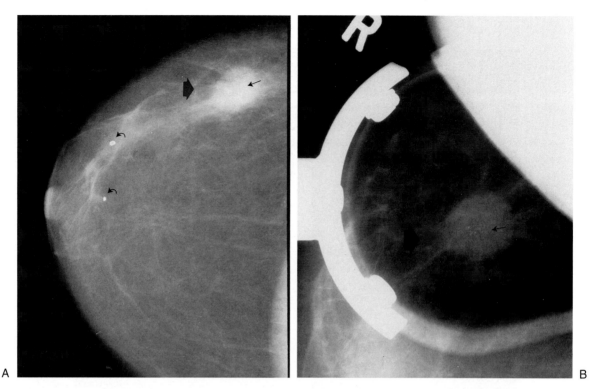

FIG. 4-6. A: Right breast craniocaudal mammogram. Carcinoma of the breast with malignant calcifications. The water density malignant mass lesion *(arrowhead)* has spiculated and poorly defined borders. The outline or border of this mass is in contrast to the sharp and well-defined border of the benign cyst in Fig. 4-4A. The malignant calcifications *(straight arrow)* are punctate and centrally located. In the same breast there are coarse benign calcifications *(curved arrows)* that are larger and more globular in appearance. **B:** Right breast spot magnification view of the lesion in Fig. 4-6A. This clearly demonstrates the classical appearance of malignant calcifications *(straight arrow)* in the mass *(arrowhead)*. Note the difference between the coarse benign calcifications in the fibroadenoma in Fig. 4-3 and the more delicate punctate malignant calcifications in this patient. Also, the spiculated and poorly defined borders are more obvious in this magnification view.

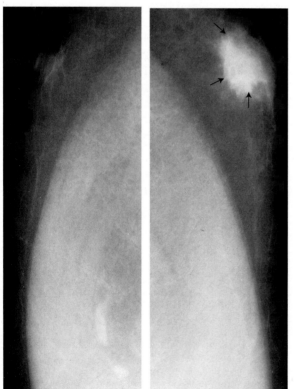

FIG. 4-7. A: Right male breast mediolateral oblique mammogram. Normal. **B:** Left male breast mediolateral oblique mammogram. Benign gynecomastia. The straight arrows indicate the typical increased subareolar soft tissue without calcification.

Key Points

- Approximately one in eight females in the United States will develop carcinoma of the breast at some time.
- Mammograms must be interpreted by qualified radiologists. Mammograms of high quality are imperative.
- A routine mammogram consists of mediolateral oblique and craniocaudal views.
- Screening mammography, monthly breast self-examination, and annual breast examinations by a physician can improve the survival rate of breast cancer.
- Mammographic findings suspect for malignancy include an irregularly outlined mass, skin retraction and/or thickening, architectural distortion (asymmetric compared to opposite breast), and/or a hypoechoic mass on ultrasonography.
- Calcifications that should be suspicious for malignancy include new calcifications with or without a mass, punctate calcifications, and branching calcifications.
- Ultrasonography is often useful to differentiate between a solid and a cystic mass.

image breast tissue surrounding an implant. Small field digital technology is used for core biopsies, and full-field digital mammography is being used in some field trials. However, any one of these technologies, including positron emission tomography (PET), might play a significant future role in breast imaging.

REFERENCES

1. Cardenosa G. *Breast Imaging Companion.* Philadelphia: Lippincott-Raven, 1997.

SUGGESTED READINGS

Cardenosa G. *Breast Imaging Companion.* Philadelphia: Lippincott-Raven, 1997.

CHAPTER 5

The Rational Selection and Interpretation of Diagnostic Tests

Paul J. Chang

I have always felt somewhat conflicted by beginning texts on radiology which, despite their usefulness and importance, seem to leave medical students and house staff with an incorrect impression regarding the true utility and role of diagnostic imaging tests as a result of this initial exposure. Such misunderstanding is understandable; after reading about and seeing scores of compelling images that elegantly demonstrate a specific disease process, it would be natural to have an exaggerated assessment of the relative performance of imaging tests in the diagnostic workup of your patients. Now this isn't really the fault of the introductory radiology textbook; after all, one must start somewhere, and showing images that reveal specific pathology is a necessary and useful starting point. However, showing images that always demonstrate the abnormality, while useful pedagogically, can result in the beginning clinician putting more faith in the performance and role of imaging tests than is warranted.

For example, I'm sure you will be impressed by the chest radiographs in this textbook that elegantly show the patient's pneumonia (down to the specific lung segment!) or the abdominal film that clearly demonstrates the tumor mass. Such examples can give anyone the false impression that radiographic studies are routinely able to detect all abnormalities all of the time. Obviously, this is not the case in the real world. If our textbooks were more realistic, they would also show a bunch of normal chest films with captions saying something like "patient with pneumonia, not evident on chest radiograph," or a few unremarkable abdominal plain films identified by statements such as "patient with large colon mass, missed by frontal radiograph kidney, ureter and bladder (KUB)."

Now I am not advocating that we waste book space and your time by showing lots of radiographs that show absolutely nothing in patients with disease. However, I think it is extremely important that we take the time to remind you that radiographic images, like all diagnostic tests, are imperfect and that this imperfect performance must be taken into account when making clinical decisions. How one takes a diagnostic test's imperfection into account when making the diagnosis is the purpose of this chapter.

HOW DIAGNOSTIC TESTS WORK: BAYES' THEOREM REVISITED

For this discussion, I am not really interested in the way diagnostic tests work with respect to their biophysical properties (e.g., how the magnetic resonance scanner generates images by listening to radio wave echoes). Rather, we need to understand how diagnostic tests work in the context of making clinical decisions. In other words, I am more interested in questions like: When should we order diagnostic tests? What tests should be ordered? How do we critically interpret the results? And how do we reliably use this frequently imperfect information to make optimal medical decisions?

A very good starting point for understanding how diagnostic tests work is to introduce (or reintroduce) a few basic concepts derived from Bayes' theorem. None of these concepts are particularly complex or challenging; most of us have been exposed to many of them in undergraduate or medical school statistics courses. However, if your biostatistics experience was anything like mine, the exposure to Bayesian analysis was pretty dry, theoretical, boring . . . and irrelevant. Although this approach was rigorous, it did not yield an intuitive understanding of the concepts. Let's try a more informal, clinically meaningful approach.

WHAT THE CLINICIAN KNOWS AND WANTS TO KNOW

Let's Start with an Example

Rather than introduce Bayesian analysis using the usual 2 × 2 tables and equations, let us approach the problem by using a typical illustrative clinical scenario:

A 35-year-old woman comes to your clinic complaining of substernal chest pain that occurs with physical exertion. She is concerned about "heart trouble." What diagnostic study should you perform to make the diagnosis of myocardial ischemia? Assume your choices are limited to (a) ECG stress treadmill, (b) thallium stress test, and (c) coronary angiography. Does your test selection change if your patient is a 65-year-old man?

For the purposes of this discussion, let us assume that you would rather not use the relatively invasive angiography test initially; the choice in this hypothetical case is therefore simplified: do we use the ECG treadmill or thallium test? (Let us also avoid potentially complex and confounding utility/economic issues by assuming naively that test cost is not an issue.) We will attempt to address this idealized clinical problem using basic Bayesian analysis.

Prior Probability

Before the selection or evaluation of a specific diagnostic imaging test is considered, it is important to un-

derstand what we are confronted with: a patient with a constellation of historical, physical, and laboratory findings, all of which suggest a tentative clinical diagnosis or differential. This leads to the important Bayesian concept of the *prior,* or *"pretest,"* *probability,* our initial (i.e., *before* the imaging test is performed) assessment of how likely it is that the patient truly has a specific diagnosis.

Many workers use the term *prevalence* interchangeably with *prior probability.* I believe that this is misleading, because the clinician usually has significantly more information than just the disease prevalence (defined as the proportion of the population with the disease at a particular point in time) before an imaging test is considered. However, disease prevalence does play an important role in deriving a reasonable prior probability and should not be ignored (e.g., your attending physician will certainly lose confidence in you if you tell her that the patient you just examined has kuru—unless, of course, the patient is from New Guinea and is gnawing on your leg).

For the purpose of our illustrative example, assume that after taking a thorough history and examining our 35-year-old female patient, we feel that a "reasonable" probability of her truly having myocardial ischemia is about 0.35. After talking to our 65-year-old man (who tells us about his long smoking history), let us assume that we feel that the probability of his having angina is significantly more likely, say 0.70. These values thus represent our prior, or pretest, probabilities.

Now one might ask, "How does one come up with the above prior probability estimates of 0.35 and 0.70?" Don't ask me. Honestly, I don't think a physician can reliably and reproducibly derive a meaningful specific number representing prior probability (or any probability for that matter) for actual patients and/or specific clinical situations. Fortunately, we don't have to come up with actual numeric estimates of probability in order to derive a great deal of benefit from Bayesian analysis; it is sufficient to estimate the 35-year-old woman's risk for myocardial ischemia as pretty low and the 65-year-old man's risk as pretty high. A few medical decision analysis advocates sincerely believe that we should explicitly and quantitatively use Bayesian analysis for each specific patient at the bedside ("Just enter our prior probabilities into our handy palm-top computer, select the test choices from the menu list, and out pops our optimal decision for the diagnostic workup for Mr. Smith and his hemoptysis!"). Although this would be convenient, I believe it would also be foolhardy and an example of "pseudo-rigor." Much like the well-known "garbage-in, garbage-out" situation, decisions derived from these unreliable probability estimates would be highly suspect. I emphasize that the above probability estimates used in our hypothetical example are explicitly stated for illustrative purposes only. As stated in the introduction, I believe that much of the power of Bayesian analysis can be realized from the clinical application of heuristics or rules of thumb learned from an intuitive understanding of the principles involved, rather than from the blind explicit use of its formulas in the clinical setting.

Action Threshold

Normatively, clinicians will institute therapy or other intervention only if they are convinced that the probability of the patient having the disease in question is beyond an "action threshold" probability. In addition, most physicians will not exclude a diagnosis unless the probability is below an "exclusion threshold." These action and exclusion thresholds represent our recognition that in the real world we will never be convinced with absolute certainty that a patient truly has a disease or not, and we should not delay medical action until this unreachable goal of absolute certainty is obtained (Fig. 5-1). In most cases, our patient's prior or pretest probability will lie somewhere between these threshold values. Therefore, we can now state that the purpose of a diagnostic test is to obtain additional information in order to update a patient's prior probability to a *posterior,* or *"posttest,"* probability (also referred to as *positive predictive value*) that is either beyond the action threshold or below the exclusion threshold.

Applying the above principles to our hypothetical example, let us assume that our action threshold is 0.80; in other words, we must be convinced that the probability of our patient truly having myocardial angina is at least 0.80 before we are willing either to begin therapy or subject our patient to more invasive or costly diagnostic procedures. Similarly, assume that our exclusion threshold is 0.05: we must believe that the probability of our patient having angina is less than 0.05 before we reject the diagnosis and reassure our patient.

Figure 5-2 demonstrates that the pretest probabilities for both our young female and older male patients lie between our defined exclusion and action thresholds.

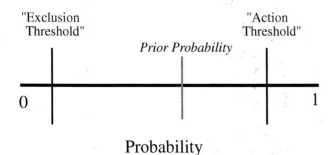

Probability

FIG. 5-1. The goal of the diagnostic test is to update the prior or "pretest" probability above or below the "action" or "exclusion" threshold, respectively. This updated "posttest" probability represents the posterior probability.

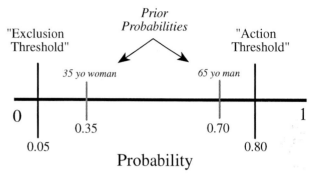

Probability

FIG. 5-2. Assumed "action" (0.80) and "exclusion" (0.05) thresholds for hypothetical example discussed in text. Prior or "pretest" probability for myocardial ischemia is significantly lower for a 35-year-old woman (0.35) than for a 65-year-old man (0.70).

Thus, we are as yet undecided about the etiology of their chest pain. We therefore need to obtain more information in order to make further clinical decisions. In Bayesian terms, our task becomes clearer: we wish to select an appropriate diagnostic test that will move our posttest probabilities beyond either the exclusion or the action threshold.

It is important to determine whether or not the clinician truly has an action and/or exclusion threshold before a test is performed; if no threshold exists, the rationality of performing any test must be questioned (e.g., the frequently encountered scenario where the results of a requested imaging test will not alter a clinician's decision to institute therapy). Similarly, if our prior probability is already beyond either the action or the exclusion threshold, the usefulness of performing any additional confirmatory tests must be questioned (e.g., if you have already decided to treat a child's sore throat with antibiotics, think twice before you order a strep culture).

This principle applies primarily to tests used for diagnosis. There are, of course, other valid indications for performing imaging tests that are not strictly for diagnostic purposes, such as providing anatomic information for surgical planning, tumor staging, evaluating treatment response, and so on.

EVALUATING TEST PERFORMANCE: HOW GOOD IS THE IMAGING TEST?

After determining the prior probability and the action and exclusion threshold values, the clinician is ready to select an appropriate diagnostic imaging test that will hopefully provide enough quality information to move the patient's prior probability to a posttest probability that is beyond either the action or the exclusion threshold. An important consideration in the selection of a test is its ability to discriminate between those who have the disease in question and those who do not. The characterization of the test's discriminating performance involves principles derived from Bayesian analysis.

The Gold Standard

The published performance of any diagnostic test (the ability of the test to distinguish between patients with and without disease) is always relative to an independent gold standard that determines who truly has the disease and who does not. This gold standard may represent pathologic and/or surgical correlation; occasionally, it may correspond to the results of another diagnostic test (i.e., pulmonary angiography for pulmonary embolism or contrast venography for deep venous thrombosis). Despite its label, the gold standard is frequently imperfect and subject to both false-positive and false-negative results. In addition, one gold standard may be replaced by another as a result of improved technology, surgical or laboratory advances, etc. Despite its imperfection, for the purposes of Bayesian analysis, the gold standard is considered to be perfect, with no false-positive or false-negative results assumed. The important point to understand is that all published test performance values are always relative to some explicitly or implicitly defined (hopefully independent) gold standard. Because the vast majority of gold standards in medicine are imperfect, published test performance values will usually overestimate the performance of diagnostic tests in the real world (where the only relevant gold standard is the actual patient outcome).

Discriminant Criteria

The criteria a diagnostic test uses to differentiate between normal and abnormal are known as discriminant criteria. Discriminant criteria are defined specific to the diagnostic test. For example, the discriminant criterion for an abnormal white cell count in the context of infection would be a specific numeric value (let's say 10,000) representing the number of white blood cells per unit volume. Discriminant criteria for the diagnosis of a malignant liver mass by computed tomography (CT) would include the size/configuration of the lesion, attenuation, contrast enhancement characteristics, etc. The experimental evaluation of test performance involves performing the test on a population (ideally in a prospective manner) and using the discriminant criterion with the classification of those with and without the disease defined independently by the gold standard (Fig. 5-3).

Positivity Criterion

Unfortunately, an overlap almost always exists between those with the disease and those without when

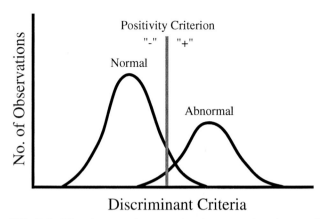

FIG. 5-3. The degree of separation between the abnormal and normal populations when a specific discriminant criterion is used determines the discriminating ability of the test. The selected positivity criterion defines a positive or negative test.

the defined discriminant criterion is used (Fig. 5-3). This is the major reason why tests are imperfect in the real world. (Actually, for most of you this is a fortunate reality because if there were no overlap between normal and abnormal patients using diagnostic tests, all diagnostic tests would be perfect and there would be no need for physicians, only technologists.) Accordingly, a threshold or "positivity" criterion is almost always selected according to which an individual is to be considered positive or negative by the test standards (Fig. 5-3).

I actually believe that this need of ours for a positivity criterion is unfortunate. This "line of death in the sand" that determines whether a test is positive or negative greatly oversimplifies the information derived from a diagnostic test. Sometimes I think it would be more instructive (and intellectually honest) if we could report test results by showing the degree of overlap between normal and abnormal distributions when using our particular diagnostic test and indicating where our particular patient's value is located relative to those two distributions. In fact, this is what many radiologists are attempting to do when they describe the findings of a particularly difficult study to a clinician. For example, suppose I am confronted with an abdominal CT examination of a patient with colon carcinoma and I see a number of equivocally enlarged lymph nodes in the retroperitoneum. Now I know that the surgeon wants to know if these nodes have tumor in them. But I also know that with CT there is a lot of overlap between normal (noncancerous) retroperitoneal lymph nodes and abnormal (cancerous) lymph nodes. What I would like to do is talk to the surgeon and, by my description of the findings, paint for him or her the overlap that exists between normal and abnormal lymph nodes by CT criteria, and then tell him or her where I think our patient is located relative to these two normal/abnormal

Sensitivity = True-Positive Rate (TPR)

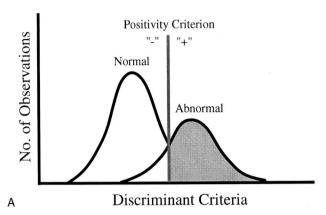

Specificity = 1 - False-Positive Rate (FPR)

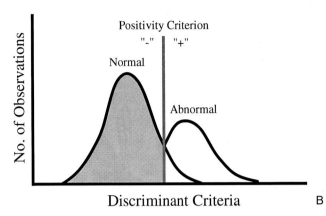

FIG. 5-4. The discriminating ability of a test using the defined discriminant and positivity criteria is characterized by the sensitivity **(A)** and the specificity **(B)**.

distributions. Unfortunately, long before I get done with my discussion, many surgeons will interrupt me by saying, "Come on, stop hedging. IS THE TEST POSITIVE OR NEGATIVE?!" This is why we need Bayes' theorem and why my hair is graying.

Sensitivity and Specificity

The discriminating power of the imaging test is characterized by the degree of overlap between the diseased and disease-free populations present when the defined discriminant and positivity criteria are used. This discriminating power can be described by the sensitivity and specificity of the test. Sensitivity is defined as the true-positive rate, the proportion of those with the disease (as defined by our imperfect independent gold standard) who test positive when the defined discriminant criteria and positivity criteria are used (Fig. 5-4A). In a similar fashion, specificity is defined as the proportion of those without disease whom we call negative (Fig. 5-4B). (Specificity can be seen to be equal to (1 minus the false-positive rate), where the false-positive rate is defined as the proportion of those without the disease whom we incorrectly call positive.)

Note the following pitfalls:

1. It is critical to realize that a test with high sensitivity does not necessarily have the capability of detecting the earliest or first manifestation of disease. High sensitivity merely means that the test is capable of correctly identifying as positive a high proportion of all patients who truly have the disease (of any stage, degree, etc.) as determined by some independent (and usually imperfect) gold standard. Unfortunately, many clinicians have the incorrect belief that high test sensitivity means high sensitivity to detect subtle or early stages of a disease.

2. It is equally important to understand that high specificity does *not* mean that a test can come up with a specific tissue (histologic) diagnosis. High specificity simply means that a test will usually correctly identify those patients who are truly normal (again by our infamous gold standard) as negative. A test with high specificity cannot, for example, tell you if a kidney mass is a cancer, an abscess, or a benign cyst. You would be surprised by the number of clinicians who have this incorrect impression.

For the purpose of our illustrative example, let us use the "reasonable" hypothetical test performance characteristic values (sensitivity and specificity) summarized in Table 5-1. Since most physicians consider coronary angiography to be the reference by which other tests are measured, angiography is defined as the gold standard. Accordingly, the sensitivity and specificity of angiography is considered to be by definition perfect (even though you and I know that that is not true). Table 5-1 also shows that the Thallium test demonstrates both superior sensitivity and specificity performance compared to the ECG stress test.

Now that we have defined our clinical problem in terms of action/exclusion thresholds and prior probabilities and have some idea of test performance, how do we use this information to select an appropriate test?

TABLE 5-1. *Test performance characteristics: (hypothetical values)*

Feature	Sensitivity	Specificity
ECG stress	0.67	0.63
Thallium	0.85	0.90
Angiogram (gold standard)	"1"	"1"

BAYES' THEOREM

Bayes' theorem models the performance of a diagnostic test as it relates to a specific clinical application by incorporating not only the discriminating power of the diagnostic test (as measured by sensitivity and specificity) but also the prior or pretest probability to derive the posterior or posttest probability. The formula for Bayes' theorem may or may not be a familiar one (Fig. 5-5); unfortunately, it is easily forgotten or blindly applied without truly understanding its underlying meaning. I do not believe that it is important to memorize this formula; it can always be looked up as needed (if ever). What is absolutely crucial to remember from Bayes' theorem is that the prior probability (or pretest clinical assessment) plays as important a role as the sensitivity and specificity of the diagnostic test in the determination of the posterior probability (the probability that the patient with a positive test truly has the disease).

The foregoing statement can be demonstrated by the use of dreary contingency tables and mathematical formulas; however, a more intuitive understanding of this principle can be achieved by a simple illustration:

Suppose a 19-year-old woman comes to the gynecology clinic worried that she might have syphilis. Assume the sensitivity of the Venereal Disease Research Laboratory (VDRL) is 0.95 and the specificity is 0.90. A VDRL is performed and is positive. What is the probability that this patient truly has syphilis?

How about it? How likely do you think it is that this patient has syphilis? An informal survey of physicians at our institution revealed that most clinicians believed the probability that this hypothetical patient had syphilis would be relatively high, say about 0.75–0.80. (After all, the sensitivity and specificity of that VDRL test looks pretty good. In fact, the sensitivity and specificity of this particular hypothetical VDRL is better than the vast majority of diagnostic tests that you will ever order!) Now consider the following additional history:

History, Take One: The woman has a past history of multiple episodes of pelvic inflammatory disease and is an IV drug abuser.

Bayes' Theorem:

$$P[D|T+] = \frac{(\text{TPR} * \text{Prior Probability})}{(\text{TPR} * \text{Prior Probability}) + [\text{FPR} * (1 - \text{Prior Probability})]}$$

FIG. 5-5. Bayes' theorem shows how the posterior probability (P[D|T+] represents the probability of having the disease if the test is positive) is a function not only of the test efficacy (as defined by the sensitivity and specificity) but also the prior probability. TPR, true-positive rate or sensitivity; FPR, false-positive rate or (1 − specificity).

Now, does that change your estimate of the likelihood that she has syphilis? Given this information, most physicians raised the probability to around 0.90–0.99. ("Yup. History, test result, everything fits.") But wait, hold on, the above bit of history was incorrect. . . . Sorry. Here's the correct history for your patient:

History, Take Two: The woman is a virgin studying to be a nun and is afraid that she might have caught syphilis by thinking "impure, immoral thoughts."

Well, do you still think your patient has syphilis? Are you ready to treat a nun for syphilis? (Hey, weren't you the medical student who thought that other patient had kuru?) Indeed, with this alternative history, all physicians surveyed dramatically lowered their estimate to less than 0.10. The important observation is that in both scenarios the performance characteristics of the test (as described by the sensitivity and specificity) did not change, nor did the test result; it was only the prior probability that changed. Clearly, the posterior probability (the probability that the patient with a positive test truly has the disease) is dependent not only on test efficacy but, to a high degree, on the prior probability. And what is prior probability in the clinical context? It is derived from such important but frequently undervalued activities as getting a full, careful history and physical examination. Only through such a solid foundation can the clinician get the best pretest assessment of how likely it is that the patient has the disease. And it is only with a reasoned, accurate pretest assessment (prior probability) that one can interpret the result of any diagnostic test.

I view Bayes' theorem as the formalization of the often heard maxim "Treat the patient, not the film." If you don't like that one, try this: "the nun with syphilis." I promise you that if you remember either statement, you will find it easier to understand Bayes' theorem than by memorizing a formula. Both statements emphasize the same critical fact: how you interpret (or trust) a test result has just as must to do with your own clinical assessment (does it make sense clinically?) as with test performance (sensitivity and specificity). In other words, don't be overly seduced by diagnostic tests (even pretty radiologic ones) or their results; your clinical assessment/judgment is just as important when it comes to determining the truth.

Here's another way to think of Bayes' theorem: it is the codification of the scientific method applied to clinical medicine. What is the scientific method? Simply put, it defines a process by which truth is sought using an iterative process of hypothesis formation, testing of the hypothesis, and reevaluation of the hypothesis. In the context of Bayes' theorem and clinical decision making, the hypothesis is our prior probability (or differential diagnosis). We generate our hypothesis by performing a careful history and physical to derive a prioritized differential diagnosis. We then test our hypothesis by performing diagnostic tests and reevaluate our differential diagnosis on the basis of the test results. The important point is that there must be first an underlying hypothesis (prior probability, differential diagnosis) before diagnostic tests are performed. Contrast this ideal behavior with what is unfortunately a frequent occurrence in the hospital: ordering expensive diagnostic tests before the patient is even examined, ordering q-am (each morning) test batteries that do not really directly address an underlying hypothesis, and so forth. Bayes' theorem shows us that this behavior is not only wasteful but irrational.

But What About Our Two Patients with Chest Pain?

Table 5-2 summarizes the resulting posterior or posttest probabilities after our hypothetical prior probability values along with test performance characteristics (as defined by test sensitivity and specificity) are incorporated into Bayes' theorem. Figure 5-6 is a graphic representation. It is interesting to note that, for our female patient, while a positive thallium test does move the posterior probability beyond our defined action threshold, a positive ECG stress test does not. Bayesian analysis clearly shows why this is: the prior probability of myocardial angina in the young woman is relatively low; the relatively poor performance characteristics of the ECG stress test are not adequate to "push" the posterior probability from this "low" pretest value to beyond the action threshold. In contrast, the relatively high performance characteristics of the thallium test can move us beyond the threshold. Therefore, our analysis suggests that we should order the thallium test for our female patient, skipping the ECG stress test entirely. The higher prior probability of angina in our older male patient is already "high enough" for even a positive ECG stress test to move the posterior probability beyond the action threshold. We therefore would be able to make the diagnosis of myocardial angina using the simpler ECG stress test in our older male patient. This example again shows that ultimate utility derived from a diagnostic test is a function of both test performance and the patient's prior probability.

I do not want to give the reader the impression that the ECG stress test has no role in the diagnostic workup of a 35-year-old woman with chest pain. A similar process can be used to determine whether or not a negative

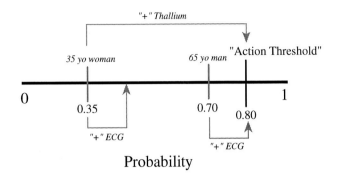

Probability

FIG. 5-6. Calculated posterior ("posttest") probabilities (also known as positive predictive values) for hypothetical example. A positive ECG stress test is not sufficient to move the posterior probability for myocardial ischemia in a 35-year-old woman beyond the action threshold. However, a positive thallium test will result in a posterior probability beyond this threshold. In contrast, a positive ECG test alone is sufficient in a 65-year-old man.

test will move our posttest probability below our exclusion threshold. In the proper clinical context (such as a patient with a relatively low prior probability and a physician more interested in excluding the diagnosis of ischemia), a negative ECG stress test may result in a posttest probability below the exclusion threshold and be quite valuable. The important point is that Bayesian analysis can be used to rationally select the appropriate test given any clinical context.

Our hypothetical example thus demonstrates how the selection of an appropriate diagnostic test depends not only on the performance characteristic of the test (as defined by sensitivity and specificity), but also to a very high degree on the prior probability of disease. Depending on the pretest probability, one may need a test with high sensitivity and/or specificity performance; alternatively, one may be able to "get away with" a test with relatively poorer performance (which is usually cheaper, simpler, or less invasive). Bayes' theorem enables us to approach test selection in an optimal manner that can be analyzed before any test is ordered, thus maximizing test utilization efficiency. Again, I do not believe that it is necessary to do the math and explicitly calculate positive predictive values from Bayes' theorem using numeric estimates of prior probability. It is enough to understand in a general way the importance of prior probability in the final determination of the positive predictive value. For example, if there is a lot of distance between your nonquantitative estimate of your patient's prior probability (pretty low) and the action threshold (which you estimate as pretty high), you will need to use a diagnostic test that has high performance (high sensitivity and specificity) in order to move your patient s positive predictive value beyond the action threshold (just like our 35-year-old woman with chest pain). However, if you estimate that the dis-

TABLE 5-2. *Posterior probabilities: hypothetical example*

	+ ECG	+ Thallium
Woman, 35 yo	0.48	0.81
Man, 65 yo	0.81	0.95

tance between your patient's prior probability and the action threshold is small, you might get away with a test (possibly less expensive or invasive) with less than great performance characteristics.

FLUIDITY OF THE POSITIVITY CRITERION: THE ROC CURVE

Now that we have a better understanding of how diagnostic tests work, let's take a closer look at what we mean by test performance. Specifically, I want to address that pesky positivity criterion again. As I stated before, I've never liked the fact that we are forced to interpret tests as either positive or negative: it is the presence of the positivity criterion that is to blame. You now know that test sensitivity and specificity is defined largely by the location of this positivity criterion (see Fig. 5-4). So where should the positivity criterion be placed? An examination of Fig. 5-7A and B demonstrates that the observed test sensitivity and specificity can be changed by moving the positivity criterion. It is very important to understand how test sensitivity and specificity change when the positivity criterion is moved.

Figure 5-7A shows that by moving the positivity criterion as shown we can maximally increase the sensitivity of our test. Unfortunately, there is no free lunch; by moving the positivity criterion to maximize sensitivity, specificity drops. Figure 5-7B shows that the same reciprocal relationship exists when moving the positivity criterion to maximize specificity; sensitivity suffers. It is important to observe that this change in test sensitivity and specificity as a function of the positivity criterion does not alter the intrinsic discriminating power of the examination (the degree of overlap between diseased and undiseased populations).

What does this mean? Well, for one thing, it means that there is no such thing as single sensitivity and specificity values for a particular diagnostic test. In reality, there are an infinite number of possible sensitivity and specificity values that one can observe for a diagnostic test; all you need to do is move the positivity criterion. Accordingly, a wide variation may be observed in test sensitivity and specificity corresponding to identical discriminant criteria and test efficacy. This sometimes makes the interpretation of published test performance expressed in terms of sensitivity and specificity alone

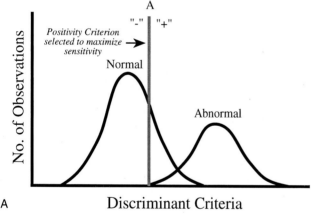

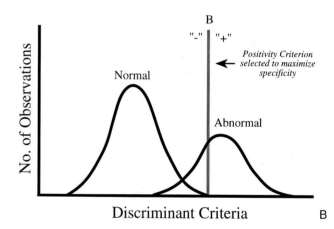

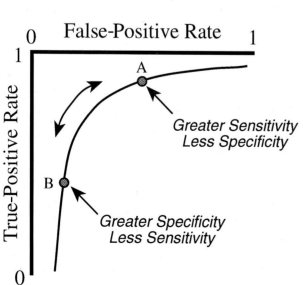

FIG. 5-7. Moving the positivity criterion can optimize either sensitivity **(A)** or specificity **(B)**. The reciprocal relationship between sensitivity and specificity as a function of changing the positivity criterion can be expressed by the receiver operating characteristic (ROC) curve **(C)**.

difficult and misleading. Clearly, citing single values for sensitivity and specificity does not adequately describe the intrinsic discriminating power of a test subject to variation in the positivity criterion. This should make you feel a little uneasy about published test sensitivity and specificity values.

The reciprocal relationship between sensitivity and specificity as a function of varying the positivity criterion can be represented more effectively by the use of the receiver operating characteristic (ROC) curve (Fig. 5-7C). This curve is a more meaningful representation of the intrinsic discriminating power of a given test and enables the direct comparison of the relative performance of different tests, especially when these tests are subject to variation in the positivity criteria (Fig. 5-8). ROC curves aren't very mysterious or complicated; they are simply plots of all of the possible true-positive (sensitivity) and false-positive rate (1 − specificity) values that one can observe as the positivity

criterion is moved. Space does not permit a discussion of the power and elegance of ROC analysis; the interested reader is directed to the excellent review by Metz (1).

The selection of the positivity criterion can, and should, be quite fluid and specific to the application, especially when the test interpretation is subjective and observer-dependent. Now that we now understand that observed test sensitivity and specificity is a function of positivity criterion placement, we can now optimally position the positivity criterion (move to an optimal position on the ROC curve) to achieve the desired test sensitivity (at the expense of specificity, of course) or specificity (at the expense of sensitivity). This can be demonstrated in any radiology department. A vague, somewhat "nodular" opacity on a chest film can be interpreted either as "worrisome for metastasis, suggest aggressive workup" (in the case of a patient with known malignancy), or as "the probable confluence of normal vascular and osseous structures" (in the case of

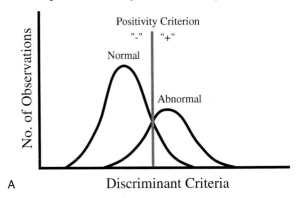

Test "A" :
More Overlap Between Normal and Abnormal
Populations = Inferior Test Performance

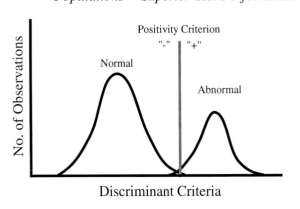

Test "B" :
Less Overlap Between Normal and Abnormal
Populations = Superior Test Performance

FIG. 5-8. Intrinsic test performance is directly related to the overlap between normal and abnormal populations. Tests with a great deal of overlap **(A)** will have inferior performance relative to tests with less overlap **(B)** irrespective of positivity criterion placement. The receiver operating characteristic (ROC) curve **(C)** is a good way to demonstrate the relative performance of diagnostic tests: the superior test ROC curve can be seen to be closer to the upper left-hand corner of the graph.

TABLE 5-3. *Selecting appropriate test performance guidelines*

- As **prior probability** *decreases,* maximize *specificity*
- As **prior probability** *increases,* maximize *sensitivity*
- As adverse consequences of missing the disease **increase,** maximize *sensitivity*
- As adverse consequences of false positives **increase,** maximize *specificity*

the "routine" preemployment chest film). This familiar example represents the shifting of the positivity criterion toward improved sensitivity (in the first patient) or specificity (in the second patient).

The foregoing discussion emphasizes the importance for accurate and thorough clinical information from the referring physician before imaging tests are selected and performed. Without adequate clinical history, the radiologist does not know where to optimally place the positivity threshold, which can result in unacceptably high false-negative or false-positive interpretations. Thorough clinical information also enables the radiologist to help the clinician select an appropriate imaging test: knowledge of the prior probability and the action/exclusion thresholds can be used with Bayes' theorem to select a test with appropriate sensitivity/specificity characteristics (2).

SELECTION OF OPTIMAL DIAGNOSTIC TEST CHARACTERISTICS

The above principles can be extended to provide guidelines with respect to the optimal selection of diagnostic test characteristics given a specific clinical problem. These guidelines are summarized in Table 5-3. The formal derivation and proof of these guidelines are beyond the scope of this introductory paper; interested readers are directed to Weinstein's text (3).

SUMMARY

This brief introduction to how diagnostic tests work in the context of medical decision making is necessarily superficial. However, even these basic concepts can help us significantly when we need to rationally select and interpret diagnostic tests and their results for a specific clinical situation. Of course, the optimal selection of diagnostic tests frequently must take into account other considerations in addition to the Bayesian concepts of prior probability and sensitivity/specificity values. Test cost, availability, degree of invasiveness, morbidity, and other issues should also be incorporated. These latter parameters, although not directly addressed by classic Bayesian analysis, can also be modeled using a variety of decision analytic tools, such as decision tree analysis, cost–benefit analysis, dynamic probabilistic analysis, etc. (3). Indeed, it is hoped that this brief discussion of diagnostic test performance will serve as an introduction to the general field of medical decision analysis and will tempt some readers to explore further.

Before we get to the pretty pictures, I want to emphasize that the above comments are applicable to all types of diagnostic tests, not just radiographic ones. I would like to finish this chapter by making a few comments concerning radiographic imaging tests in particular:

Radiographic tests are usually much better at detecting *structural* abnormalities than *functional* abnormalities. Radiologists usually need to see the abnormality in order to make the diagnosis. Accordingly, we do best when the disease process manifests itself by some morphologic change (mass lesion, contour deformity, opacity, etc.). It is important to realize that many important disease processes do not manifest structural, morphologic, or anatomic changes; radiographic studies of patients with these diseases will frequently be negative. Important exceptions to the above statement include nuclear medicine, positron emission tomography, and some advanced magnetic resonance examinations; these tests can sometimes give very useful functional, physiologic information.

The majority of radiographic tests cannot give specific histologic diagnoses. For example, many times a mass seen on an image is just that: a mass. Frequently, we will not be able to tell you whether that mass is a neoplasm, an abscess, or even a congenital anomaly. Similarly, an area of lung parenchymal opacity may represent pneumonia, blood, pulmonary edema, or even cancer. This is where your refined clinical assessment (prior probability) comes in, saves the day, and helps to generate a prioritized differential diagnosis.

The interpretation of radiographic tests is almost always subjective. This means that we are constantly shifting the positivity criterion around, hopefully to optimize sensitivity or specificity. What this also means is that you must give the radiologist enough clinical history (prior probability) in order for him or her to rationally place the positivity criterion. At least be legible when you fill out those radiology requisition forms!

Improved test performance usually is associated with increased cost and/or risks. In the context of increasing external and economic constraints, this is becoming an important consideration. As shown earlier, Bayes' theorem can sometimes help pick the most appropriate (and possibly most cost-effective) test.

Try to keep these principles in mind while studying the images and commentary herein; they have been carefully assembled to show normal and abnormal anatomy in the clearest possible fashion. This clarity is not a luxury with which you will be blessed at all times and in all places.

REFERENCES

1. Metz CE. Basic principles of ROC analysis. *Semin Nucl Med* 1978;8:283–298.

2. Doubilet P. A mathematical approach to interpretation and selection of diagnostic tests. *Med Decis Making* 1983;3:177–195.
3. Weinstein MC, Fineberg HV, et al. *Clinical Decision Analysis.* Philadelphia: WB Saunders, 1980.

SECTION II

Diagnostic Radiology

CHAPTER 6

Chest

William E. Erkonen

Patients often complain of chest problems, and their symptoms might include shortness of breath, pain, cough, and hemoptysis or bloody sputum. The workup or investigation of these symptoms usually begins with a chest radiograph, so that it is not surprising that the chest radiograph has become the most common imaging consultation requested by clinicians. The main purpose of this chapter is to demonstrate a simple way to approach chest radiographs.

TECHNIQUE

Fortunately, the amount of radiation required for a routine chest examination is extremely small and not a threat to the patient. The chest radiographic examination is usually accomplished in a radiology department, and a routine study consists of posteroanterior (PA) and lateral views. When the patient is unable to tolerate these routine views, a portable anteroposterior (AP) view is obtained with the patient either standing, sitting, or supine. PA and lateral radiographs should be re-

quested whenever possible because they are less expensive and give far more information than a portable study. Illustrations for these radiographic techniques have been previously demonstrated in Chapter 1 (Figs. 1-1 to 1-4).

Chest radiographs should not be requested to evaluate suspected problems in the ribs, shoulders, or the dorsal spine. When bone disease is suspected, the specific bone radiographs should be requested.

HOW TO VIEW THE PA AND AP
CHEST RADIOGRAPH

Step 1 is to place the radiograph correctly on the viewbox, and the ability to do this is an immediate confidence builder. There is nothing more pathetic, yet humorous, than watching somebody pontificate before a radiograph that is upside down or reversed side to side on the viewbox. *A significant part of the art and practice of medicine is just learning the jargon, lingo, routines, and rituals.*

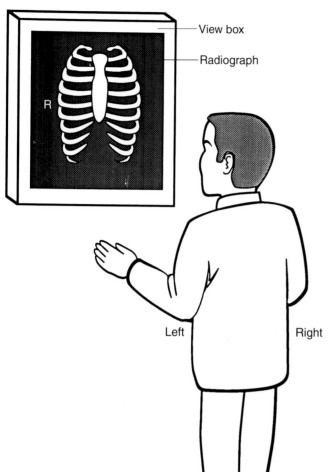

FIG. 6-1. The correct positioning of a chest radiograph on a viewbox. The patient's right side on the film should always be opposite the viewer's left side.

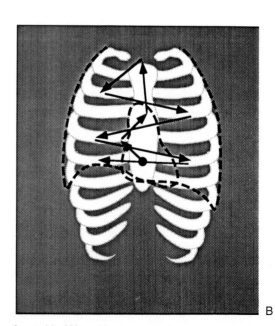

$$\frac{(AB)}{CD} = \text{Cardiothoracic}$$

FIG. 6-3. Method for determining the cardiothoracic ratio.

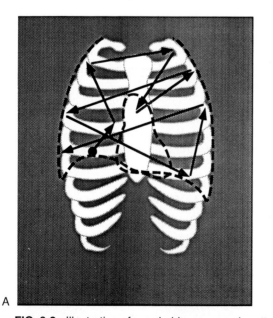

FIG. 6-2. Illustration of a probable eye search pattern of a rookie (A) and by someone with a systematic approach (B) to a radiograph. Note that the rookie's search pattern is highly disorganized.

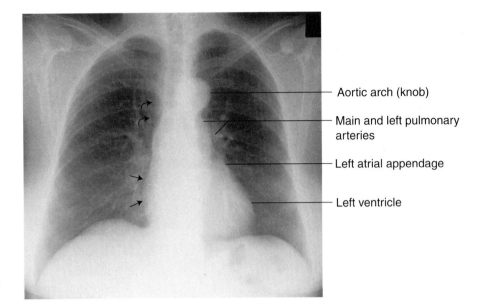

FIG. 6-4. Chest posteroanterior (PA) radiograph. Normal. The convex right cardiac border is formed by the right atrium (*straight arrows*), and the curved arrows indicate the location of the superior vena cava. The left cardiac and great vessels border might be considered as four skiing moguls. From cephalad to caudad the moguls are the aortic arch, the main and left pulmonary arteries, the left atrial appendage, and the left ventricle.

Aortic arch (knob)

Main and left pulmonary arteries

Left atrial appendage

Left ventricle

Obviously, the R and L markers on the film indicate the patient's right and left side, respectively. Position the radiograph on the viewbox with the R film marker opposite your left side and the L film marker opposite your right side (Fig. 6-1). This routine applies to all AP and PA chest radiographs as well as nearly all other radiographs and images. Of course, the patient's head should be oriented to the top of the radiograph.

Step 2 is to approach and evaluate the radiograph by casually glancing at the entire image for any obvious abnormality that might jump out at you, such as a huge heart or a baseball-sized lung mass. *Remember to always look at all four corners of the image.*

Step 3 is to evaluate the radiograph systematically. Unfortunately, there is no single generally accepted or standardized system for evaluating a chest radiograph, so develop your own comfortable system. After all, even a veteran commercial pilot will use a checklist just prior to take-off. The list might consist of such things as flaps down, brakes on, and check the fuel gauges. The pilot checklist is necessary, as it is virtually impossible to remember everything when preparing for takeoff. Similarly, a mental checklist or system is needed to review a chest radiograph. So program your internal computer with a *systematic checklist* to avoid overlooking important areas or structures, as many of the errors made in medicine are errors of omission. The following suggested system can be used for a lifetime or until you develop your own system.

The arrows in Fig. 6-2A roughly approximate the haphazard visual pathway of a rookie viewing a chest radiograph. If you persist with this rookie approach, errors of omission are inevitable! The arrows in Fig. 6-2B demonstrate how someone with a system might approach a chest radiograph. On the other hand, a highly experienced radiologist generally views a radio-

graph in a more circumferential and peripheral manner.

After a general once-over glance at the entire image, use the water density cardiac silhouette as your starting point. First, determine the cardiac size. The transverse diameter of the cardiac silhouette should not exceed 50% of the transverse diameter of the thoracic cage measured or estimated at the same level. This is called the *cardiothoracic ratio* (Fig. 6-3). The exception to the cardiothoracic ratio is that the cardiac silhouette will appear larger on an AP view than on a PA view on the same patient. Because the heart is an anterior thoracic structure, it lies farther from the radiographic film on an AP radiograph than on a PA. Consequently the heart casts a larger shadow on the AP view than on the PA. *The greater the distance between an anatomic structure and the radiographic film, the more the magnification.* Also, when the patient's inspiration is poor, the diaphragms will be elevated, causing the heart to appear larger than it is.

Cardiac contour and size are best evaluated by gross eyeballing, and generally a ruler is not needed. When you are waiting at the bus stop, you can instantly determine if a passerby is obese, tall, short, or acting strangely. Your visual-cerebral computer automatically concludes these facts based on prior experiences. After you have viewed many more chest radiographs, your evaluations of cardiac size and shape will become easier.

Next evaluate the cardiac shape. What actually determines the cardiac shape? The convex right cardiac border is formed by the water density right atrium, and just cephalad or superior to the right atrium is the straight-bordered superior vena cava. The cardiac apex is formed primarily by the left ventricle, and the left atrium contributes to the superior left cardiac border (Fig. 6-4). The right ventricle is superimposed on the left ventricle and

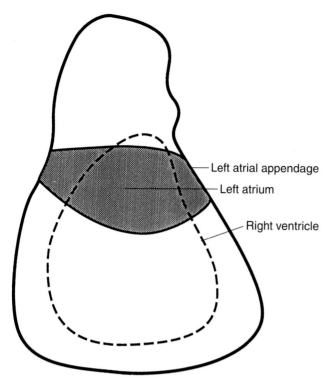

FIG. 6-5. The approximate location of the left atrium and right ventricle on a normal PA or AP chest radiograph. These cardiac chambers cannot be delineated on normal studies. However, the left atrial appendage can occasionally be seen in normal hearts.

is not visualized as such on normal PA or AP radiographs. Also, a normal left atrium is not visible on the PA or AP radiograph (Fig. 6-5). As the left ventricle enlarges, the cardiac apex moves to the patient's left. As the right atrium enlarges, the cardiac silhouette enlarges to the patient's right (Fig. 6-6).

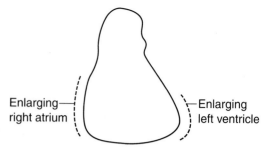

FIG. 6-6. Cardiac silhouette changes during right atrium and left ventricle enlargement. As the right atrium enlarges, the convex right heart border enlarges to the patient's right. As the left ventricle enlarges, the cardiac apex moves to the patient's left and downward.

Next your visual pathway takes you to the aortic arch, pulmonary arteries, and the main stem bronchi. The left and right pulmonary arteries and the main stem bronchi form the hilar shadows (Fig. 6-7). On normal chest radiographs the left hilum is more cephalad than the right hilum approximately 70% of the time, and the hila will be at the same level 30% of the time. The normal right hilum is rarely cephalad to the left hilum. The *aortopulmonary window* is the air density space between the water density aortic arch knob and the water density left pulmonary artery (Fig. 6-7). When the aortopulmonary window fills in with a water density, you should be suspicious of a mass occupying this space such as a primary or secondary neoplasm. The water density pulmonary arteries and their branches emanate outward from the hila. The main pulmonary artery segment tends to be more prominent in the young and athletic, especially in females, and this prominence usually disappears with age. It is important to remember that in the elderly patient the aorta becomes tortuous, and this can be seen

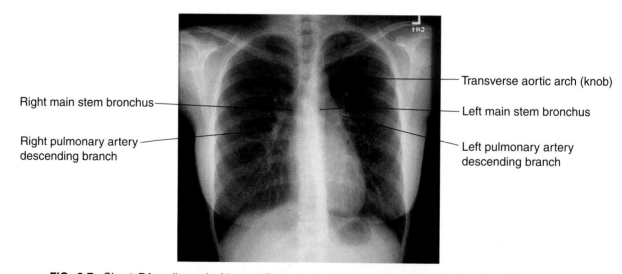

FIG. 6-7. Chest PA radiograph. Normal. The air density aortopulmonary window *(straight arrow)* is situated between the water density aortic arch knob and the superior aspect of the water density left pulmonary artery. It is important to note that the air-filled main stem bronchi appear black, whereas the blood-filled pulmonary arteries appear white. See Table 1-1 in Chapter 1.

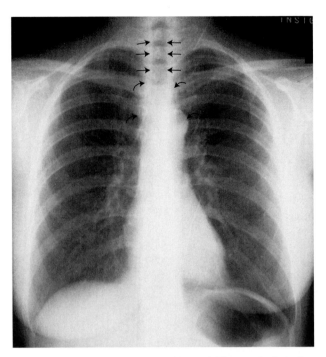

FIG. 6-8. Chest PA radiograph. Normal. The vertical air density trachea *(straight arrows)* should always be midline. The narrow mediastinum is water density *(curved arrows).*

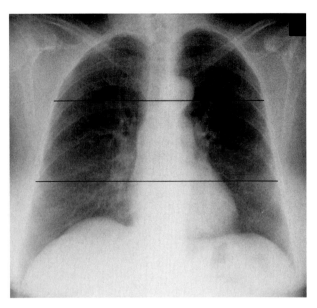

FIG. 6-9. Chest PA radiograph. Normal. Divide the PA or AP chest radiograph into horizontal thirds and compare the right and left lung fields moving in a head-to-foot direction. Note the aortopulmonary window *(straight arrow).*

on frontal as well as lateral views. On frontal views a tortuous aorta often over rides or obliterates the superior vena cava.

Now your gaze should be directed to the water density mediastinum and evaluate it for widening, and again this is based on experience. Most of the mediastinum water density is caused by the great vessels or the vascular pedicle. The vascular pedicle

entends from the thoracic inlet cephalad to the base of the heart caudally. The right border of the pedicle is the superior vena cava and the left border is the aortic knob near the origin of the subclavian artery. The air density or black trachea should be in the midline (Fig. 6-8). Now divide the lungs into horizontal thirds and compare the right and left lung fields (Fig. 6-9). Evaluate the domed curvilinear diaphragms, the costophrenic angles, and the gastric air bubble (Fig. 6-10).

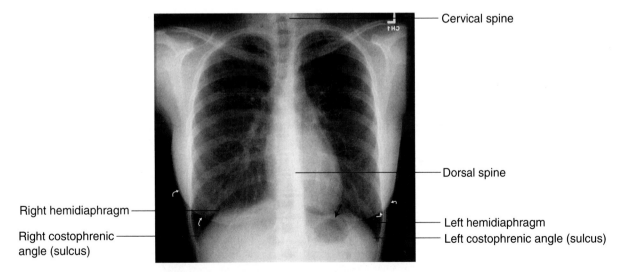

Cervical spine

Dorsal spine

Right hemidiaphragm

Right costophrenic angle (sulcus)

Left hemidiaphragm
Left costophrenic angle (sulcus)

FIG. 6-10. Chest PA radiograph. Normal. After comparing the lung fields, you next view the diaphragms, costophrenic angles, and lower dorsal spine. Note the close proximity of the gastric fundus air to the left hemidiaphragm *(arrow).* Always remember to identify the breast shadows in female patients *(curved arrows).*

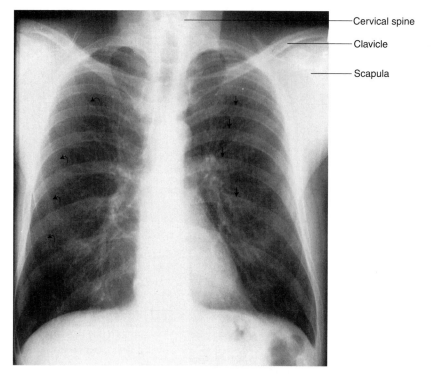

Cervical spine

Clavicle

Scapula

FIG. 6-11. Chest PA radiograph. Normal. The posterior ribs *(straight arrows)* are horizontal and anterior ribs *(curved arrows)* are angled caudad or inferiorly. All of these osseous structures must be included in your checklist as well as the shoulder girdles, cervical and dorsal spine areas.

Next, examine the visible bones such as the cervical spine, dorsal spine, clavicles, shoulders, and ribs (Figs. 6-10 and 6-11). Ribs are tough to evaluate, so you need to visually trace each one or use your fingertip. On a PA radiograph the horizontal portions of the ribs are the posterior arcs, and the anterior ribs are usually angled downward (see Fig. 6-11). As always, you should compare the right and left sides. The amount of cervical and dorsal spine visible on a radiograph is variable.

HOW TO VIEW THE LATERAL CHEST RADIOGRAPH

Now position the lateral chest radiograph on the view-box with the patient's head oriented to the top of the film. There is no hard and fast rule about the direction that the patient should be facing, but we commonly have the patient facing to the viewer's left (Fig. 6-12). Once again, begin the radiograph evaluation by casually viewing the entire image so that something obvious can jump out at you. As on PA and AP radiographs, begin by estimating the size and shape of the anteriorly located heart. The right ventricle forms the anterior border of the cardiac silhouette. The left ventricle forms the major portion of the inferior-posterior cardiac border, and the left atrium forms the superior-posterior cardiac border

(see Fig. 6-12). On the majority of lateral chest radiographs the inferior vena cava *(straight arrows)* can be seen as it enters the right atrium posteriorly and inferiorly (Fig. 6-12). The left ventricle is considered enlarged if it is more than 2 cm posterior to the inferior vena cava. The right atrium is not visualized as such on the lateral view.

Now look at the hilar structures and the trachea (Fig. 6-13). Then observe the sternum and search the retrosternal and retrocardiac spaces for abnormal or pathologic water and air densities (Fig. 6-14). On the lateral view, the retrosternal lungs are primarily the upper lobes, whereas the right middle lobe and the lingular segments of the left upper lobe project over the cardiac silhouette. The lower lobes are located in the retrocardiac space (Fig. 6-14B). It is important to understand these pulmonary lobe spatial relationships to assist in locating pulmonary pathologic processes that usually are water density.

Finally, observe the contours of the diaphragms and the posterior costophrenic angles or sulci. Note that the right hemidiaphragm can be seen in its entirety because black air in the right lower lobe abuts the gray right hemidiaphragm and liver. However, the water density left hemidiaphragm abuts the water density heart anteriorly, and as a result the left hemidiaphragm disappears anteriorly (Fig. 6-15). *Whenever two abutting ob-*

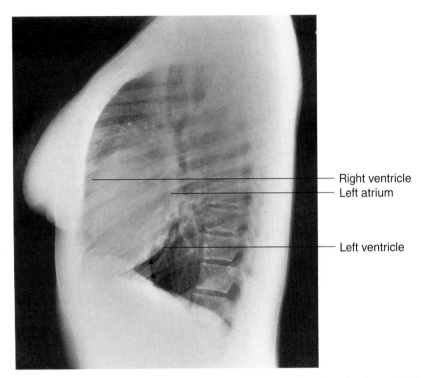

Right ventricle
Left atrium

Left ventricle

FIG. 6-12. Chest lateral radiograph. Normal. The radiograph is positioned on the viewbox with the patient facing either to your left or right. Note that the cardiac silhouette is an anterior structure and makes an excellent starting point for your evaluation. The faint vertical water density line *(straight arrows)* represents the inferior vena cava.

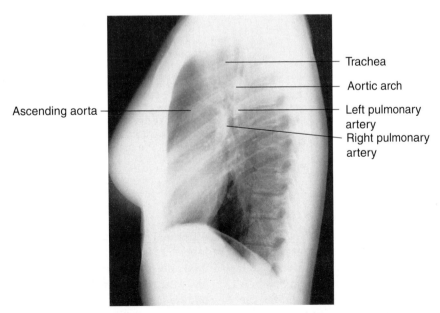

Trachea

Aortic arch

Left pulmonary
artery
Right pulmonary
artery

Ascending aorta

FIG. 6-13. Chest lateral radiograph. Normal. Note that the oval shaped right pulmonary artery lies anterior and inferior relative to the left pulmonary artery. The left pulmonary artery crosses cephalad over the left main stem bronchus and it lies inferior to the aortic arch.

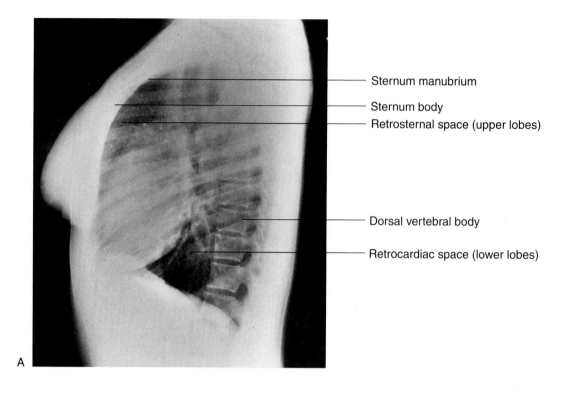

Sternum manubrium

Sternum body

Retrosternal space (upper lobes)

Dorsal vertebral body

Retrocardiac space (lower lobes)

A

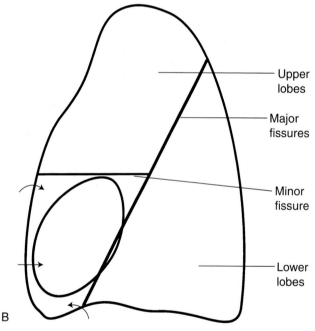

Upper lobes

Major fissures

Minor fissure

Lower lobes

B

FIG. 6-14. A: Chest lateral radiograph. Normal. The anterior and posterior osseous structures should always be routinely viewed. The spine appears darker or more dense as you proceed caudally as there is more air in the lower lungs. **B:** Illustration of the spatial relationships of the pulmonary lobes on the lateral view. Note that the right middle lobe and the lingular segments of the left upper lobe *(curved arrows)* project over the heart *(straight arrow)*. The lower lobes are primarily posterior structures. The major fissures extend approximately up to the T4 level.

jects are of similar density, it is difficult to identify their boundaries or silhouettes. This very important principle is called the *silhouette sign,* and it is a powerful and important radiologic tool. Since most pulmonary pathology is water density, the silhouette sign facilitates the detection and location of water density pathology. For example, if a diaphragm cannot be seen on the PA view and it is obliterated posteriorly on the lateral view, then water density pathology must be suspected in the lower lobe. Furthermore, since the right middle lobe is situated anteriorly and adjacent to the right cardiac border, any water density pathologic process involving the right middle lobe will obliterate the anteriorly located right cardiac border on a PA or AP radiograph. Therefore, whenever the right cardiac border is obscured or indistinct on a PA or AP radiograph, a right middle lobe

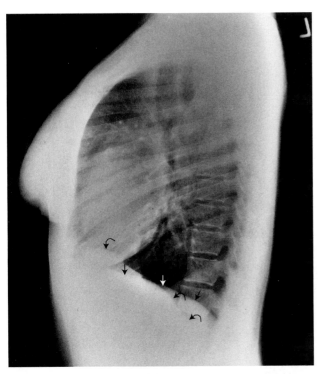

FIG. 6-15. Chest lateral radiograph. Normal. Note that the anterior aspect of the left hemidiaphragm *(straight arrows)* is not visible anteriorly where it abuts on the water density heart. On the other hand the entire right hemidiaphragm *(curved arrows)* is visible. This is an excellent example of the silhouette sign.

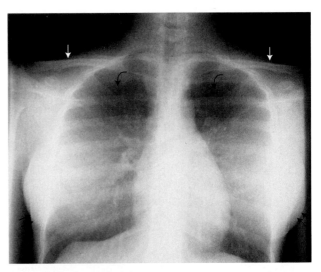

FIG. 6-16. Chest AP lordotic radiograph. Normal. This view is obtained with the patient leaning backwards a few degrees. Note how the clavicles *(straight arrows)* project cephalad to the pulmonary apices allowing an improved view of the upper lobes *(curved arrows)*. The scapulae project somewhat lower than on the standard AP or PA radiograph. The breasts are indicated by the double straight arrows.

water density pathologic process such as pneumonia, atelectasis, tumor, blood, and infarction must be strongly suspected. Similarly, when the left cardiac border is obliterated on a PA or AP radiograph, pathology must be suspected in the anteriorly situated lingular segments of the left upper lobe.

AP LORDOTIC CHEST

There are occasions when disease is suspected in the pulmonary upper lobes; however, the ribs and clavicles may be obscuring the lesion. In these situations an AP lordotic radiograph (Fig. 6-16) is helpful to view the upper lobes without overlying clavicles. In general, the appearance of the lordotic AP radiograph is somewhat similar to that of a routine AP radiograph (Fig. 6-17).

NORMAL THORACIC SECTIONAL ANATOMY

The images in Figs. 6-18 through 6-26 demonstrate thoracic sectional anatomy in the axial, coronal, and sagittal planes. *The anatomy does not change, but the densities or appearances of anatomic structures change depending on the imaging modality utilized.*

text continues on page 90

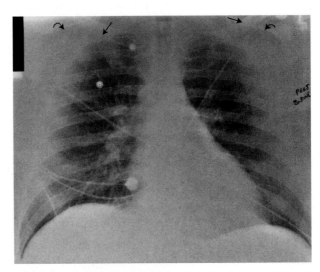

FIG. 6-17. Chest AP portable supine radiograph. Normal. Compare the position of the clavicles *(straight arrows)* and scapulae *(curved arrows)* to those in the AP lordotic radiograph in Fig. 6-16. The white lines overlying the thorax are wires attached to monitoring electrodes. The AP radiograph is similar in appearance to the PA radiographs shown earlier in this chapter. Although the cardiac silhouette may appear larger than normal, it is within normal limits for an AP view.

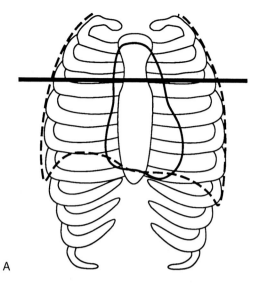

FIG. 6-18. A: Approximate axial anatomic level through the aortic arch for B–D. **B:** Axial cadaver radiograph of the sectioned chest at the aortic arch level. Normal. A frozen cadaver was sectioned and then radiographed. **C, D:** Chest CT images at the aortic arch level with mediastinal windows (C) and parenchymal windows (D). Normal. The patient is scanned once, and the mediastinal windows and parenchymal windows are the result of technical adjustments. Note how well the pulmonary vessels *(straight arrow)* are visualized with the parenchymal window technique compared to the mediastinal window technique in C.

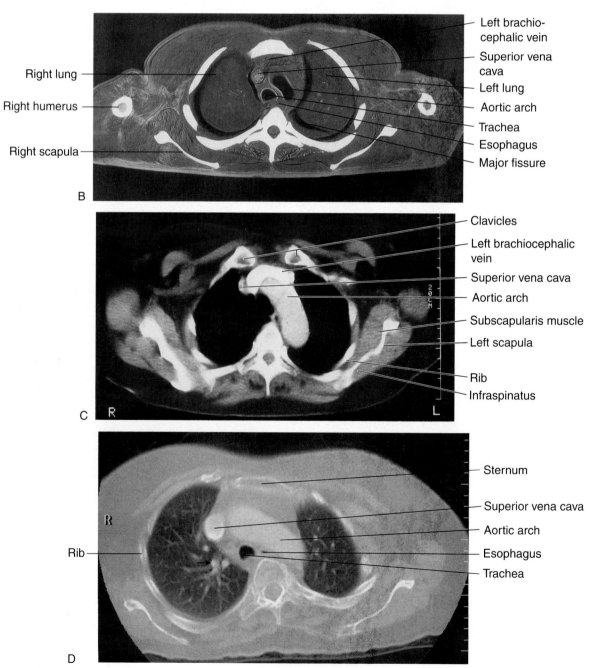

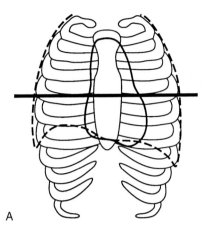

A

FIG. 6-19. **A:** Approximate axial anatomic level through the pulmonary arteries for B–E. **B:** Axial cadaver radiograph of the sectioned chest at the level of the pulmonary arteries. Normal. **C, D:** Chest axial CT images at the level of the pulmonary arteries with mediastinal (C) and parenchymal windows (D).

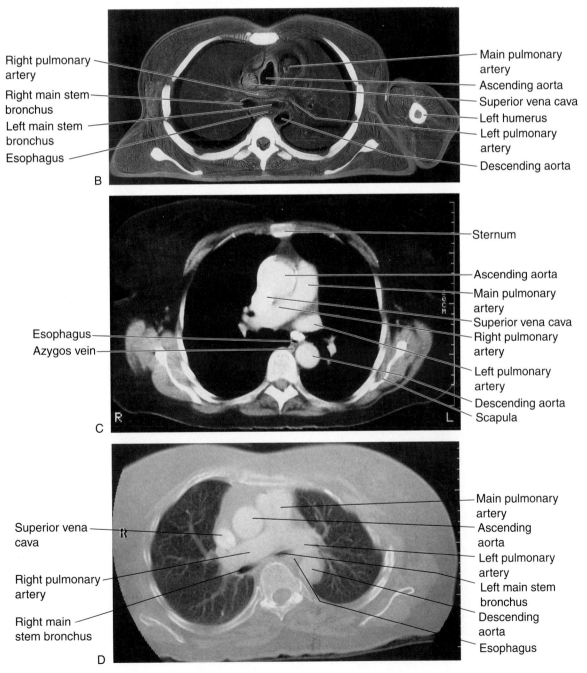

Right pulmonary artery

Right main stem bronchus

Left main stem bronchus

Esophagus

B

Main pulmonary artery

Ascending aorta

Superior vena cava

Left humerus

Left pulmonary artery

Descending aorta

Sternum

Ascending aorta

Main pulmonary artery

Superior vena cava

Right pulmonary artery

Left pulmonary artery

Descending aorta

Scapula

Esophagus

Azygos vein

C

Superior vena cava

Right pulmonary artery

Right main stem bronchus

D

Main pulmonary artery

Ascending aorta

Left pulmonary artery

Left main stem bronchus

Descending aorta

Esophagus

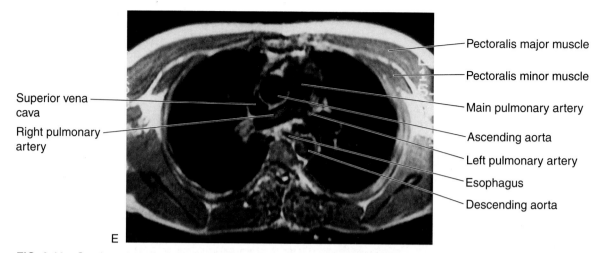

Pectoralis major muscle

Pectoralis minor muscle

Superior vena cava

Main pulmonary artery

Right pulmonary artery

Ascending aorta

Left pulmonary artery

Esophagus

Descending aorta

E

FIG. 6-19. *Continued.* Normal. **E:** Chest axial MR image at the level of the pulmonary arteries. Normal.

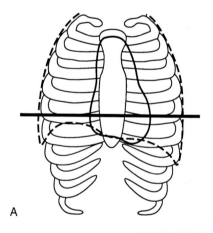

A

FIG. 6-20. A: Approximate axial anatomic level through the right and left atria for B–E. **B:** Axial cadaver radiograph of the sectioned chest at the level of the right and left atria. Normal.

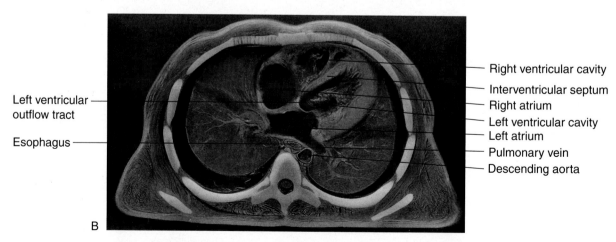

Left ventricular outflow tract

Esophagus

Right ventricular cavity

Interventricular septum

Right atrium

Left ventricular cavity

Left atrium

Pulmonary vein

Descending aorta

B

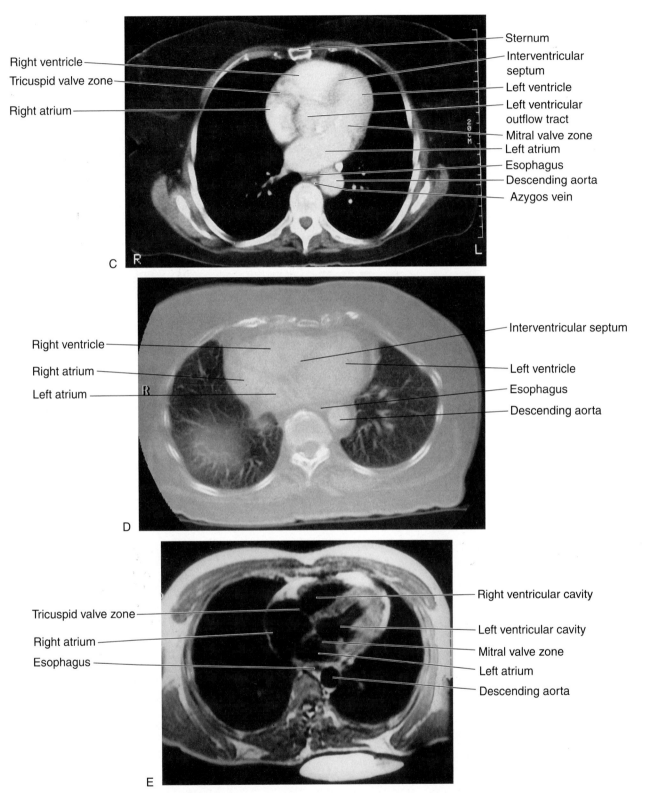

FIG. 6-20. *Continued.* **C, D:** Chest axial CT images at the level of the atria with mediastinal (C) and parenchymal (D) windows. Normal. **E:** Chest axial MR image at the level of the atria. Normal.

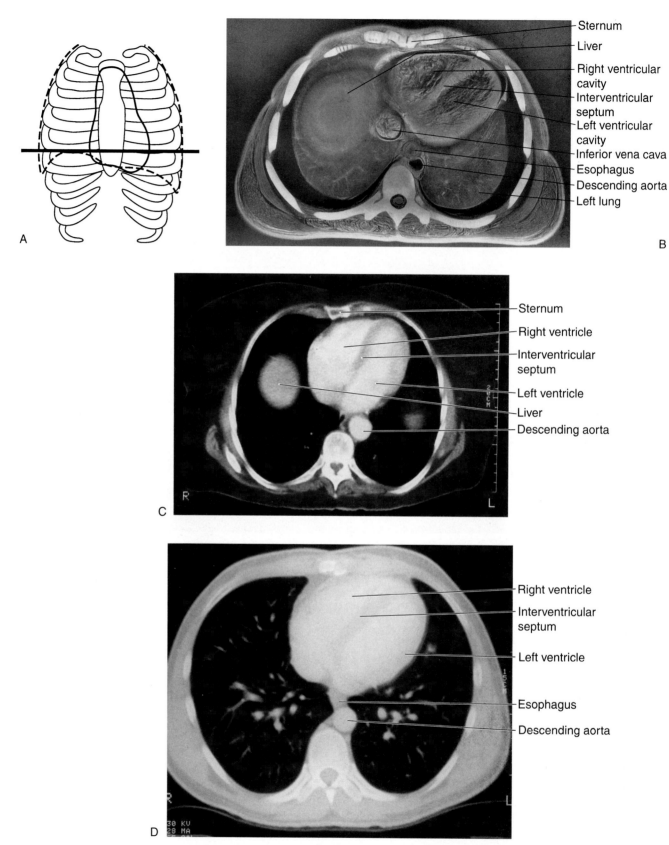

FIG. 6-21. A: Approximate axial anatomic level through the right and left ventricles for B–E. **B:** Axial cadaver radiograph of the sectioned chest at the level of the ventricles. Normal. **C, D:** Chest axial CT image through the ventricles with both mediastinal (C) and parenchymal (D) windows. Normal.

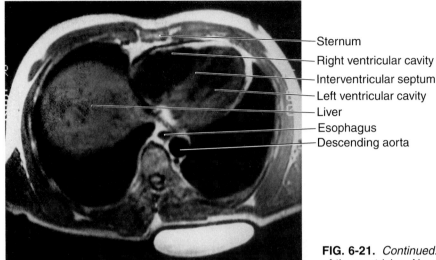

Sternum
Right ventricular cavity
Interventricular septum
Left ventricular cavity
Liver
Esophagus
Descending aorta

E

FIG. 6-21. *Continued.* **E:** Chest axial MR image at the level of the ventricles. Normal.

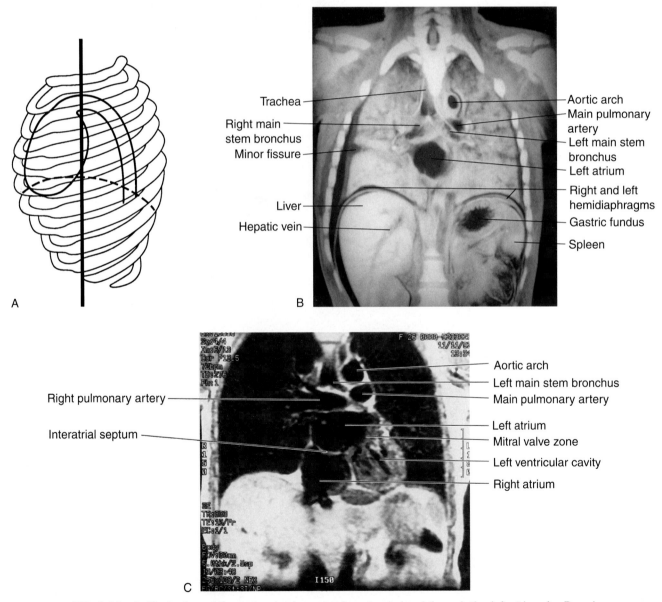

Trachea
Right main stem bronchus
Minor fissure
Liver
Hepatic vein

Aortic arch
Main pulmonary artery
Left main stem bronchus
Left atrium
Right and left hemidiaphragms
Gastric fundus
Spleen

A

B

Right pulmonary artery
Interatrial septum

Aortic arch
Left main stem bronchus
Main pulmonary artery
Left atrium
Mitral valve zone
Left ventricular cavity
Right atrium

C

FIG. 6-22. A: Illustration of the approximate coronal anatomic level through the left atrium for B and C. **B:** Coronal cadaver radiograph of the sectioned chest through the level of the left atrium. Normal. **C:** Chest coronal MR image through the right and left atria. Normal.

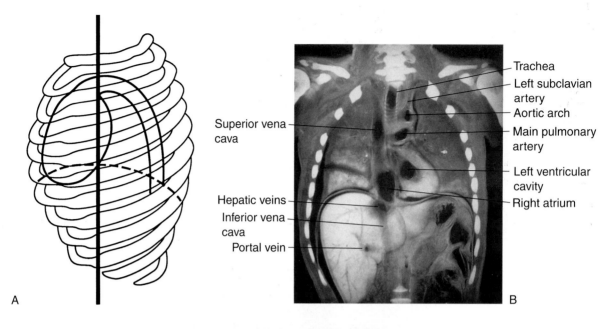

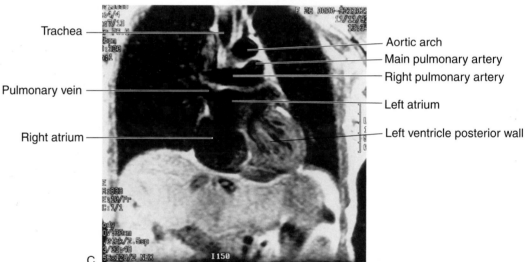

FIG. 6-23. **A:** Approximate coronal anatomic level through the right atrium and left ventricle for B and C. **B:** Coronal cadaver radiograph of the sectioned chest through the level of the right atrium and left ventricle. Normal. **C:** Chest coronal MR image through the atria and left ventricle. Normal.

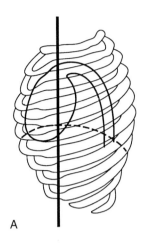

A

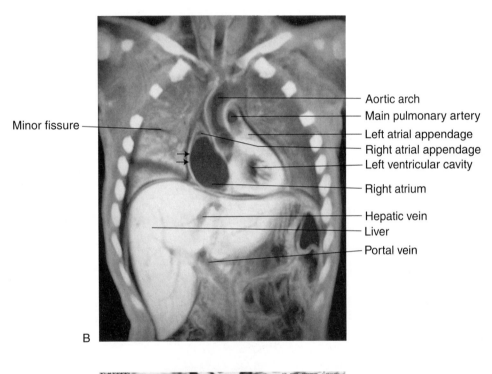

Minor fissure —

— Aortic arch
— Main pulmonary artery
— Left atrial appendage
— Right atrial appendage
— Left ventricular cavity

— Right atrium

— Hepatic vein
— Liver
— Portal vein

B

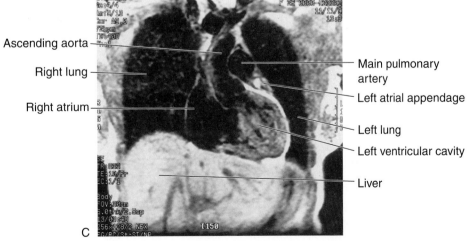

Ascending aorta —

Right lung —

Right atrium —

— Main pulmonary artery

— Left atrial appendage

— Left lung

— Left ventricular cavity

— Liver

C

FIG. 6-24. A: Illustration of the approximate coronal anatomic level through the left ventricle and the ascending aorta for B and C. **B:** Coronal cadaver radiograph of the sectioned chest through the left ventricle and the ascending aorta. Normal. Note that the convex right cardiac border is due to the right atrium *(straight arrows).* **C:** Chest coronal MR image through the left ventricle and the ascending aorta. Normal.

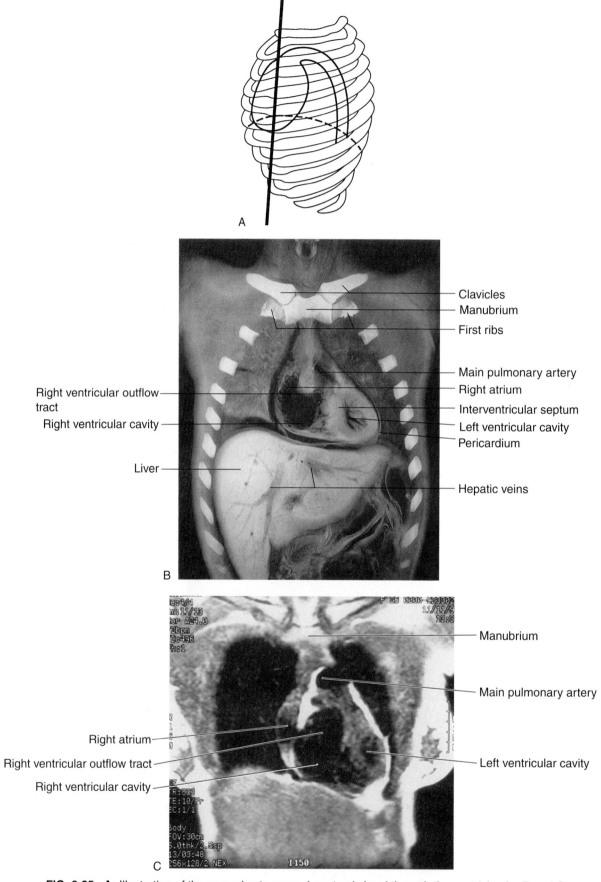

FIG. 6-25. A: Illustration of the approximate coronal anatomic level through the ventricles for B and C. **B:** Coronal cadaver radiograph of the sectioned chest through the ventricles. Normal. **C:** Chest coronal MR image through the ventricles. Normal.

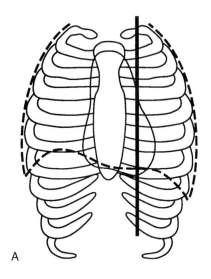

A

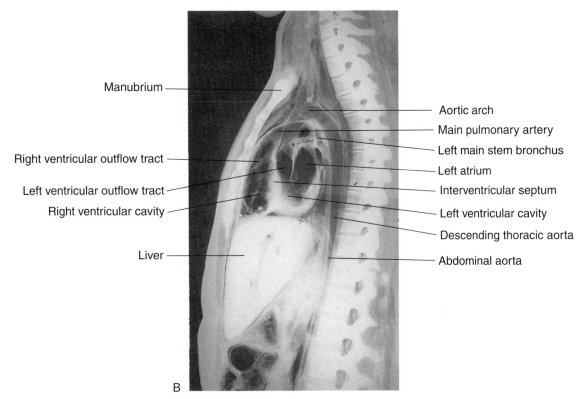

Manubrium —

Aortic arch

Main pulmonary artery

Left main stem bronchus

Right ventricular outflow tract —

Left atrium

Left ventricular outflow tract —

Interventricular septum

Right ventricular cavity —

Left ventricular cavity

Descending thoracic aorta

Liver —

Abdominal aorta

B

FIG. 6-26. **A:** Illustration of the approximate sagittal anatomic level for B. **B:** Sagittal cadaver radiograph of the sectioned chest through the right ventricular outflow tract and the right ventricle. Normal.

CHEST ANGIOGRAPHY

Nearly all of the thoracic arteries and veins can be imaged via angiography. Examples of common thoracic angiographic images are shown in Fig. 6-27.

ANOMALIES

Numerous congenital anomalies involve the sternum, clavicles, bronchi, lungs, heart and great vessels, and diaphragms. There are many more, but only a few are demonstrated. The majority of thoracic congenital abnormalities are detected in infancy or early childhood.

Pectus excavatum or funnel chest (Fig. 6-28) is a common and usually asymptomatic abnormality of the chest wall that may be associated with other congenital abnormalities such as Marfan's syndrome, scoliosis, and Poland's syndrome (1). Therapy is usually not indicated.

Pectus carinatum or pigeon breast (Fig. 6-29) can be either a congenital or an acquired abnormality wherein the sternum projects more anterior than normal. The acquired form may occur in patients with untreated congenital heart disease. The patients are usually asymptomatic, and therapy is usually not indicated (1).

Another osseous abnormality is the congenital absence of the clavicles (Fig. 6-30). It is uncommon but very dramatic. This abnormality may be associated with cleidocranial dysostosis, which is a disease manifested by delayed or incomplete calvarial ossification, hypoplasia or aplasia of the clavicles, and many other associated osseous abnormalities (2).

When the azygos vein fails to migrate to its normal position just above the right main stem bronchus, the azygos fissure subtends a variable amount of the right

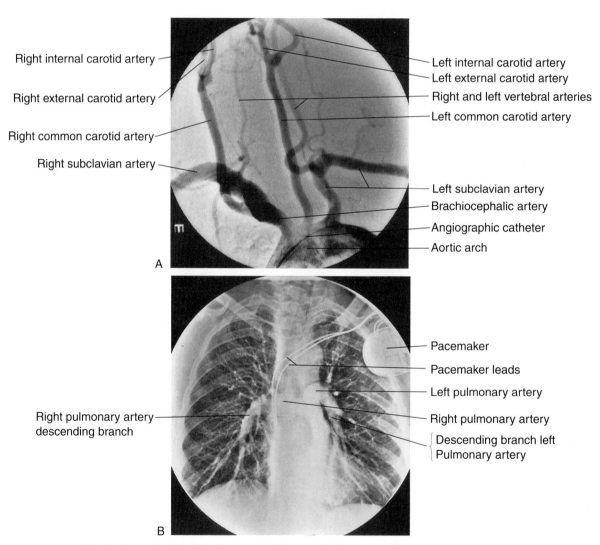

FIG. 6-27. A: Aortic arch angiogram. Normal. **B:** Pulmonary arteriogram. Normal.

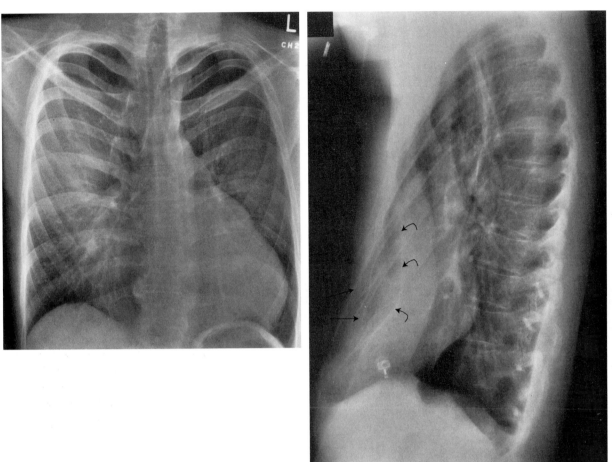

FIG. 6-28. Chest PA **(A)** and lateral **(B)** radiographs. Pectus excavatum. Note that on the PA view the cardiac silhouette is rotated and displaced to the patient's left, and the left cardiac border is straight simulating mitral valve disease. There is mild deformity of the ribs bilaterally on the PA view. The extent of the defect is best appreciated on the lateral view where the anterior ribs *(straight arrows)* project anterior to the sternum *(curved arrows)*.

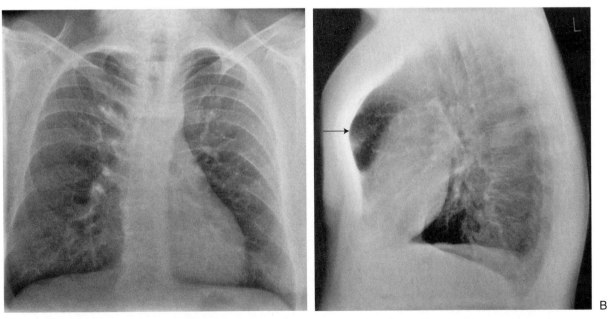

FIG. 6-29. Chest PA **(A)** and lateral **(B)** radiographs. Pectus carinatum. The PA view is essentially normal with mild dorsal spine scoliosis. The exaggerated anterior projection of the sternum *(straight arrow)* is best appreciated on the lateral view.

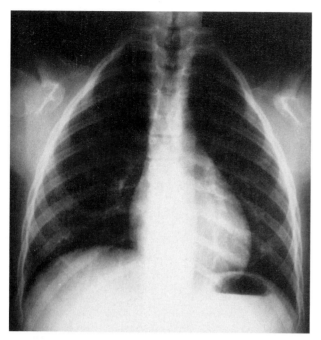

FIG. 6-30. Chest AP radiograph. Cleidocranial dysostosis with bilateral absence of the clavicles. This was a routine chest radiograph in an asymptomatic 20-year-old woman.

upper lobe to form the azygos lobe (Fig. 6-31). The azygos fissure is best visualized on the PA radiograph as a thin curvilinear arc made up of two layers of visceral and two layers of parietal pleura. The azygos lobe is not particularly susceptible to disease.

The inferior accessory, or cardiac, lobe (Fig. 6-32) is another common pulmonary accessory lobe. It can occur on the left but is most commonly found on the right side. It is of no clinical significance.

The most common aortic arch anomaly is a right aortic arch with a left descending aorta wherein the aortic arch crosses the midline posterior to the esophagus to reach the left side (Fig. 6-33). There are five types of right aortic arch, and the classification is based on the arrangement of the arch vessels (3). Right-sided arches are also found in tetralogy of Fallot and other congenital heart problems. On the PA radiograph the right-sided arch often appears more cephalad than a normal left-sided arch.

Another vascular anomaly is coarctation or stenosis of the proximal descending aorta. The degree of coarctation is variable, and the signs, symptoms, and physical findings vary with the location and degree of stenosis. Blood pressures in the upper body may be normal or above normal, whereas in the lower body they may be below normal. Even the upper extremities blood pressures may be unequal depending on the location of the stenosis relative to the left subclavian artery. Also, the presence of murmurs, cardiac enlargement, and aortic pre- and poststenotic dilatation depends on the location and severity of the stenosis. Often the site of stenosis can be identified on routine chest radiographs (see Fig. 6-34). Rib notching can occur along the inferior aspect of the ribs secondary to increased collateral flow through the intercostal arteries bypassing the aortic stenosis.

CONFUSING EXTRATHORACIC CONDITIONS

On occasion there are objects outside the thorax that can be confused with intrathoracic pathology (Figs. 6-35 text continues on page 96

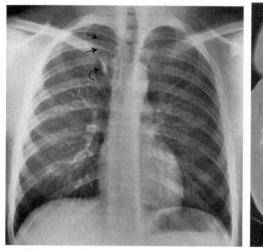

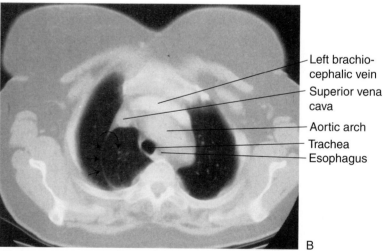

Left brachio-cephalic vein
Superior vena cava
Aortic arch
Trachea
Esophagus

FIG. 6-31. **A:** Chest PA radiograph. Azygos lobe. The azygos lobe is outlined with straight arrows. The curved arrow indicates the azygos vein that is located more cephalad and lateral to its normal position near the right main stem bronchus. **B:** Chest axial CT image in a different patient. Azygos lobe. The image is through the level of the aortic arch and nicely demonstrates the azygos lobe fissure *(straight arrows)* and the azygos lobe *(curved arrow).*

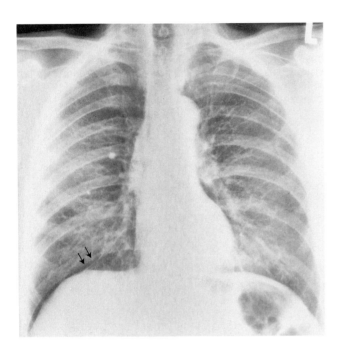

FIG. 6-32. Chest PA radiograph. Inferior accessory or cardiac lobe. The inferior accessory lobe projects over the right medial lung base *(straight arrows)*.

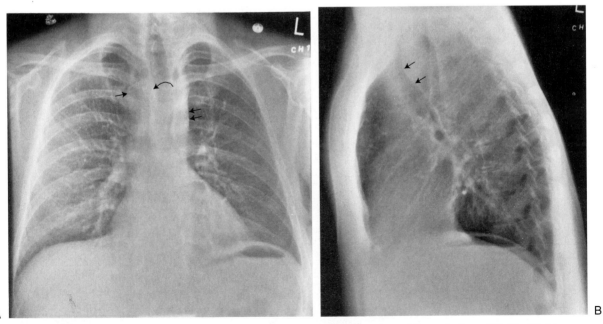

A   B

FIG. 6-33. Chest PA **(A)** and lateral **(B)** radiographs, barium swallow **(C)**, and chest CT **(D)**. Right-sided aortic arch and left descending thoracic aorta. This 42-year-old male smoker was suspected of having cancer of the lung. A neoplastic mass was suspected on the PA radiograph (A) but this proved to be an ill-defined aortic knob to the right of the midline *(straight arrow)*. The right aortic arch is indenting the right side of the trachea *(curved arrow)*. The double straight arrows are on the descending aorta that descends on the left side. The right-sided aortic arch indents the posterior aspect of the trachea *(straight arrows)* on the lateral radiograph (B).

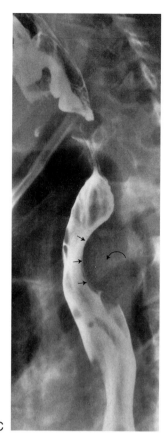

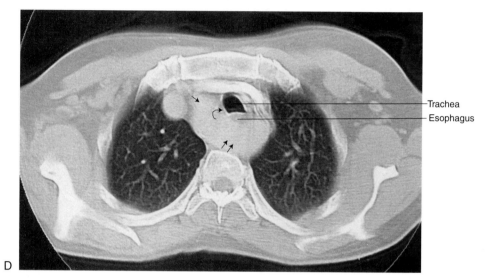

FIG. 6-33. *Continued.* Barium swallow (C) confirms a significant indentation on the posterior aspect of the barium-filled esophagus *(straight arrows)* secondary to the crossing aortic arch *(curved arrow).* The diagnosis is confirmed on chest CT (D) that shows the right-sided aorta *(single straight arrow)* passing posterior to the esophagus and trachea *(double straight arrows)* to reach the left side of the thorax. Again, note the indentation on the right side of the trachea *(curved arrow)* secondary to the right-sided aortic arch.

Trachea
Esophagus

C

D

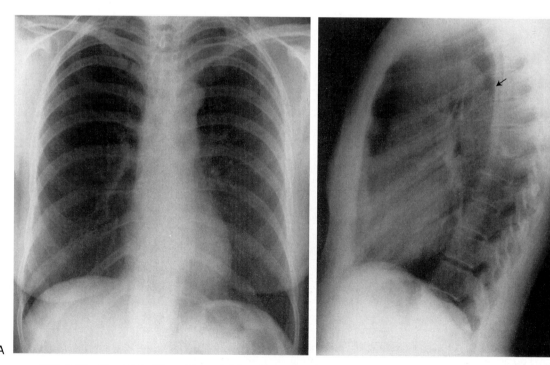

A

B

FIG. 6-34. Chest PA **(A)** and lateral **(B)** radiographs. Coarctation of the aorta. The classical PA radiographic appearance is an indentation *(arrow)* involving the lateral aspect of the proximal descending aorta (A) and a posterior indentation *(arrow)* involving the posterior aspect of the proximal descending aorta on the lateral radiograph (B). These indentations represent the site of stenosis or coarctation in the proximal descending aorta. There is no evidence of rib notching and the cardiac size is normal.

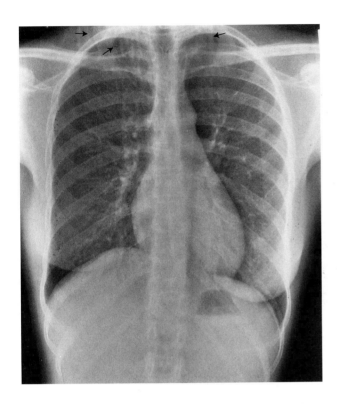

FIG. 6-35. PA chest radiograph. Hair artefacts *(straight arrows)* projecting over the upper lobes. Hair, hair braids, ponytails, and ribbons can project over the upper lobes and should not be confused with a pathologic process.

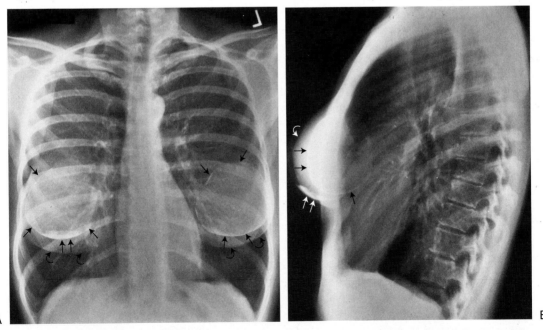

A

B

FIG. 6-36. Chest PA **(A)** and lateral **(B)** radiographs. Bilateral breast augmentations or implants. The breast implants *(straight arrows)* are partially opaque, and the native breasts are indicated by the curved arrows. Note the benign postoperative calcification on both the PA and lateral views *(double straight arrows)* in the inferior aspect of the right breast. The hyperinflated lungs are probably within limits.

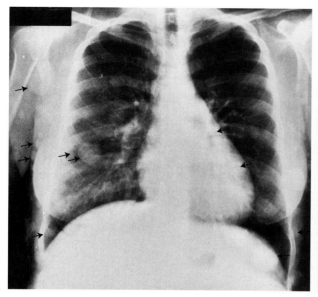 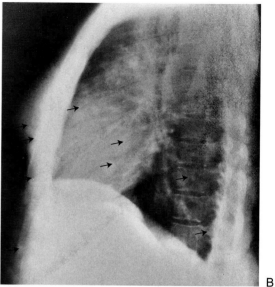

FIG. 6-37. Chest PA **(A)** and lateral **(B)** radiographs. Multiple soft tissue nodules projecting over the thorax. Multiple subcutaneous soft tissue nodules *(arrows)* project over the thorax and must not be mistaken for pulmonary nodules.

to 6-37). It is important to keep such possibilities in mind at all times.

FOREIGN BODIES, LINES, AND TUBES

Another pitfall on chest radiographs that must be kept in mind is the presence of intrathoracic foreign bodies (see Fig. 6-38). Some foreign bodies are intentionally placed within the thorax such as lines and tubes. It is very important to recognize the typical appearances of these commonly used lines and tubes, especially when caring for patients in acute care areas. The normal and some abnormal locations of these lines and tubes are demonstrated in Fig. 6-39.

POSTOPERATIVE CHEST PROBLEMS

It is important to recognize some common radiographic findings that may be present on postoperative chest images (Fig. 6-40).

Air in the Wrong Places

An important chest problem encountered in medicine is pneumothorax (air in the pleural space). Pneumothorax can be secondary to trauma or disease, or it may be spontaneous. Some of its etiologies are listed in Table 6-1. Spontaneous pneumothorax most commonly occurs in young male adults but does involve female

patients as well. These patients typically present with a sudden onset of unilateral chest pain that can be accompanied by varying degrees of breathing difficulties. The radiographic diagnosis of pneumothorax is made by identifying the *visceral pleura line* (Fig. 6-41A), and varying degrees of pneumothorax are demonstrated in Fig. 6-41. A *tension pneumothorax* is when the pressure within the pneumothorax becomes elevated enough to cause cardiac and respiratory problems (see Fig. 6-41C). Tension pneumothorax requires immediate therapy in the form of a chest tube or syringe aspiration of the air.

text continues on page 101

TABLE 6-1. *Partial list of pneumothorax etiologies*

Traumatic
1. Accidents, e.g., motor vehicle
2. Iatrogenic
   a. Thoracoscopy
   b. Thoracentesis
   c. Placement of central line
   d. Artificial ventilation
   e. Postthoracic surgery
   f. Transthoracic and bronchoscopic biopsy

Spontaneous
1. Rupture of a bleb or bullae
2. Secondary to underlying pulmonary disease
3. Secondary to pneumomediastinum

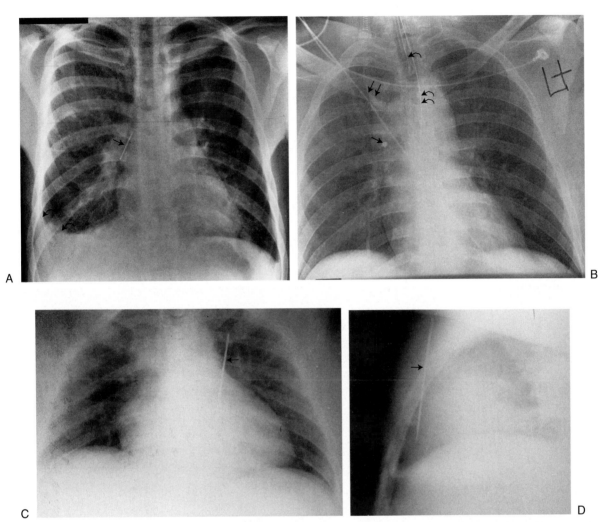

FIG. 6-38. A: Chest PA radiograph. Straight pin *(straight arrow)* in the right intermediate bronchus. This 26-year-old mentally impaired male had a tendency to swallow everything in sight. He suddenly sneezed and apparently aspirated the pin into the bronchial tree. The pin was removed at bronchoscopy. Note the right pleural effusion *(curved arrows)*. It has been estimated that there must be at least 125 cc of pleural fluid before it is recognized on PA and AP views. **B:** Chest portable AP radiograph. Tooth fragment *(straight arrow)* in the right bronchial tree. The patient was involved in a motor vehicle accident and a portion of a tooth was missing. The chest radiograph shows the tooth fragment projecting over the right upper bronchial tree. The tooth fragment was removed at bronchoscopy. Note the endotracheal tube tip *(single curved arrow)* lies to the patient's right of the nasogastric tube *(double curved arrows)*. An azygos lobe is present, and the double straight arrows indicate the position of the azygos vein that is more lateral and cephalad than normal. **C, D:** Chest AP (C) and lateral (D) radiographs. Darning needle lodged in the right ventricle. The child of this young mother accidentally stabbed her with a darning needle. Note that the needle *(straight arrows)* projects over the right ventricle region in both views. The needle was successfully removed at thoracotomy, and recovery was uneventful.

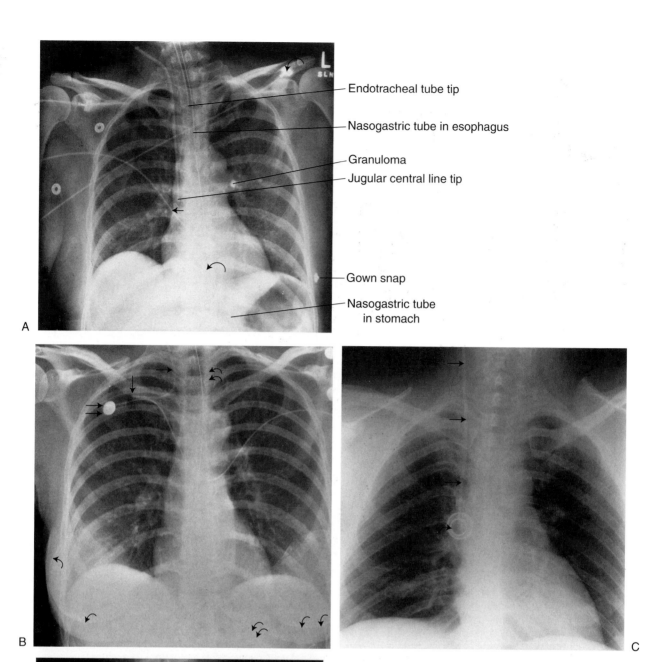

Endotracheal tube tip

Nasogastric tube in esophagus

Granuloma

Jugular central line tip

Gown snap

Nasogastric tube in stomach

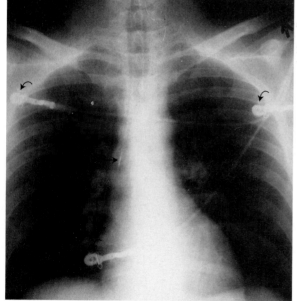

FIG. 6-39. A: Chest AP radiograph. Normal tube and line positions. The tip of the central line via a right jugular vein approach projects over the superior vena cava. Note that the central line tip lies cephalad to the junction *(straight arrow)* of the straight bordered superior vena cava and the convex right atrium. The curved arrows point to monitoring electrodes that lie on the skin of the patient's thorax. **B:** Chest AP radiograph. Right jugular central line inadvertently passed into the right subclavian vein *(single straight arrows)*. Bilateral breast augmentations or implants are present *(single curved arrows)*. A monitoring electrode *(double straight arrows)* and a nasogastric tube *(double curved arrows)* are also present. **C:** Chest AP radiograph. A right jugular Hickman line passing cephalad. The Hickman line *(straight arrows)* with an infusaport *(curved arrow)* is directed cephalad in the jugular vein rather than caudad toward the superior vena cava. The tip of the line is beyond the edge of the radiograph. **D:** Chest AP radiograph. Endotracheal tube *(arrow)* inadvertently placed in right intermediate bronchus. External monitoring electrodes are present *(curved arrows)*.

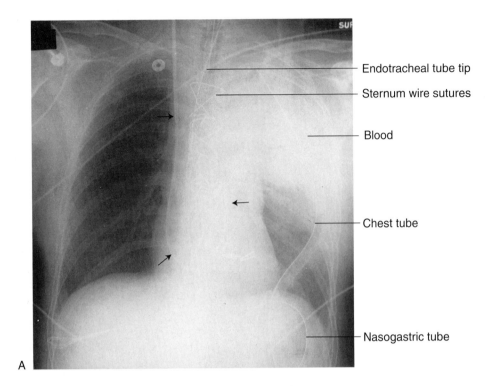

- Endotracheal tube tip
- Sternum wire sutures
- Blood
- Chest tube
- Nasogastric tube

A

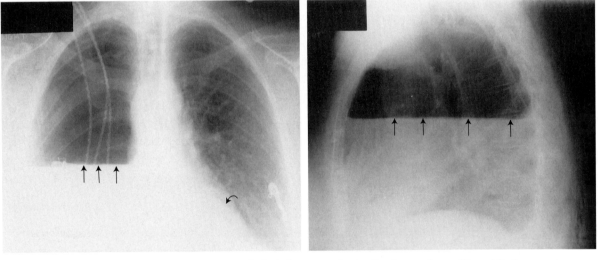

B

C

FIG. 6-40. A: Chest AP supine radiograph. Left thorax postoperative hemorrhage. The white homogeneous density in the region of the left upper lobe represents active bleeding in the thorax 2 hours following coronary artery bypass grafting. The patient was reoperated to evacuate the blood and control the bleeding. Infection, atelectasis, and tumor could give a similar appearance, but the history made the diagnosis obvious. The straight arrows indicate a right jugular Swan-Ganz catheter. **B, C:** Chest AP (B) and lateral (C) radiographs. Right pneumonectomy. The straight arrows indicate the presence of an air–fluid level that is a common finding following pneumonectomy. Gradually over a period of days the vacant right thorax will fill with fluid that will eventually fibrose. Left lower lobe atelectasis is manifest by the retrocardiac double density *(curved arrow)*, and there is obliteration of the medial aspect of the left hemidiaphragm (silhouette sign). Left lower lobe atelectasis is common following thoracic surgery.

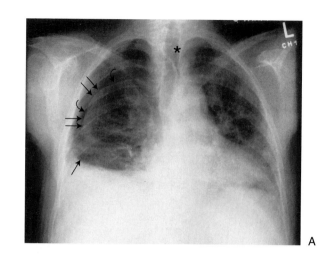

FIG. 6-41. A: Chest PA radiograph. Mild to moderate right pneumothorax. A thoracentesis was performed to remove right pleural fluid *(straight arrow)*, but it resulted in a right pneumothorax. The visceral pleura is outlined by the curved arrows. There is air in the pleural space *(double straight arrows)* lying between the visceral pleura and the parietal pleura or chest wall. The result is a partially collapsed or atelectatic right lung. Note that the trachea (*) is midline. **B:** Chest AP radiograph. Moderate right pneumothorax. While on the ventilator this patient developed right chest pain and shortness of breath. There is a moderate-sized right pneumothorax. The right lateral costophrenic sulcus or angle is very deep and lucent compared to the left, and this is called the "deep sulcus sign." A deep sulcus sign should always make you suspicious for pneumothorax. Note the double density behind the cardiac silhouette *(straight arrows)* and the associated obliteration of the left hemidiaphragm medially *(curved arrow)* represent the atelectatic left lower lobe. The left hemidiaphragm is obliterated because the water density collapsed left lower lobe is in juxtaposition to the water density left hemidiaphragm making it impossible to differentiate between diaphragm and collapsed left lower lobe. These findings are typical of left lower lobe atelectasis. The inability to find a border between two abutting water densities is called the silhouette sign. **C:** Chest AP radiograph. Right tension pneumothorax. This patient was on the ventilator and developed right chest pain and hypotension. There is a large right pneumothorax with complete atelectasis of the right lung, and the straight arrows indicate the visceral pleural line. Note the right deep sulcus sign *(curved arrow)*. The heart is displaced to the left compatible with a tension pneumothorax.

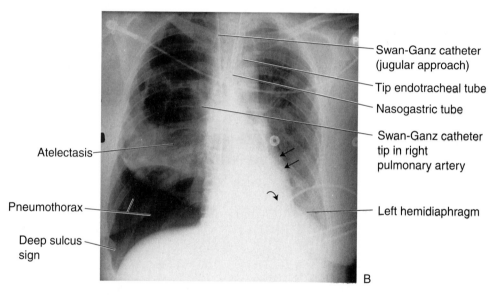

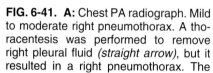

Swan-Ganz catheter (jugular approach)

Tip endotracheal tube

Nasogastric tube

Swan-Ganz catheter tip in right pulmonary artery

Atelectasis

Pneumothorax

Left hemidiaphragm

Deep sulcus sign

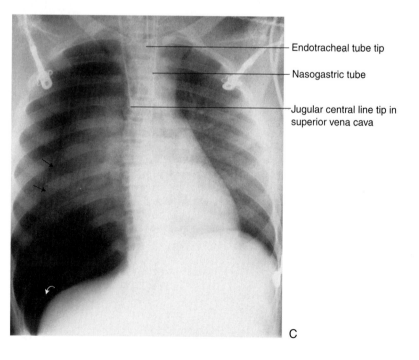

Endotracheal tube tip

Nasogastric tube

Jugular central line tip in superior vena cava

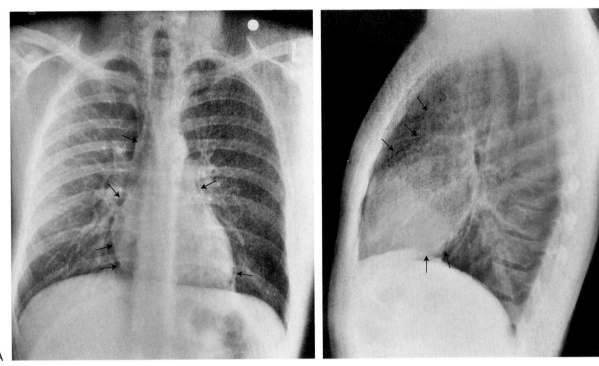

A   B

FIG. 6-42. Chest PA **(A)** and lateral **(B)** radiographs. Pneumomediastinum. This patient had routine chest radiographs for vague chest pain, and surprisingly the radiographs revealed mediastinal air *(straight arrows).* The etiology was never found, and the air resolved spontaneously.

Pneumomediastinum (Fig. 6-42) has a number of etiologies as shown in Table 6-2, and it may be accompanied by thoracic and/or cervical subcutaneous emphysema.

When a patient has experienced chest trauma, lacerations of the lungs are generally unsuspected and consequently go undetected. Routine chest radiographs are usually negative or may show water density contusions. Nevertheless, lacerations of the lung should always be suspected when there has been chest trauma. Often pulmonary lacerations are incidental findings when chest CT imaging is performed for some other reason (Fig. 6-43).

Other Air Accumulations In and Around the Chest

Abnormal air accumulations may occur within the thorax secondary to esophageal hiatal hernias (Fig. 6-44). They represent a portion of the stomach herniated through the esophageal hiatus and their size is variable. They may be asymptomatic or be associated with mild to severe chest pain.

TABLE 6-2. *Some etiologies of pneumomediastinum*

Traumatic
1. Closed chest trauma
2. Secondary to chest and neck surgery
3. Esophageal perforation
4. Tracheobronchial perforation
5. Vigorous exercise
6. Asthma
7. Ventilator

Spontaneous
1. No apparent etiology

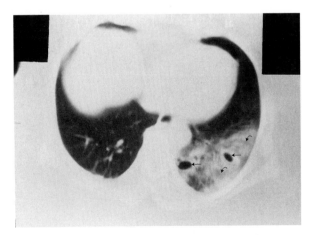

FIG. 6-43. Chest axial CT through the lung bases. Lung parenchymal lacerations *(straight arrows)* in the left lower lobe. The lacerations are surrounded by water density contused lung parenchyma *(curved arrows).*

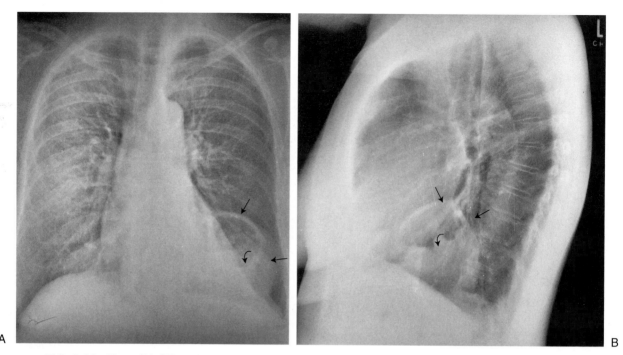

A

B

FIG. 6-44. Chest PA **(A)** and lateral **(B)** radiographs. Esophageal hiatal hernia. The straight arrows indicate the large esophageal hiatal hernia that contains air–fluid levels *(curved arrows)*. The chest is otherwise normal.

Abscesses can occur within the soft tissues surrounding the thorax, and they should be recognized as such (Fig. 6-45). Usually there is an air–fluid level that projects outside of the thorax on at least one of the views. If the air–fluid level projects over the lungs in both the PA and lateral view, then the abscess must by definition lie within the lungs.

Pneumoperitoneum is a significant abnormal air accumulation in the abdomen that often can be identified on chest radiographs (Fig. 6-46). As little as a

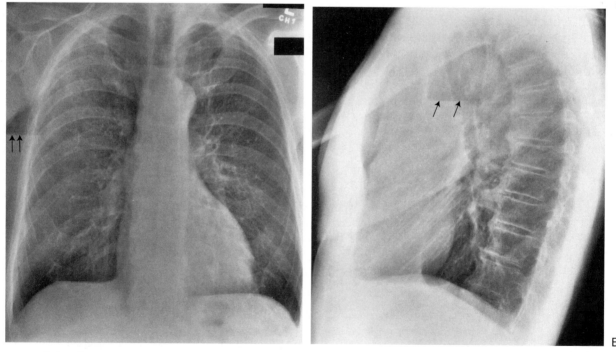

A

B

FIG. 6-45. Chest PA **(A)** and lateral **(B)** radiographs. Right axillary abscess. This patient was postoperative following a right axillary node dissection. A right axillary air–fluid level *(straight arrows)* is well visualized on both the PA and lateral views. The abscess was subsequently drained.

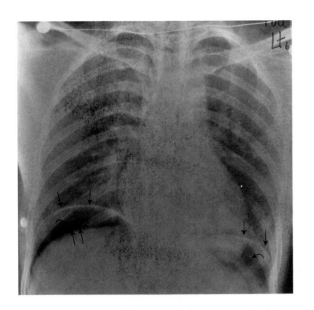

FIG. 6-46. Chest AP radiograph. Pneumoperitoneum. The patient experienced sudden onset of severe abdominal pain, and physical examination revealed a board-like rigidity of the abdomen. The patient proved to have a perforated duodenal ulcer at surgery. The *straight arrows* indicate the diaphragms bilaterally and the *curved arrows* delineate free subdiaphragmatic air secondary to the perforated ulcer. The dome of the liver is indicated by the *double straight arrows*, and the chest is otherwise normal.

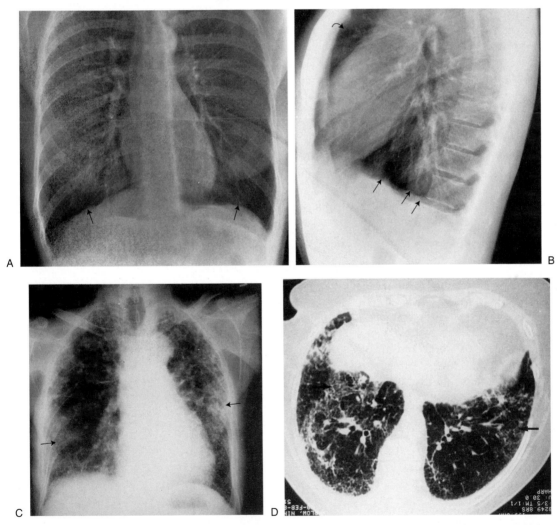

FIG. 6-47. Chest PA **(A)** and lateral **(B)** radiographs. Chronic obstructive pulmonary disease (COPD). The lungs are hyperlucent and markedly overexpanded. The diaphragms are flat on the lateral view and nearly flat on the PA radiographs *(straight arrows)*. The retrosternal air space is overexpanded *(curved arrow)*, and the AP dimension of the chest is greater than normal. **C, D:** Chest PA radiograph (C) and axial prone chest CT (D). Idiopathic pulmonary fibrosis. This 79-year-old man had a long history of shortness of breath. On the PA chest radiograph (C) there are typical peripheral white linear streaks *(straight arrows)* that represent fibrosis. The lungs are normally inflated. On CT **(D)**, the fibrosis is mainly peripheral *(straight arrow)* and there is an overall honeycomb appearance to the lung parenchyma.

TABLE 6-3. *Partial list of COPD etiologies*

1. Cigarette smoking
2. Air pollution
3. Childhood infections
4. Heredity

few cubic centimeters of air may be detected on upright radiographs of the lower chest and upper abdomen.

Too Much Air in the Lungs

Chronic obstructive pulmonary disease (COPD) (Fig. 6-47A, B) is a significant health problem that is the fifth commonest cause of death (1), and it has become an important reason for work incapacity. The terminology surrounding lung disease is confusing and includes chronic bronchitis, emphysema, and COPD. COPD is airway obstruction without a specific known pathophysiology. Table 6-3 lists some of the COPD etiologies. On the other hand, emphysema is enlargement of the airspaces distal to the terminal bronchioles without fibrosis (1).

On the other hand, idiopathic pulmonary fibrosis (Fig. 6-47C, D) is a disease characterized by normal inflation or hypoinflation (less than normal ventilation) with associated pulmonary fibrosis that is usually peripheral. It is fortunate the disease is not common because its etiology is unknown.

ATELECTASIS, PULMONARY EMBOLI, AND INFECTIONS

It is important to remember that most pathologic conditions such as pneumonia, tumor, infarct, and atelectasis will appear as water densities or shades of gray on radiographs. So think water density or gray when viewing radiographs and concentrate less on the

TABLE 6-4. *General etiologies of atelectasis*

1. Bronchial obstruction
   a. Tumor
   b. Foreign body
   c. Infection
2. Postoperative
3. Extrinsic pressure
   a. Pleural fluid
   b. Pneumothorax
4. Restrictive motion
   a. Trauma
   b. Neuromuscular diseases
   c. Infections

TABLE 6-5. *Radiographic signs of atelectasis*

Primary
a. Loss of volume of involved segment, lobe, or lung
b. White-appearing airless lung
   1. Air bronchograms
   2. Displaced bronchi and vessels
Secondary
a. Elevation of the hemidiaphragm
b. Mediastinal shift
c. Rib narrowing
d. Indistinct hilum and hilar displacement

black. After all, black densities in the lungs represent air.

Atelectasis

Atelectasis (Figs. 6-48 and 6-49) is the incomplete expansion or loss of volume of a portion of a the lung that ranges from complete collapse of a lung to discoid or plate-like atelectasis. Atelectasis is not a primary disease but a sign of disease or abnormality (3). The general etiologies are listed in Table 6-4 and the radiographic signs are listed in Table 6-5.

Discoid atelectasis (Fig. 6-48) is probably the most common linear opacity found on chest radiographs. It is generally believed that discoid atelectasis results from several factors including decreased diaphragmatic movement, cough-inhibiting factors, and the pooling of secretions. Radiographically discoid atelectasis appears as a horizontal linear density measuring a few millimeters in width and 5–10 cm in length.

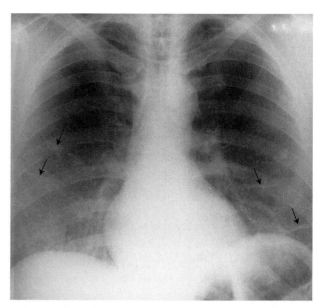

FIG. 6-48. Chest PA radiograph. Bilateral discoid (plate-like) atelectasis. The straight arrows indicate the typical appearance of this abnormality that is commonly found in postoperative, posttrauma, severely ill, and debilitated patients.

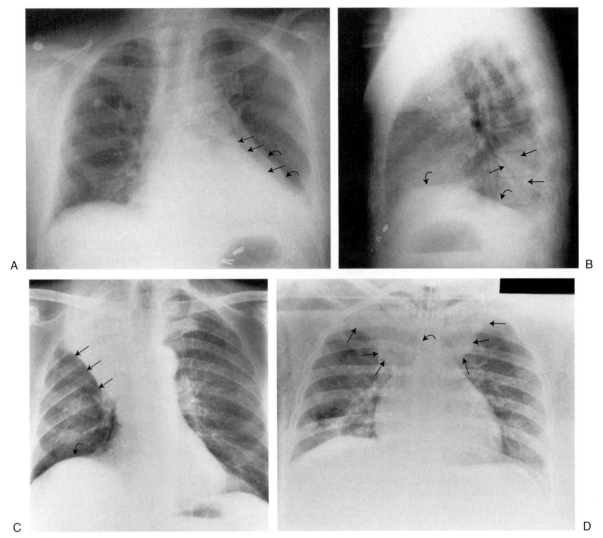

FIG. 6-49. A: Chest PA radiograph. Postoperative left lower lobe atelectasis. There is a double density in the cardiac silhouette, and the straight arrows indicate the edge of the atelectatic left lower lobe whereas the curved arrows indicates the left cardiac border. The left hemidiaphragm is poorly visualized because the water density atelectatic left lower lobe is in juxtaposition to the left hemidiaphragm or a silhouette sign. The patient is mildly rotated to the left. **B:** Chest lateral radiograph. Same patient as in A. There is a positive spine sign *(straight arrows)*. Remember that on the lateral view the spine should appear darker as you proceed caudad because there is more lung in the lower thorax. When a water density disease process like atelectasis or pneumonia is present in the lower lobes, the spine will appear whiter as you proceed caudad rather than darker (spine sign). The left hemidiaphragm cannot be seen as it is silhouetted by the atelectasis in the left lower lobe, but the entire right hemidiaphragm can be seen *(curved arrow)*. **C:** Chest AP radiograph. Right upper lobe atelectasis. There is a water density appearance to the atelectatic right upper lobe, the minor fissure is elevated *(straight arrows)*, the right pulmonary artery and the ascending aorta are silhouetted by the water density atelectasis, and the right hemidiaphragm *(curved arrow)* is elevated. **D:** Chest AP radiograph. Bilateral upper lobe atelectasis *(straight arrows)*. This 30-year-old woman developed bronchospasm in the operating room. Both upper lobes are airless, collapsed, and the mediastinum is silhouetted. The curved arrow indicates the tip of an endotracheal tube.

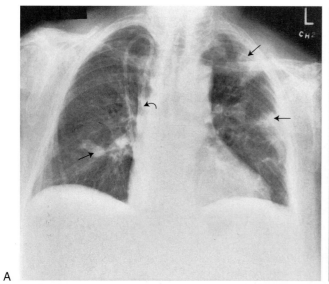

A

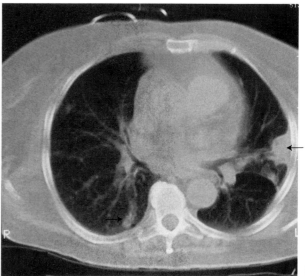

B

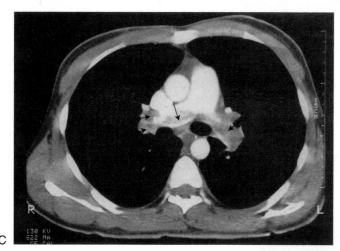

C

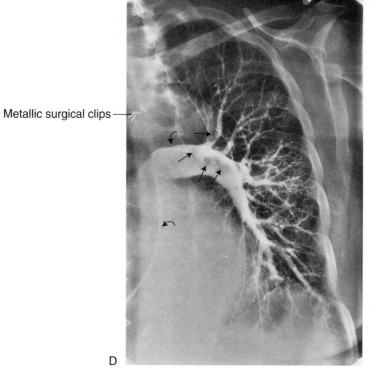

External monitoring electrode

Metallic surgical clips

D

TABLE 6-6. *Common etiologies of pulmonary embolic disease*

1. Venous thromboembolism
   a. Postsurgical
   b. Bed rest
   c. Trauma
   d. Neoplasm
2. Foreign body
   a. Bone marrow post–long bone fracture
   b. Amniotic fluid
3. Septic emboli
4. Air

TABLE 6-7. *Some general etiologies of pneumonia*

1. Infections
   a. Bacterial
   b. Viral
   c. Fungal
   d. Parasitic
2. Aspiration
3. Radiation
4. Chemical

Pulmonary Emboli

Pulmonary emboli have a number of etiologies as shown in Table 6-6. For example, central lines can become infected and septic pulmonary emboli may result (Fig. 6-50A, B).

Pulmonary thromboembolus is an exceedingly common and important clinical problem that often occurs in hospitalized and inactive patients, and the thrombus usually originates in the lower extremity and/or pelvic veins. Pulmonary thromboembolus is the presence of a thrombus or a fragment of thrombus in the pulmonary arterial tree, and the thromboembolus can result in infarction, atelectasis, hemorrhage, or increased pulmonary arterial pressure. The radiographic signs in these patients are highly variable and range from normal to grossly abnormal. Eventually some radiographic abnormality is usually present. A CT study (Fig. 6-50C) may make the diagnosis and eliminate the need for an invasive pulmonary angiogram. However, in some instances a pulmonary angiogram is necessary when radionuclide studies and CT imaging are indeterminate (Fig. 6-50D).

Pulmonary Infections

Pulmonary infections have many etiologies, some of which are listed in Table 6-7. These patients often present with fever and cough, and the cough may or may not be productive. If the cough is productive, the sputum may be colored and even contain blood. Pleuritic and general chest pain may be present. If a pneumonia is mild, the patient may walk into your office, whereas other pneumonias can be severe enough to cause death. The radiographic appearances of pneumonia are highly variable and often it is impossible to determine the etiology of a pneumonia based on the radiologic appearance alone. The radiographic findings vary from a small, ill-defined infiltrate to complete unilateral or bilateral opacification of the lungs (Figs. 6-51 to 6-55). Some pneumonias progress resulting in complications such as empyema, pleural fluid, and abscess formation (Fig. 6-56). Pneumonias can be easily confused with blood, fluid, atelectasis, and even tumor, as they are all water density.

There are many patients who are immune-suppressed secondary to disease or therapy, and they are susceptible to pulmonary tuberculosis (Fig. 6-57). Consequently, pulmonary tuberculosis continues to be a problem dis-

text continues on page 112

FIG. 6-50. A: Chest PA radiograph. Bilateral septic emboli secondary to an infected Hickman catheter. The chest radiograph is grossly abnormal with multiple bilateral water densities *(straight arrows)* secondary to septic emboli and the differential diagnosis would include: pneumonia, emboli, atelectasis, and hemorrhage. The tip of the Hickman catheter *(curved arrow)* is in the superior vena cava. **B:** Chest axial CT through the level of the left atrium in the same patient as A. Bilateral pulmonary septic emboli from the infected Hickman catheter. The emboli *(straight arrows)* are commonly peripheral, wedge-shaped, homogeneous density, and pleural-based. **C:** Chest axial CT through the pulmonary arteries in a different patient than A and B. Bilateral pulmonary artery thromboemboli secondary to lower extremity deep vein phlebothrombosis. This 30-year-old man developed bilateral lower extremity edema and shortness of breath following a long automobile trip. There are filling defects *(straight arrows)* in the right and left pulmonary arteries created by the thromboemboli. These findings necessitated pulmonary embolectomy, anticoagulation, and the placement of a Greenfield filter in his inferior vena cava. As a result of his pulmonary emboli he had pulmonary hypertension. **D:** Left pulmonary arteriogram. Multiple left pulmonary artery embolic thrombi *(straight arrows)* within the left main pulmonary artery and its branches secondary to bilateral lower extremity deep vein phlebothrombosis. This 72-year-old woman was 72 hours postcoronary artery bypass grafting and developed shortness of breath and hypoxia. Radionuclide studies showed probable thromboemboli. The angiographic catheter *(curved arrows)* is visible in the left pulmonary artery.

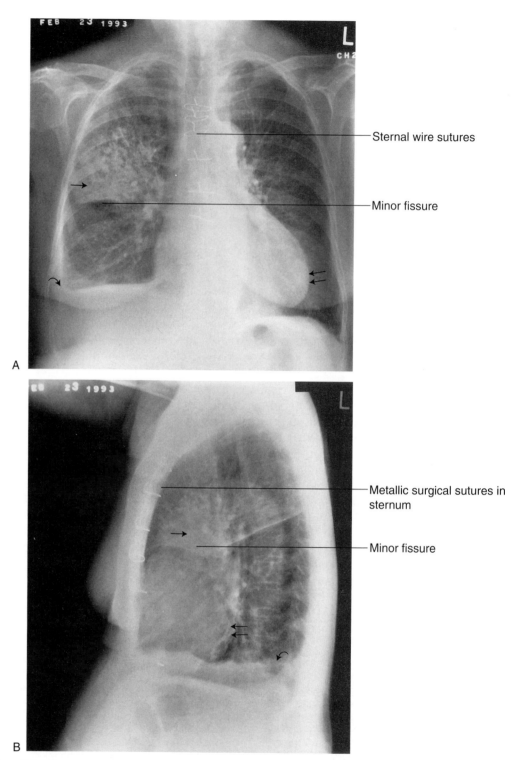

Sternal wire sutures

Minor fissure

Metallic surgical sutures in sternum

Minor fissure

FIG. 6-51. Chest PA **(A)** and lateral **(B)** radiographs. Right upper lobe partially confluent pneumonia *(straight arrows)*. On the PA and lateral views there is a small amount of right pleural fluid *(curved arrows)* and mild left ventricular enlargement *(double arrows)*. Note that the pneumonia is located in the upper lobe above the minor fissure.

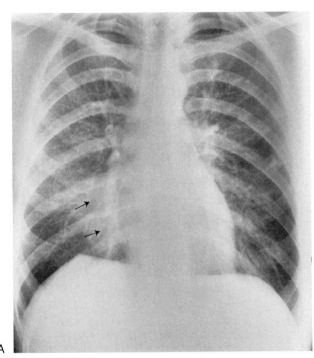

A

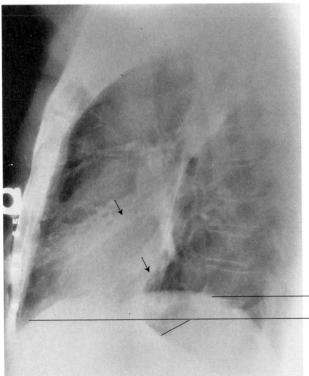

B

FIG. 6-52. Chest PA **(A)** and lateral **(B)** radiographs. Right middle lobe pneumonia *(straight arrows)*. On the PA radiograph the right cardiac border is not visible (silhouette sign) as both the right middle lobe infiltrate and the right atrium are water density and anterior structures. Also, note that the right hemidiaphragm is clearly visible and not silhouetted on the PA view. On the lateral view the pneumonia projects over the heart and partially silhouettes the right anterior hemidiaphragm.

Left hemidiaphragm

Right hemidiaphragm

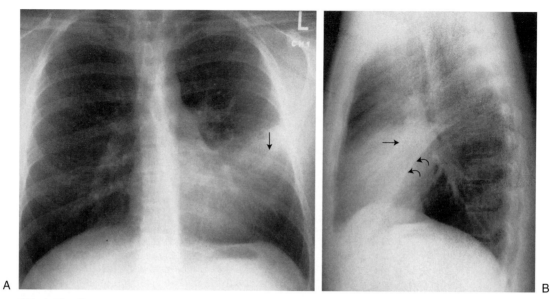

FIG. 6-53. Chest PA **(A)** and lateral **(B)** radiographs. Left upper lobe lingular segments pneumonia *(straight arrows)*. On the PA radiograph the left cardiac border is not visible (silhouette sign) as both the left upper lobe lingular infiltrate and the heart are anterior water densities. Also, note that the left hemidiaphragm is clearly visible (not silhouetted) on the PA view. The curved arrows on the lateral view indicate the left major fissure, and note that the pneumonia projects over the heart.

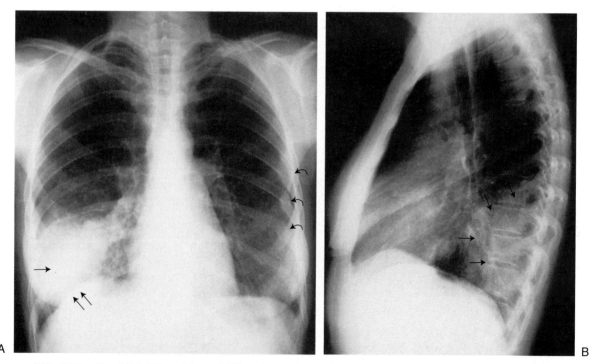

FIG. 6-54. Chest PA **(A)** and lateral **(B)** radiographs. Right lower lobe pneumonia *(straight arrows)*. On the PA radiograph the right cardiac border is clearly visible and the right hemidiaphragm is partially silhouetted *(double straight arrows)*. These findings indicate that the infiltrate is posterior or in the right lower lobe as confirmed on the lateral radiograph *(straight arrows)*. Also, there are old healed left rib fracture deformities *(curved arrows)*. There is a positive spine sign on the lateral radiograph as the spine appears whiter as you proceed down the spine. Normally, the spine appears darker as you descend cephalad to caudad on the lateral view.

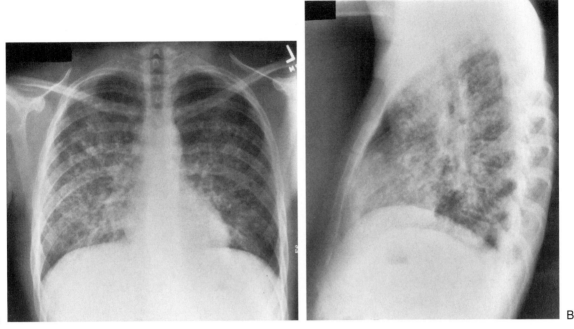

A B

FIG. 6-55. Chest PA **(A)** and lateral **(B)** radiographs. Bilateral varicella (chicken pox) pneumonia. There are diffuse nodular infiltrates throughout both lung fields. These patients are usually critically ill, and the skin lesions help to make the diagnosis.

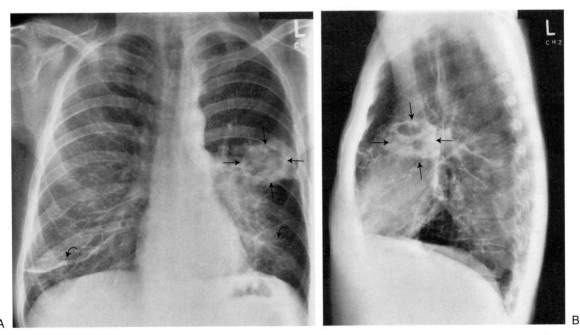

A B

FIG. 6-56. Chest PA **(A)** and lateral **(B)** radiographs. Left upper lobe lingular abscess *(straight arrows)*. There is air within the abscess cavity. Minimal infiltrates are present in the lower lung fields *(curved arrows)*.

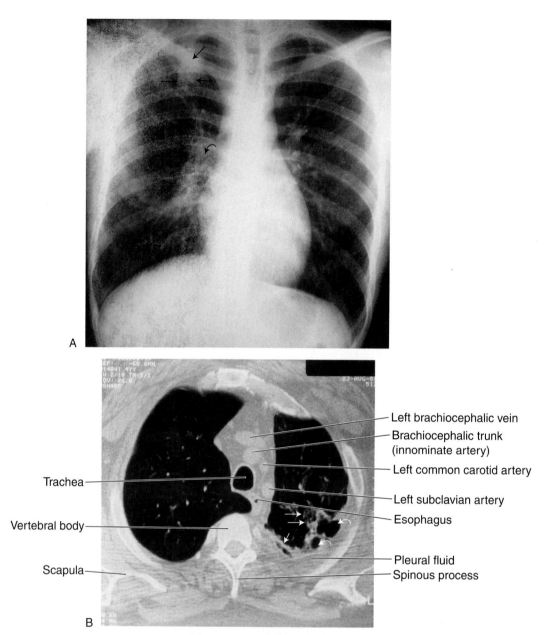

FIG. 6-57. A: Chest PA radiograph. Right upper lobe tuberculosis. The tuberculous infiltrate in the right upper lobe *(straight arrows)* is partially obscured by the right clavicle. There is fullness in the right hilum compatible with hilar lymphadenopathy *(curved arrows).* **B:** Chest axial CT through the upper thorax. Cavitary tuberculosis of the left upper lobe with associated left pleural fluid. The cavitation *(curved arrows)* is surrounded by the tuberculous infiltrate *(straight arrows).*

ease in spite of new therapies and improved public health measures. Tuberculosis should be considered in many pulmonary parenchymal differential diagnoses (Table 6-8).

Tuberculosis patients present with a variety of symptoms ranging from vague fatigue to fever, cough, weight loss, or hemoptysis. Also, the chest radiographic findings vary from a poorly defined infiltrate to obvious infiltrate with or without cavitation. *Remember that the diagnosis must be confirmed by laboratory findings.*

TUMORS

A wide variety of pulmonary nodules and/or tumor masses may be encountered on chest radiographs. These widely located lesions can be single, multiple, calcified, noncalcified, poorly or well defined. One approach to their diagnosis is to divide them into benign and malignant categories (Table 6-9).

Multiple benign granulomas usually do not present much of a diagnostic problem. Solitary granulomas

TABLE 6-8. *Differential diagnosis of pulmonary tuberculosis*

1. All other pneumonias
2. Hemorrhage
3. Emboli
4. Tumor

TABLE 6-9. *A partial list for the differential diagnosis of pulmonary masses*

Benign
1. Granuloma (histoplasmoma, tuberculoma)
2. Adenoma
3. Hamartoma
4. Round pneumonia
5. Bronchogenic and pericardial cysts
6. Arteriovenous malformation
7. Pulmonary infarction

Malignant
1. Primary malignant tumors
   a. Squamous cell carcinoma (epidermoid carcinoma)
   b. Adenocarcinoma
   c. Alveolar cell carcinoma (bronchiolar carcinoma)
   e. Bronchial adenoma
2. Lymphoma
3. Metastatic neoplasm

are easy to diagnose if they contain typical dense calcifications. These calcifications are variable in appearance including a diffusely homogeneous pattern, a centrally located nidus, multiple foci, or laminated. When such calcifications are present a fairly confident diagnosis of benign granuloma can be made (Fig. 6-58). When the presence of calcification is not a certainty, CT imaging can be utilized to measure the density of the mass. When a pulmonary nodule

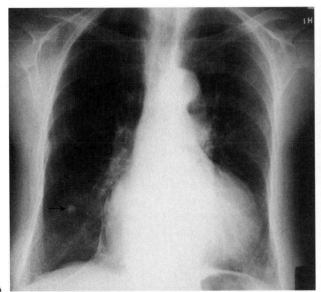

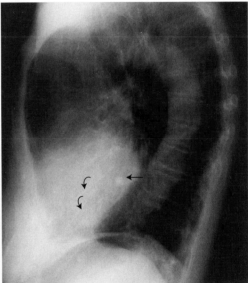

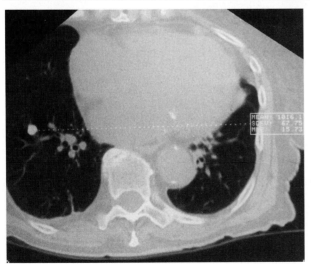

FIG. 6-58. Chest PA (A) and lateral (B) radiographs. Calcified granuloma *(arrows)* in the right lower lobe. The homogeneous high-density appearance of this small nodule strongly suggests calcification and that makes the diagnosis of granuloma fairly certain, and no further workup was probably needed. Its location is assisted by the identification of the major fissures *(curved arrows)* on the lateral view. Incidentally, there is mild cardiomegaly and hyperinflation of the lungs due to chronic obstructive pulmonary disease. C: Chest axial CT through the left atrium level. The lesion in the right lower lobe is very dense and calcific in appearance, and the lesion measures 1016 Hounsfield units. These findings indicate a high probability that it is a benign granuloma.

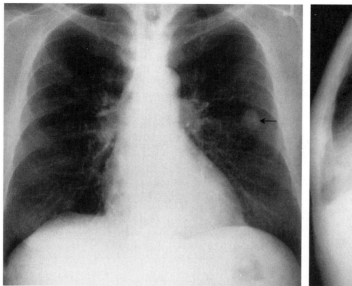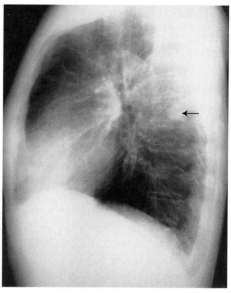

A   B

FIG. 6-59. Chest PA **(A)** and lateral **(B)** radiographs. Histoplasmoma superior segment left lower lobe *(arrows)*. This noncalcified solitary nodule was seen on a routine chest radiograph on this 58-year-old asymptomatic man. The differential diagnosis of a solitary noncalcified pulmonary nodule was entertained, and malignancy could not be excluded. Thoracotomy and resection of the lesion resulted in the diagnosis of a benign histoplasmoma.

measures greater than 200 Hounsfield units on a CT study, there is a very high probability that the lesion is a calcified benign granuloma or hamartoma and no further workup is necessary. A noncalcified mass does require further evaluation, and the workup varies with the clinical circumstances. A solitary noncalcified nodule that does not change in size or appearance in 2 years is probably benign (Fig. 6-59). This rule should be applied with caution, as there are exceptions.

In addition to noncalcification, other factors that are suspicious for malignancy include poorly defined margins, rapid growth pattern, pleural fluid, atelectasis, bone destruction, and a long history of cigarette smoking. The workup of these suspicious masses range from obtaining old radiographs and follow-up radiographs to CT imaging, percutaneous biopsy, and actual thoracotomy.

The location of a mass is sometimes useful in arriving at a diagnosis, especially if the mass is determined to be in the mediastinum. Classically, the mediastinum can be divided into three general areas, and the following is an easy and simplified method to remember these mediastinal compartments. The anterior mediastinum lies between the sternum anteriorly and the anterior aspect of the pericardium and aorta. Tumor masses found in this area can be characterized by the letter T that represents a differential diagnosis of thyroid masses, teratoma, thymus masses, and tortuous or aneurysmal vessels (Fig. 6-60A, B). The middle mediastinum includes the heart, pericardium, the great vessels, and

the proximal bronchi (Fig. 6-60C, D). The posterior mediastinum (Fig. 6-60E, F) extends from the posterior aspect of the pericardium to the dorsal spine vertebral bodies and includes the paravertebral gutters (1). A differential diagnosis can be made for a radiographic mass in each of these compartments (Table 6-10). Again, the silhouette sign will help to locate the mass depending on which structure borders are obscured by the mass. Notice that lymph nodes are found in all parts of the mediastinum, so that a lymphoma may occur in any thoracic location (Fig. 6-61).

TABLE 6-10. *Differential diagnosis for mediastinal masses*

Anterior mediastinum
1. Thyroid and parathyroid masses
2. Thymus masses (Fig. 6-60A, B)
3. Teratoma
4. Tortuous vessels such as aneurysm of ascending aorta (Fig. 6-66A, B)
5. Lymph nodes

Middle mediastinum
1. Pericardial fat pad and pericardial cyst (Fig. 6-61A, B)
2. Bronchogenic cyst and bronchogenic carcinoma
3. Lymph nodes
4. Diaphragm hernia (Morgagni)
5. Dilated great vessels including aneurysms

Posterior mediastinum
1. Neurogenic tumors
2. Duplication cysts
3. Lymph nodes
4. Esophageal lesions including esophageal hiatal hernia (Fig. 6-44A, B)

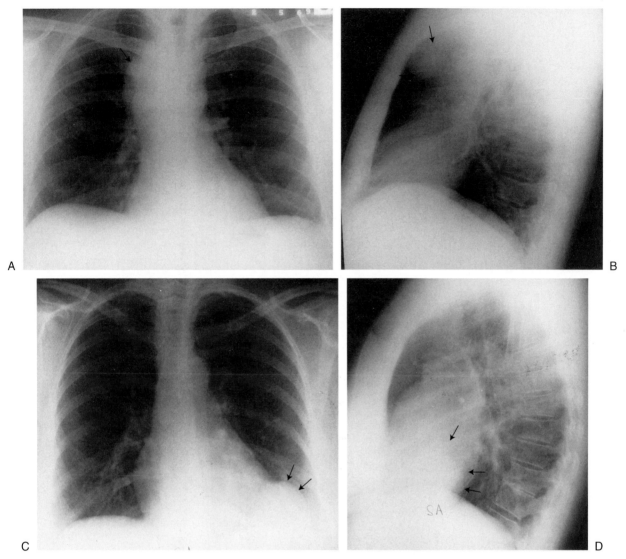

FIG. 6-60. Chest PA **(A)** and lateral **(B)** radiographs. Thymoma *(straight arrows)*. The lesion clearly lies in the anterior mediastinum. **C, D:** Chest PA **(C)** and lateral **(D)** radiographs. Pericardial cyst *(straight arrows)*.

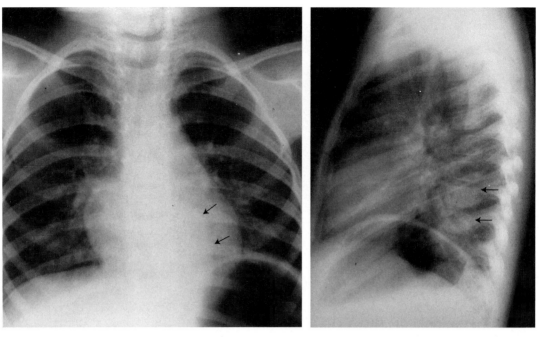

E   F

FIG. 6-60. *Continued.* This lesion was found on a routine chest radiograph in an asymptomatic 54-year-old female patient. These oval masses usually are on the right side at the cardiohepatic angle. This left-sided pericardial cyst lies near the apex of the cardiac silhouette on the PA view and projects over the heart on the lateral view. The differential diagnosis was left ventricle aneurysm, bronchogenic cyst, Morgagni hernia, and diaphragmatic tumor. The diagnosis can sometimes be made by ultrasound or CT imaging. In this case the diagnosis was made at thoracotomy. **E, F:** Chest PA (E) and lateral (F) radiographs. Neuroblastoma. In the PA view the mass can be seen through the cardiac shadow *(straight arrows)*. The lateral view shows the mass to be posterior as there is loss of distinction of the lower dorsal spine vertebral bodies and a positive spine sign.

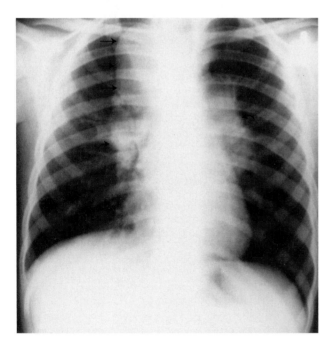

FIG. 6-61. Chest PA radiograph. Lymphoma. This young adult male was admitted because of an abnormal white blood count. There is a large mediastinal mass *(straight arrows)* with associated bilateral hilar lymphadenopathy *(curved arrows)*. The mass resides within the anterior and middle mediastinum. This is a typical appearance of lymphoma of the chest.

Although some chest masses are difficult to detect, the visualization of most masses is fairly straightforward. A tumor mass can cause secondary signs that may be the first indication of a mass. Some secondary signs or complications suggesting the presence of tumor are atelectasis, malignant pleural effusions, cavitation of the

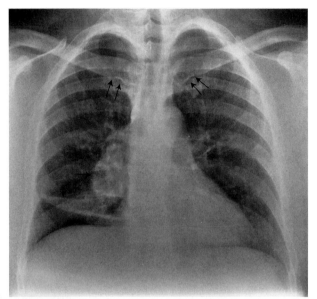

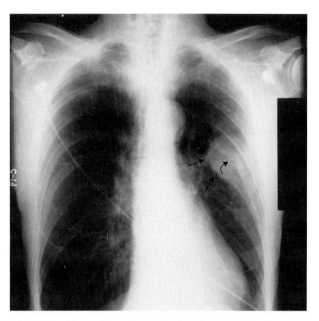

FIG. 6-63. Chest AP radiograph. Carcinoma of the lung with rib destruction. The moderately sized primary carcinoma in the left upper lobe *(straight arrows)* has partially destroyed the left 7th rib *(curved arrow)*. Note how overexpanded the lungs are, probably secondary to chronic obstructive pulmonary disease. A monitoring electrode runs across the thorax from left to right.

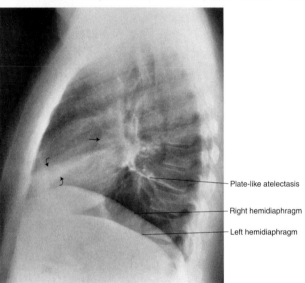

Plate-like atelectasis

Right hemidiaphragm

Left hemidiaphragm

FIG. 6-62. Chest PA **(A)** and lateral **(B)** radiographs. Right infrahilar primary neoplasm *(straight arrows)* causing right middle lobe atelectasis *(curved arrows)*. The right hemidiaphragm is mildly elevated secondary to the right middle lobe atelectasis. Note on the lateral view how nicely you can see the right and left hemidiaphragms. The right hemidiaphragm can be seen in its entirety whereas the left hemidiaphragm is silhouetted anteriorly by the heart. The double arrows indicate bilateral infraclavicular notching or rhomboid fossae. These fossae are a variation of normal, and they give origin to the costoclavicular or rhomboid ligaments. [1]

tumor, hilar nodal enlargement, and local bone destruction (Figs. 6-62 to 6-64).

Detecting metastatic disease to the lungs is extremely important when caring for patients with primary neoplasms. Routine chest radiographs and CT imaging are used extensively to detect metastatic disease (Fig. 6-65).

CARDIAC AND GREAT VESSELS

Unfortunately, the radiographic appearance of cardiac chambers does not correlate with their function. Echocardiography, magnetic resonance imaging, and cine CT allow not only improved cardiac anatomy visualization but physiologic and motion imaging such as ejection fractions and valve movement. However, this section is confined to static imaging.

Aneurysms, Enlarged Vessels, and Vascular Calcifications

An aneurysm of the thoracic aorta is a significant acquired abnormality. These aneurysms may present as a mass in any of the three mediastinal areas depending on their exact location (Fig. 6-66). Of course, aneurysms can occur in the pulmonary arteries or any other thoracic artery. On occasion, there are clinical situations wherein the central pulmonary arteries become markedly en-

text continues on page 121

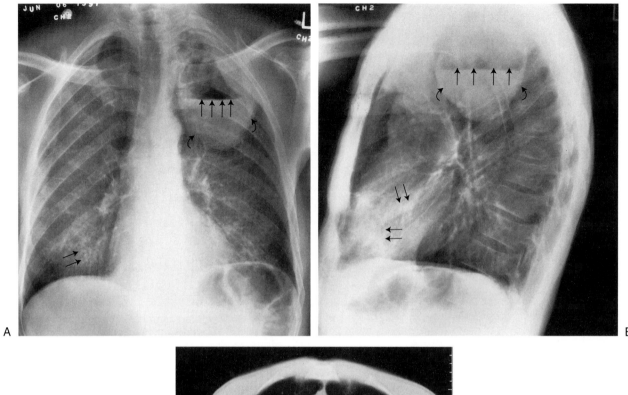

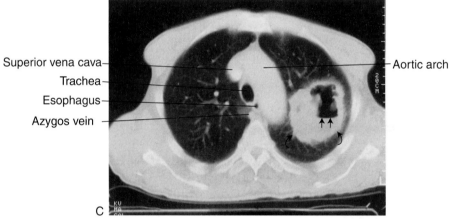

FIG. 6-64. Chest PA **(A)** and lateral **(B)** radiographs and a chest axial CT image **(C)** through the level of the aortic arch. Cavitating primary squamous cell carcinoma of the left upper lobe. The large tumor mass *(curved arrows)* contains an air–fluid level *(straight arrows)* that is secondary to necrotizing tumor. There is a partially confluent pneumonia in the right middle lobe *(double straight arrows)*.

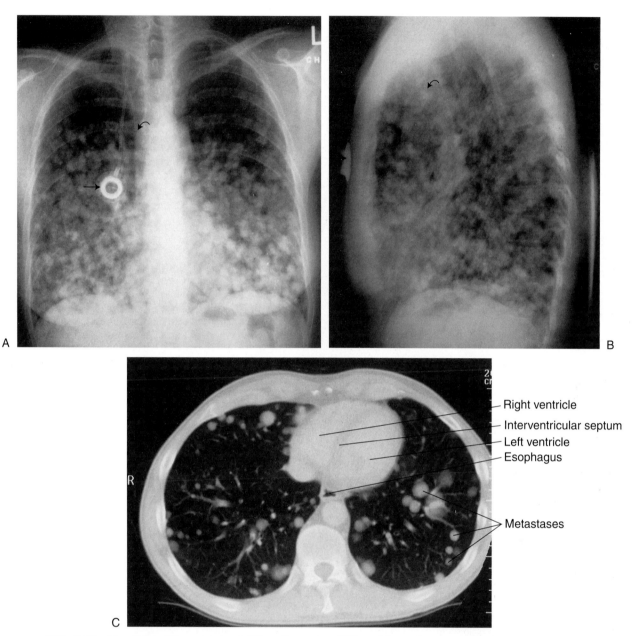

FIG. 6-65. Chest PA **(A)** and lateral **(B)** radiographs. Diffuse bilateral metastases. The metastatic lesions are not calcified and typically are variable in size. The infusaport *(straight arrows)* is used to administer medications. The tip of the infusaport catheter *(curved arrows)* projects over the superior vena cava in both views. **(C)** Chest axial chest CT through the level of the ventricles. The multiple widespread metastases are variable in size.

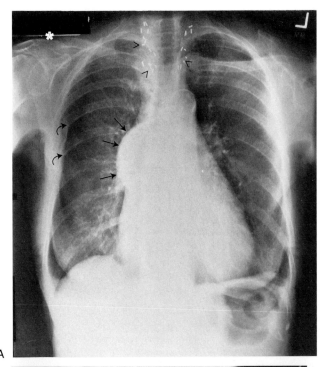

A

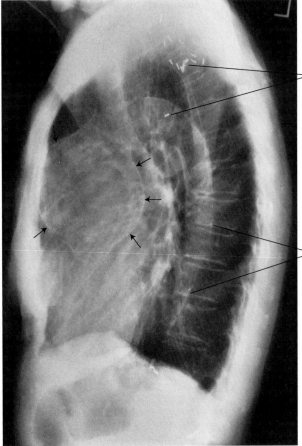

B

FIG. 6-66. Chest PA **(A)** and lateral **(B)** radiographs. Large calcified ascending thoracic aorta aneurysm *(straight arrows)*. The aneurysmal calcification is faint on both views. On the PA radiograph the heart appears enlarged but on the lateral view it is within normal limits. Note the old healed right 6th and 7th rib fracture deformities *(curved arrows)*. The lungs are hyperinflated. Note the surgical clips *(arrowheads)* and the artefact (*) appearing on the right shoulder.

Surgical metallic clips

Calcified descending thoracic aorta

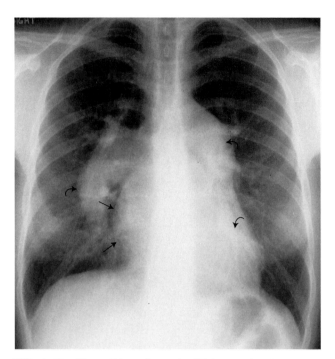

FIG. 6-67. Chest PA radiograph. Right atrial enlargement and large pulmonary arteries. The right atrium is enlarging to the patient's right side *(straight arrows)*, and the pulmonary arteries are larger than normal *(curved arrows)*. The etiology in this patient is unknown.

larged (Fig. 6-67), and a partial differential diagnosis is listed in Table 6-11.

Calcification of thoracic vessels does occur and should be recognized as such on radiographs and CT images (Fig. 6-68).

Pulmonary Edema

Pulmonary edema (Fig. 6-69) is a common and extremely important problem encountered by the primary physician and almost all health care providers. There are many etiologies for pulmonary edema (Table 6-12). The most common etiology is left-sided cardiac disease that results in an increased pulmonary venous pressure. These patients may complain of dyspnea on exertion, orthopnea, paroxysmal nocturnal respiratory distress, weight gain, lower extremity edema, cough, and, on occasion, hemoptysis.

TABLE 6-12. *Etiologies of pulmonary edema*

1. Cardiogenic
2. Neurogenic
3. Increased permeability
   a. Toxic inhalation
   b. High-altitude sickness
   c. Aspiration
   d. Contusion
   e. Fat embolism

It is important to appreciate and recognize the wide variety of radiographic presentations that may occur in this clinical problem (Table 6-13). The first radiographic sign of pulmonary edema is generally considered to be a redistribution of the blood flow to the upper lobes. Normally the lower lobe vessels are three times larger than the upper lobe vessels. As the pulmonary venous pressure increases, patchy infiltrates appear representing fluid in the acini. These infiltrates may have a bat wing appearance around the hilum and are usually more predominant in the lower lung fields due to a gravitational effect. Kerley B lines or thickening of the interlobular septa and pleural effusions eventually appear secondary to the increased venous and lymphatic pressures. As edema surrounds the pulmonary vessels, they tend to become indistinct with surrounding cuffs. Pleural effusions are common in pulmonary edema and have a variety of appearances as seen in Fig. 6-69. Occasionally chest decubitus views (the patient lies on their side) are obtained when pleural effusions are suspected or if it is important to know if the pleural fluid is free flowing (see Fig. 5-69E).

Widening of the vascular pedicle can occur when there is too much fluid and salt circulating as in fluid overload and pulmonary edema. The vascular pedicle width is measured from the superior vena cava as it crosses the right main stem bronchus to the aortic arch where approximately the subclavian artery arises. The azygos vein lies lateral to the right main stem bronchus and tends to enlarge in similar situations.

In situations characterized by increased capillary permeability as in adult respiratory distress syndrome, the edematous pattern is more diffuse and more patchy and tends to change very slowly.

TABLE 6-11. *Partial differential diagnosis of enlarged pulmonary arteries*

High-volume situations
1. Left-to-right shunts
2. High cardiac output situations (anemias, thyrotoxicosis)

Peripheral arterial narrowing and occlusion
1. Thromboembolic disease
2. Idiopathic pulmonary hypertension

TABLE 6-13. *Radiographic findings in pulmonary edema*

1. Redistribution (increase size of vessels to the upper lobes)
2. Patchy infiltrates (bat wing and gravitational)
3. Kerley B lines
4. Interlobar fissure thickening
5. Pleural fluid
6. Parahilar zone bronchial cuffing
7. Parahilar vessels less distinct

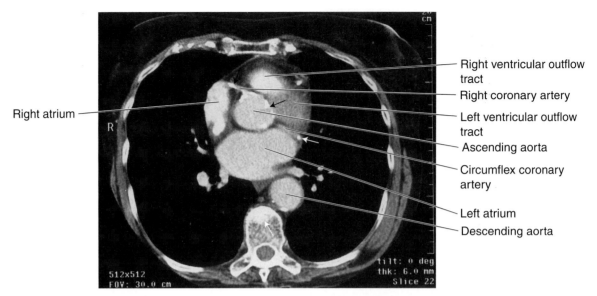

FIG. 6-68. Chest axial CT image through the level of the left atrium. The right coronary artery, the circumflex coronary artery, ascending and descending aorta all contain calcifications *(straight arrows)*.

Valvular Heart Disease

Acquired and congenital cardiac valve diseases have the potential to cause chamber enlargement and pulmonary edema. Valve disease can obstruct the flow of blood out of a chamber (stenosis) or the valve may allow retrograde flow (regurgitation). Either situation can result in increased pressure and size in the involved cardiac chamber. Two good examples of this type of problem are found in diseases of the mitral valve (Fig. 6-70) and the aortic valve (Fig. 6-71).

As the left atrium enlarges, it can create a double density along the right heart border as the enlarged left atrium projects through the right atrium. Also, the enlarging left atrium may widen the tracheal bifurcation and elevate the left main stem bronchus. As the left atrium and/or atrial appendage enlarge, they create a bulge along the left upper cardiac border (Fig. 6-70A).

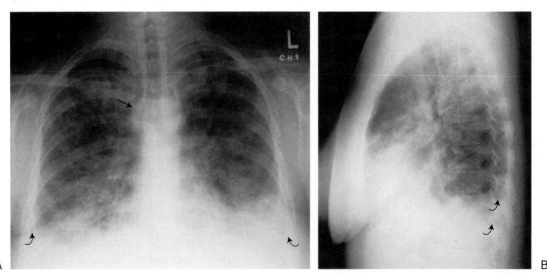

FIG. 6-69. Chest PA **(A)** and lateral **(B)** radiographs. Congestive heart failure or pulmonary edema. The azygos vein *(straight arrow)* is enlarged. The pulmonary vasculature is increased on both views, especially toward the bases (gravitational). The pulmonary vessels are indistinct, and there are bilateral pleural effusions *(curved arrows)*. It is interesting to note that the cardiac size is within normal limits suggesting a sudden onset of pulmonary edema.

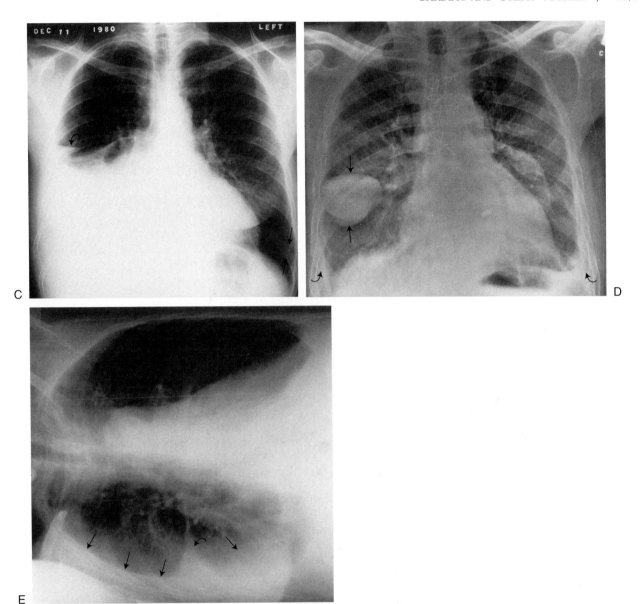

FIG. 6-69. *Continued.* **(C)** Chest PA radiograph. Congestive heart failure with Kerley B lines. This 42-year-old woman had a myocardial infarction 2 months prior to these chest radiographs and now complains of orthopnea. Kerley B lines are the white horizontal lines in the lateral lung bases *(straight arrows)*, and they represent fluid in the lymphatics. These lines are another radiographic sign of pulmonary edema. There is a large right pleural effusion and some of the fluid is entering the minor fissure *(curved arrow)*. The pleural effusion silhouettes or obliterates the right hemidiaphragm, as well as the right cardiac border, making it difficult to assess the cardiac size. **D:** Chest PA radiograph. Pseudo-tumor sign and congestive heart failure. There is mild to moderate cardiomegaly and bilateral pleural effusions *(curved arrows)*. Pleural fluid secondary to the pulmonary edema has accumulated in the minor fissure *(straight arrows)* mimicking a tumor, hence the term pseudo-tumor. This nicely demonstrates that the fissures are contiguous with the pleural space. **E:** Chest right lateral decubitus radiograph. Moderate amount of free-flowing right pleural fluid. The free-flowing pleural fluid *(straight arrows)* flows cephalad in the dependent right pleural space. Some of the pleural fluid flows into the minor fissure *(curved arrow)*.

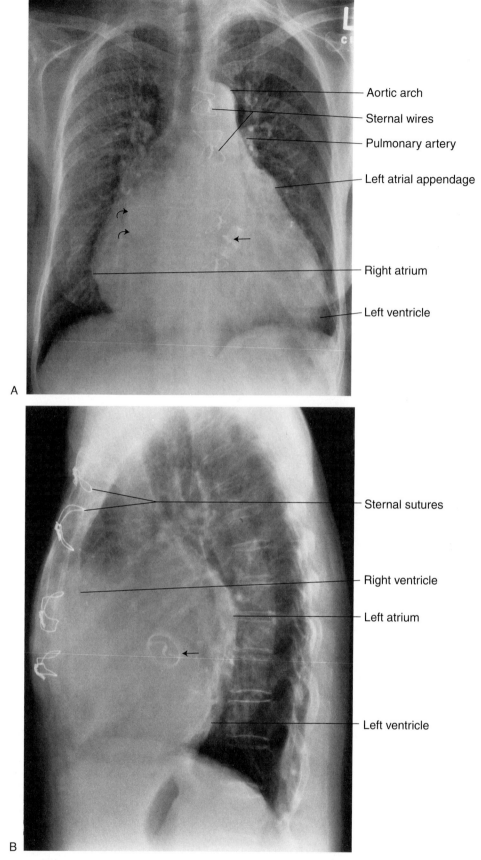

FIG. 6-70. Chest PA **(A)** and lateral **(B)** radiographs. Severe cardiomegaly and a prosthetic mitral valve *(straight arrows).* The patient had mitral valve stenosis and regurgitation that necessitated a prosthetic mitral valve. All of the cardiac chambers are enlarged. On the PA view the enlarged left atrium creates the double density indicated by the curved arrows, and the left atrial appendage is prominent along the left cardiac border. Also, on the PA view there is right atrial and left ventricular enlargement. On the lateral view enlargement of the right ventricle results in fullness of the retrosternal space. Also, on the lateral view there is enlargement of the left atrium and ventricle.

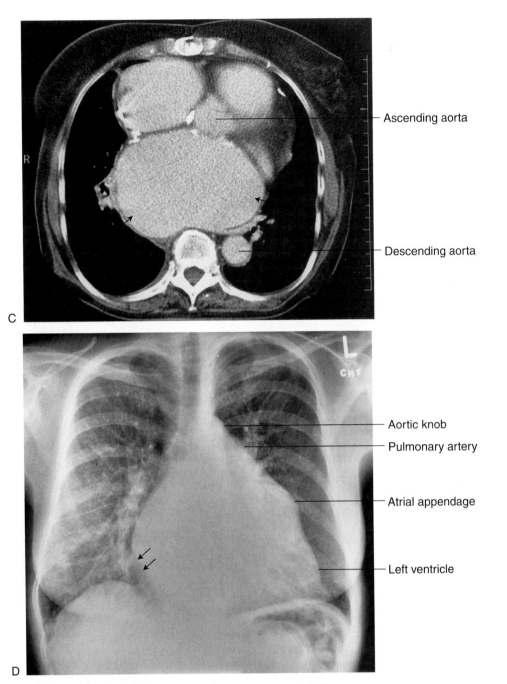

— Ascending aorta

— Descending aorta

C

— Aortic knob
— Pulmonary artery

— Atrial appendage

— Left ventricle

D

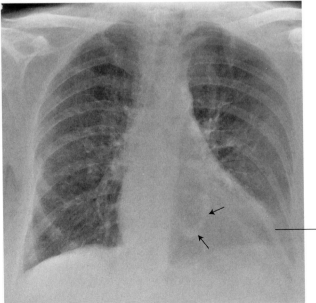

— Left ventricle

E

FIG. 6-70. *Continued.* **C:** Chest axial CT image through the atrium level. Left atrial enlargement *(straight arrows).* This is a different patient from that in A and B. This patient also had mitral stenosis resulting in left atrial enlargement. **D:** Chest PA radiograph. Mitral stenosis and cardiomegaly. There is a nice demonstration of the classic moguls in mitral stenosis that are visible along the left cardiac border consisting of the aortic knob, a prominent left pulmonary artery, the enlarged left atrial appendage, and the left ventricle. Also, the double density of an enlarged left atrium *(straight arrows)* can be identified. **E:** Chest PA radiograph. Mitral annulus calcification *(straight arrows).* This patient was asymptomatic and the calcified mitral annulus was an incidental finding on a routine chest study. There is mild cardiomegaly with mild enlargement of the left ventricle.

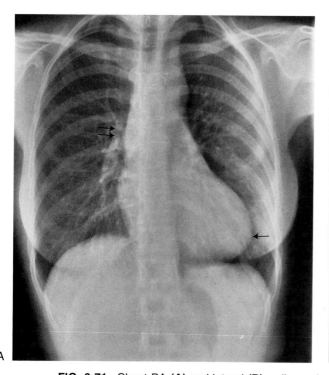 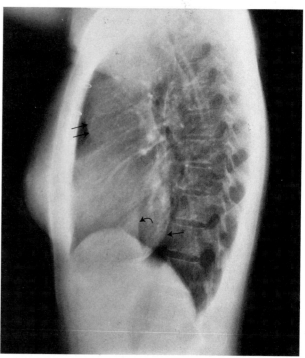

FIG. 6-71. Chest PA **(A)** and lateral **(B)** radiographs. Aortic valve stenosis and regurgitation. Systolic and diastolic aortic valve murmurs were discovered during a routine physical examination. There is left ventricular enlargement *(straight arrows)* manifest by rounding of the cardiac apex on the PA view, and on the lateral view the enlarged left ventricle projects more than 2 cm posterior to the inferior vena cava *(curved arrow)*. The latter finding is a fairly reliable sign for left ventricular enlargement. The ascending aorta shows poststenotic dilatation *(double straight arrows)*, and this is often found in aortic stenosis.

Key Points

- PA and lateral views are the routine standard chest radiographs.
- AP is the standard portable chest radiograph.
- If thoracic bone imaging is necessary, it is best to order the specific radiographs such as ribs, shoulders, or dorsal spine.
- Position chest radiographs on the viewbox with the patient's labeled right side opposite the viewer's left hand, and this generally applies to almost all other images.
- Develop a simple systematic approach for viewing chest radiographs to avoid errors of omission.
- The cardiac transverse diameter should not exceed 50% of thoracic cage transverse diameter. This is called the *cardiothoracic ratio.*
- Cardiac size estimation is most generally accomplished by gross eyeballing and becomes easier with experience.
- Cardiac size appears larger on the AP than the PA view due to magnification.
- The right atrium forms the convex right cardiac border, and the left ventricle forms the cardiac apex on AP or PA radiographs.
- On a chest radiograph look for water densities, as most chest radiographic pathology is water density.
- Excessive black density on a chest radiograph generally indicates too much air, and its location will help make the diagnosis.
- When two similar densities abut each other, it is virtually impossible to differentiate their borders on a radiograph. This is called the "silhouette sign."

REFERENCES

1. Fraser RS, Pare JA, Fraser RG, Pare PD. *Synopsis of Diseases of the Chest,* 2nd ed. Philadelphia: WB Saunders, 1994.
2. Edeiken J. *Roentgen Diagnosis of Diseases of Bone*, 4th ed. Baltimore: Williams and Wilkins, 1990.
3. Juhl JH, Crummy AB. *Paul and Juhl's Essentials of Radiologic Imaging*, 6th ed. Philadelphia: JB Lippincott, 1993.

FURTHER SUGGESTED READINGS

El-Khoury GY, Bergman RA, Montgomery WJ. *Sectional Anatomy by MRI*, 2nd ed. New York: Churchill Livingstone, 1995.

CHAPTER 7

Pediatric Chest Radiology

Wilbur L. Smith

NORMAL

Children are not merely small adults. Surely the body parts (hearts, eyes, noses) are the same, but the fact that children are growing and changing, subjects them to different diseases as well as to different structural appearances. Chest radiographs of young children, for instance, feature that ubiquitous, often misdiagnosed, anterior mediastinal mass, the thymus (Fig. 7-1). This organ, important in the immune response, usually becomes inconspicuous by age 5 or so; however, its involution is extremely variable, and it is not uncommon to find thymic remnants on chest CT scans up to age 20 years (Figs. 7-2 and 3). The thymus is a living piece of tissue that changes its configuration in a number of ways. In response to stress, it may shrink. When indented by the ribs, it may form a wavy border and in pathologic conditions, such as a pneumomediastinum, it may even be displaced superiorly and laterally over the lung fields (Figs. 7-4 to 7-6). The first rule in looking at children's radiographs is, expect change and variation and consider those factors before inventing a disorder that isn't real.

NEONATAL CHEST

The newborn's chest radiograph is a complex study with a substantial number of differences from that of an adult (Fig. 7-7). All babies have to change from an intrauterine environment where their lungs are fluid-filled to one where they are breathing air. This transformation, which must occur within moments of birth, involves interaction of the pulmonary lymphatics, capillary vessels, and chest compression. This normal biologic process is not always smooth. In fact, many babies, if not all, have some very short-lived tachypnea in the first minute or two after being born, owing to the vagaries of clearing their normal in utero lung fluid. The physiologic phenomenon is reflected as the pleural effusions and streaky densities seen in the lungs on radiographs taken shortly after birth. In an insignificant number of babies, it takes longer than a few moments to clear all of the in utero lung fluid. This condition has been aptly termed *transient tachypnea of the newborn* (TTN) (Fig. 7-8). TTN should resolve clinically and radiographically within 24 hours, leaving behind a normal chest. In the first hours of life, however, this picture leads to a great clinical quandary because the radiograph of the neonate with TTN is indistinguishable from the radiograph of early neonatal pneumonia. There are a few clues, such as the presence of a large pleural effusion, which favors pneumonia; however, a definitive distinction can never be made. Here is a classic health care conundrum. TTN is much more common than neonatal pneumonia; however, conventional diagnostic tests cannot separate the two. The outcome of an untreated neonatal pneumonia is dire, so what do you do? Most prudent physicians bite the bullet and treat, knowing that in many instances the antibiotics are unnecessary.

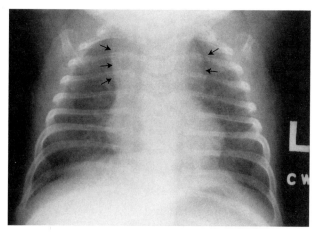

FIG. 7-1. The large superior mediastinal mass that bulges both to the right and to the left is the thymus in this normal 3-month-old infant.

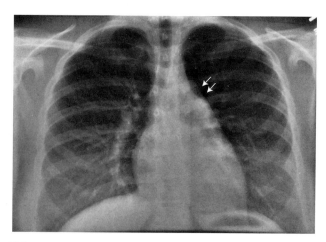

FIG. 7-2. This teenager has a clearly visible thymic edge *(arrows)* on chest x-ray. Visualization of the thymus in normal teenagers is an unusual, but not rare, finding.

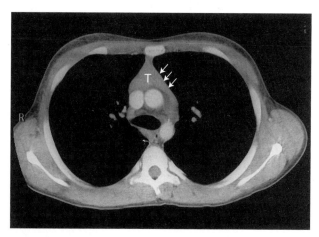

FIG. 7-3. Chest CT of a 16-year-old patient shows a large thymus anterior to the opacified vessels. Note how the left lobe of the thymus (T) sticks out to abut the lung *(arrows)*.

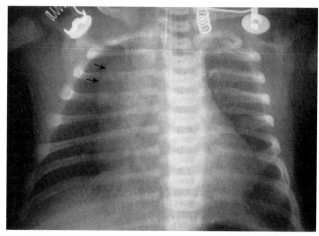

FIG. 7-4. The large anterior mediastinal mass with the irregular margin *(arrows)* is the thymus. The thymic wave sign or undulating thymic border occurs because the costal cartilages are made of more firm tissue than the thymus itself; therefore, the thymus itself is indented. This is a normal finding.

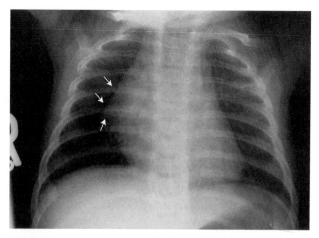

FIG. 7-5. The so-called thymic sail sign shows the sharp edge of the thymus, somewhat like a boat sail, projected against the lung.

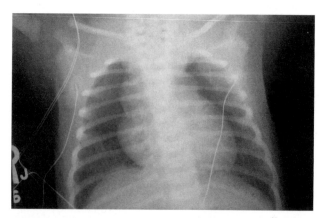

FIG. 7-6. The large superior mediastinal mass in this otherwise well-term neonate is the thymus. If you call anything in the anterior superior mediastinum of a neonate normal thymus, you will be right 99% of the time.

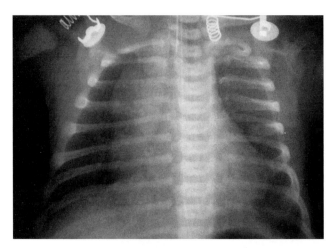

FIG. 7-7. A normal newborn infant's chest. Notice the very different appearance from an adult chest. First the heart and thymus are much larger than the cardiomediastinal silhouette of an adult. If you measure the heart and thymus (cardiothymic structures) and compare it to the diameter of the chest, often a baby's cardiothymic ratio will exceed 60% of the chest diameter. This is still normal. Notice also that the bones are very different with a number of growth plates and other variants owing to infant development.

This situation demonstrates the principle that if the perceived severity of possible outcome is great, it alters the treatment choice when diagnosis is ambiguous. In other words, if you cannot tell, but the patient might die if you don't treat, overtreating is often acceptable.

There are other neonatal lung diseases that exhibit radiographs showing bilateral streaky densities. Transient tachypnea of the newborn is the prototype for this appearance; however, neonatal pneumonia, neonatal venous stasis, and neonatal congestive heart failure can be mimicked. A few points of differentiation are possible. A large pleural effusion usually favors pneumonia and specifically *reactive* pneumonia, owing to group B streptococcal infection (Fig. 7-9). Most neonatal pneumonias are acquired during the birth process, so that these pneumonias start small and tend to get dramatically worse over the first few days of life. If the streaky densities are associated with marked overaeration of the lungs, one might think of meconium aspiration. This disorder occurs when the newborns release their sphincters, spilling meconium into the amniotic fluid. This sphincter release, a response to stress, usually occurs in utero and the meconium is aspirated as the child begins to try to breathe. This is a particularly nasty pneumonia because the meconium is both irritating and viscous, so that it obstructs the airways as well as causing the reactive pneumonia. One of the tips for diagnosing meconium aspiration is the massive hyperinflation of the lungs usually seen on the chest x-ray (Fig. 7-10).

Babies can get congestive heart failure for a number of reasons, some of which involve intrinsic heart disease and many of which do not (Fig. 7-11). Arrhythmias, anemia, and arteriovenous shunts can cause high-output failure that is indistinguishable by chest x-ray from the failure caused by intrinsic heart lesions such as hypoplastic left heart. The best clue that the streaky density pattern you are looking at on the chest x-ray is owing to heart disease is cardiomegaly. Beyond that it is difficult to be more precise. The most important thing is to remember heart failure in your differential diagnosis.

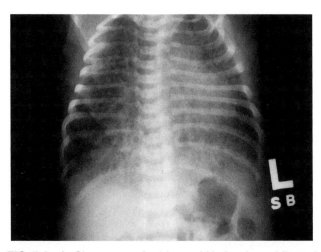

FIG. 7-8. A: Chest x-ray of a 4-hour-old baby shows bilateral streaky densities whose distribution is asymmetric. Note that the lungs are also very hyperinflated. All this cleared within 24 hours and the findings were due to transient tachypnea of the newborn. On this film alone, however, you cannot exclude pneumonia. It is necessary to have the follow-up film to confirm the diagnosis of transient tachypnea.

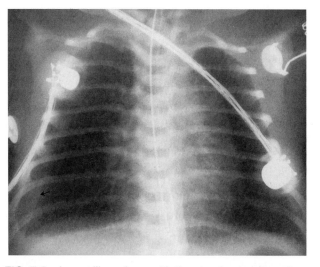

FIG. 7-9. A very ill newborn with the streaky density pattern in both lungs and a large pleural effusion *(arrow)* on the right. Pneumonia plus a pleural effusion usually means group B strep infection in neonates.

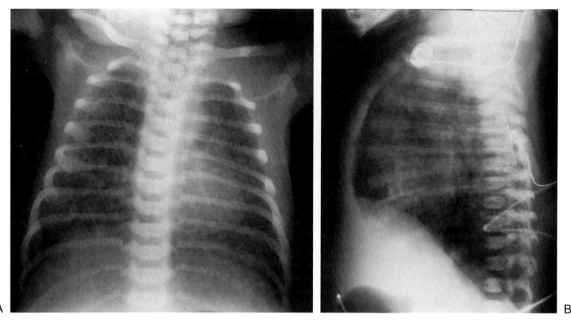

FIG. 7-10. The anterior posterior radiograph **(A)** and lateral radiograph **(B)** of a 1-day-old infant with severe meconium aspiration, showing marked hyperinflation of the lungs and bilateral streaky densities in both lung fields consistent with meconium aspiration. Notice on the lateral view (B) how flat the diaphragms are and how prominent the anterior posterior diameter of the chest is. Meconium aspiration is highly associated with air block phenomenon.

HYALINE MEMBRANE DISEASE

A common disorder of neonates is hyaline membrane disease (HMD). Here the clinical information helps a lot as most of these infants are premature and most do not have respiratory distress immediately after birth. The other good news is that the radiographs are virtually diagnostic in the vast majority of cases (Fig. 7-12). The HMD radiograph shows four characteristic features: (a) diffuse granularity, (b) uniform disease, (c) air bronchograms, and (d) a relatively small lung volume. Not all radiographs will show all of these features, but most will have at least three. HMD occurs owing to a lack of the lipid chemical surfactant that is synthesized by the alveolar lining cells of term infants. These type 2 alveolar lining cells develop and mature during the third trimester of pregnancy; therefore, they are deficient among premature infants. Surfactant works by lowering the surface tension of the alveoli, allowing them to remain expanded. A simple analogy is that of a child's bubble pipe. You have to add soap to the water in the pipe in order to change the surface tension or you cannot blow many bubbles! If the surfactant is not present in the neonate's lung, the bubbles (alveoli) collapse. There you have it: the radiology of HMD is predominantly the radiology of profound atelectasis on an alveolar rather than a segmental level. In fact, some of the more forward-thinking clinicians propose changing the name of this disease to surfactant deficiency disorder.

SURGICAL CONDITIONS

Pediatric surgical disease of the chest of a neonate can be roughly defined as anything that needs prompt intervention (Table 7-1). By this definition, for example, a tension pneumothorax needing treatment with a chest tube is surgical disease. In assessing the newborn child's chest radiograph when surgical disease is suspected you must take two steps. First, identify which side is the more abnormal (most surgical conditions are unilateral). Second, determine the direction of shift of the mediastinum. This is best done by looking at the trachea, but the position of the heart and thymus can also be second-

TABLE 7-1. *Common surgical chest conditions in neonates*

Pneumothorax
Diaphragmatic hernia
Lobar emphysema
Cystic adenomatoid malformation
Pleural effusions (large)

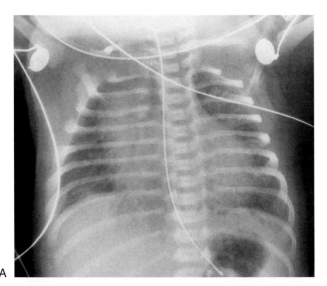

A

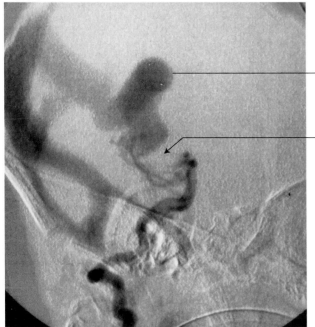

Vein

Posterior cerebral branch

B

FIG. 7-11. A: Cardiomegaly with pulmonary congestion in a child with congestive heart failure. The findings are nonspecific, and failure can occur due to multiple causes. **B:** A lateral arteriogram of the head of the baby shown in A shows the carotid artery branches *(arrows)* connecting to a large venus sinus, creating an arterial venous fistula. This condition is called a vein of Galen aneurysm. The baby is in high-output congestive heart failure.

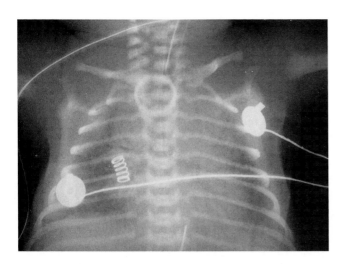

FIG. 7-12. Classic radiograph of a patient with hyaline membrane disease. Note that the lungs are relatively small in volume.

ary clues (Fig. 7-13). As a general (99%) rule, surgical conditions will displace the mediastinum *away* from the more abnormal side. For example, in the instance of a diaphragmatic hernia (a condition owing to an in utero defect that allows the abdominal contents to protrude into the chest), the heart and mediastinum are clearly shifted away from the side of the hernia by the mass of the protruding guts (Fig. 7-14). Therefore, if you look at the x-ray and decide that the side with the bowel in the chest is the abnormal side, and then look at the mediastinal position, you can readily deduce that this is a surgical condition and an emergency. When you are deciding on the more abnormal lung in neonates, remember that birth is a time of transition. In our example of a diaphragmatic hernia, in utero the bowel is filled with fluid. It isn't until the infant begins to breathe and swallow air that the gut assumes its normal postnatal air-filled condition. Therefore the first film in a neonate may show a fluid density filling the chest, but within a few moments the normal swallowing of air results in replacement of this fluid density by the bubbly appearance of air-filled bowel.

In some conditions this transition to an air-filled mass can be even further delayed until 2 or 3 days after birth. This usually occurs in situations where the connection between the lung and the tracheobronchial tree is abnormal, and it can take a considerable period of time, up to several days, for the normal in utero lung fluid to empty out and the air to fill the lung anomaly. A good example of this is lobar emphysema, a condition

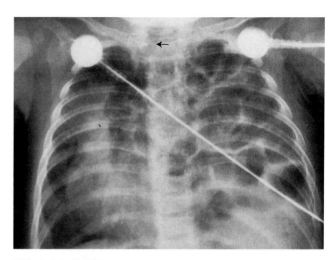

FIG. 7-14. Bubbly material fills the left chest, displacing the heart and mediastinum far to the right. These bubbles actually are air-filled bowel. Notice the trachea area. Position of the trachea is the single best indicator of mediastinal displacement.

whereby the tracheobronchial airway connects abnormally to a lobe of the lung, allowing air to flow in but not out. The lobe, therefore, hyperinflates, becoming a tumor in the chest. Babies don't breathe air in utero; their lungs are fluid-filled. Right after birth this abnormally connected lobe is full of lung fluid as is the rest of the lung. The same mechanics that do not allow air to freely escape also do not allow the fluid to freely escape; therefore, it takes a long time for turnover of the fluid to take place, and the initial chest x-ray looks like a solid (water) density mass with mediastinal displacement (Fig. 7-15). In a sense it doesn't make any difference because criteria 1 and 2 for diagnosing a surgical condition are met no matter what the status of the mass; however, it's always nice to make a precise diagnosis.

CYSTIC FIBROSIS

When you are studying pediatric patients it is always important to remember that the prevalence of congenital or heritable abnormalities is higher among the pediatric population than the adult population. Therefore, in looking at the x-rays of a child with recurrent pneumonias, you should think about heritable conditions that predispose the child to pneumonia, an example being cystic fibrosis. Cystic fibrosis, the most prevalent lethal genetic disease among the Caucasian population, begins with recurrent pneumonias but also has a number of features that allow a specific diagnosis from the x-rays (Fig. 7-16). The lungs are usually hyperexpanded, due to the blockage of many of the smaller bronchi by mucous plugs. The presence of mucoid impactions, branch-shaped collections of intrabronchial mucus, is very sug-

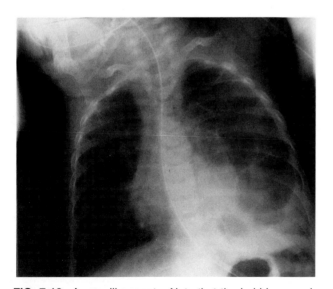

FIG. 7-13. A very ill neonate. Note that the bubbly mass in the left lung base causes the heart and mediastinum to be shifted from left to right. First you decide which lung is abnormal (in this case, clearly the left). If the heart and mediastinum are shifted away from the abnormal lung, it is almost always surgical disease of the chest. Incidentally, the mass in this case is a cystic adenomatoid malformation, a benign tumor of the lung caused by abnormal budding of the foregut.

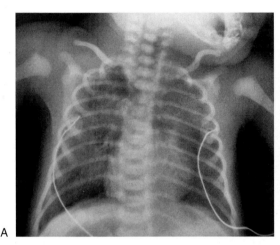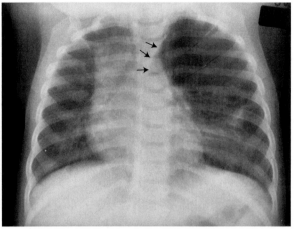

A   B

FIG. 7-15. A: A neonatal chest film shows mediastinal shift from left to right and a partially opaque fluid density in the left upper lobe. This is a patient with congenital lobar emphysema and only partial emptying of the fluid from the emphysematous lobe. **B:** The same patient at age 11 months demonstrates findings more typical of lobar emphysema with the markedly hyperinflated upper lobe herniated across the midline *(arrows)*. The principle for surgical disease remains valid; mediastinal shift away from the abnormal side needs rapid intervention.

gestive of cystic fibrosis. Generally, the children have very prominent hili, due to the combination of the inflamed lymph nodes and pulmonary artery enlargement resulting from pulmonary hypertension caused by lung destruction. The last common finding of cystic fibrosis is that of peribronchial cuffing, or thickening of the walls of the bronchus, due to the intense inflammatory change induced by the disease (Fig. 7-17). None of these signs are pathognomonic for cystic fibrosis; however, all of these signs taken in combination make the likelihood of this disease very high.

ESOPHAGEAL ATRESIA

Our discussion so far has focused on lung disease, but of course there are other significant organs in the pediatric chest, including the heart and the esophagus.

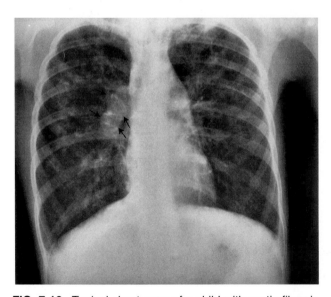

FIG. 7-16. Typical chest x-ray of a child with cystic fibrosis. Patchy infiltrates are present in both lung fields. The right hilus is very large and irregular owing to a combination of enlarged pulmonary artery and lymph nodes *(arrows)*. Note also that the heart is very small because of markedly overly expanded lungs. The pulmonary arteries are large due to a pulmonary hypertension. This is a very typical appearance for cystic fibrosis.

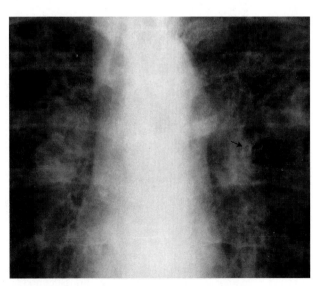

FIG. 7-17. A close-up of the lung showing peribronchiolar thickening. Note that the bronchus appears as a black dot amidst a white cuff. This cuff is edema and inflammatory cage in the bronchial wall.

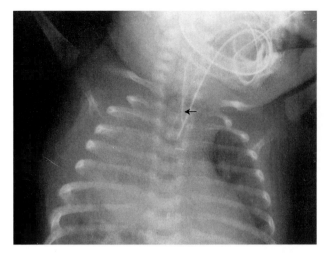

FIG. 7-18. This very ill infant choked upon being fed his first bottle. The chest radiograph shows a very dense right upper lobe infiltrate because of aspiration pneumonia. Note that the nasogastric tube won't go any further than the upper esophagus *(arrows)*. A surgical clip was placed to identify the site of the tracheoesophageal fistula as this infant was too ill to undergo primary repair of the esophageal atresia and a first-step procedure, ligating and dividing the fistula, was undertaken to protect his lungs. Survival of children with tracheoesophageal fistula correlates directly with the amount of lung disease owing to aspiration.

Esophageal abnormalities that are of importance in children are usually related to esophageal atresia. The most common form of esophageal atresia is a blind-ending proximal esophagus with a fistula extending from the trachea or left main stem bronchus to a blind distal esophagus. Inhaled air travels through the fistula and into the rest of the GI tract; therefore, the initial films can look superficially normal. The clues are that the GI tract is more distended by air than usual, and the proximal esophageal pouch is very dilated. Clinicians become alerted to this condition when the child chokes on feedings and the pediatrician cannot pass a nasogastric tube into the stomach (Fig. 7-18).

There are two less prevalent, but still frequent variants of esophageal abnormalities. The first is esophageal atresia without fistula, in which case the abdomen is gasless because the infant cannot swallow any air to displace the fluid that is in the abdomen in utero (Fig. 7-19). Such infants are usually quite ill and need emergent surgery. The second variant is tracheoesophageal fistula without esophageal atresia. This so-called H-type fistula can be a difficult diagnosis. The nasogastric tube test is normal, so that the diagnosis is not readily apparent to the clinician. The child usually presents frequent

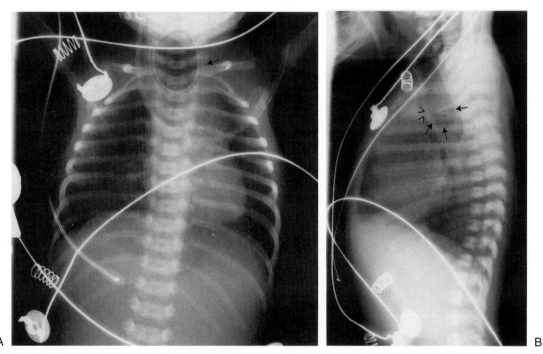

FIG. 7-19. A: A typical x-ray of a child with esophageal atresia. Note the nasogastric tube *(arrow)* coiled in the upper esophagus. There are two major differences between this film and the child shown in Fig. 18. First, this child has not gotten aspiration pneumonia because this abnormality was recognized earlier and the child was not fed. Second, note that there is no gas in the abdomen. Patients with tracheoesophageal fistula always have the very distended stomach as each breath pumps air into that organ. The absence of gas in the abdomen makes the diagnosis of esophageal atresia without fistula. **B:** Lateral view of the same patient shows the very dilated proximal esophagus *(arrows)*. Note that the dilated esophageal pouch displaces the airway anteriorly *(arrowheads)*. These infants will often have abnormalities of the airway that accompany the abnormalities of the esophagus.

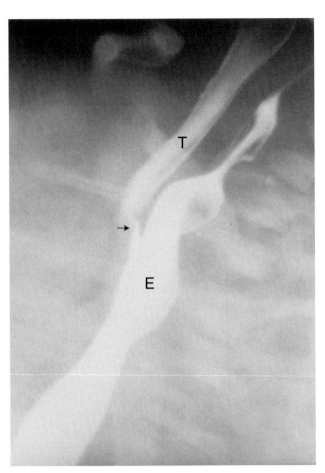

FIG. 7-20. A barium esophagram on a baby with recurrent pneumonia shows a connection between the esophagus and the trachea, a so-called H-type tracheal-esophageal fistula. This abnormality can sometimes be extremely difficult to detect.

pneumonias because each time the infant eats, some of the material goes into the lung. Whenever you have an infant with frequent and recurrent pneumonia, this entity, along with cystic fibrosis, needs to be considered (Fig. 7-20). A barium esophagram is necessary to confirm the diagnosis.

CONGENITAL HEART DISEASE

Serious congenital heart disease has a prevalence of approximately 1 per 1000 live-born infants, and therefore is a disease that you will likely encounter if you care for children. Although plain film is valuable for screening for congenital heart disease, it takes a tremendous amount of experience (and luck) before you can be specific as to the type of congenital heart disease. Several principles are very important. The first is that heart size in infants and children is more difficult to estimate than that in adults. The rule of thumb of 50% cardiothoracic ratio is not valid in children. When you're looking for cardiomegaly in a child, you need to be sure that you are not looking at thymus, *that the film has been taken on a good breath, and that lateral views are used extensively.* If the heart protrudes significantly beyond the visible airway on lateral view, the heart is usually enlarged. If on an anteroposterior (AP) view the heart appears large while on the lateral view, it is normal, then you are usually dealing with a deceiving thymus (Fig. 7-21).

The second rule is that children can have very serious heart disease and a normal-sized heart. This is particularly true in conditions where blood flow to the lungs is insufficient because of right-to-left shunting. As a

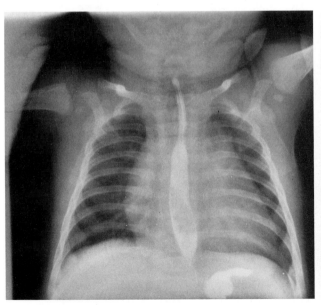
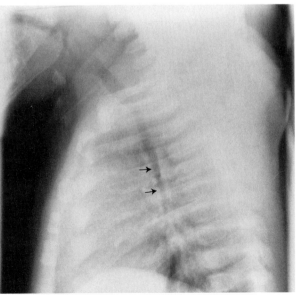

A

B

FIG. 7-21. A: This child's heart measures over 60% of the transverse diameter of the chest on the radiograph. In an adult, this would be a large heart; however, this is a normal child with a large thymus simulating cardiomegaly. **B:** Note that on lateral view, the heart does not protrude posterior to the airway *(arrows).*

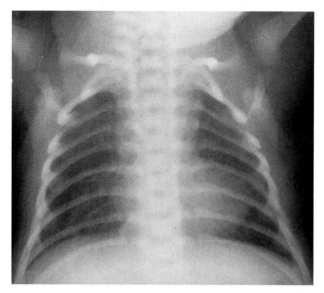

FIG. 7-22. This cyanotic, extremely ill child has a relatively small but boot-shaped heart. The pulmonary vascularity is normal due to the presence of a patent ductus arteriosis. The findings are characteristic of a variant of tetralogy of Fallot.

good general rule, children's hearts, being resilient, tend to dilate owing to a volume rather than a pressure over-load. Conditions that cause right-to-left shunting, like tetralogy of Fallot, do not give you an enlarged heart because the volume of blood traversing the heart is actually diminished (Fig. 7-22). A truly cyanotic neonate with a normal chest x-ray (including heart size) usually has some variant of tetralogy of Fallot.

Rule number three is that if you think the pulmonary vascularity is increased in a patient suspect for congenital heart disease, you are probably right; however, if you think it is decreased, you are probably wrong. For some reason, it is much easier for humans to perceive an increase in vascularity than a decrease in vascularity in a chest x-ray, probably because of the way our brains are wired. An enlarged heart and increased vascularity in an older child who is not cyanotic usually means some form of left-to-right shunt such as a ventricular septal defect (Fig. 7-23).

Rule number four is applicable to neonates. We have already talked about the fact that being born is the ultimate time of transition. When you are in utero, very little blood goes through the pulmonary artery circuit. To understand this, think about physiology. In utero the baby is not breathing air; therefore, there is no need for blood to bring oxygen to the baby from the lungs. Immediately following birth, the baby breathes air and the situation changes dramatically. It takes some time for the pulmonary arterial flow to reach adult levels of blood flow through the lungs. All neonates, therefore, have a relative state of pulmonary hypertension. Early on, lesions that should have increased vascularity, such as transposition of the great vessels are not revealed by x-ray (Fig. 7-24). The same logic explains why most left-to-right shunt lesions are not manifest until about 6 weeks of age (see rule 3) when the pulmonary artery pressure has fallen significantly.

With those rules to consider, it is possible to set out a systematic approach to looking at the chest x-

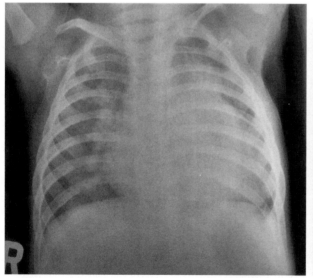
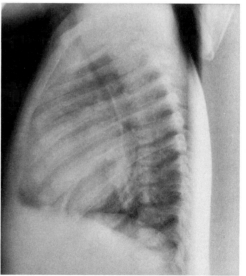

FIG. 7-23. The AP **(A)** and lateral **(B)** radiographs of a 2-month-old infant with respiratory distress when feeding, but no evidence of cyanosis, shows a markedly increased pulmonary vascularity and a large heart. This combination in a child is characteristic of a congenital left-to-right shunt. The most common left-to-right shunt is a ventricular septal defect or a communication between the right and left ventricles.

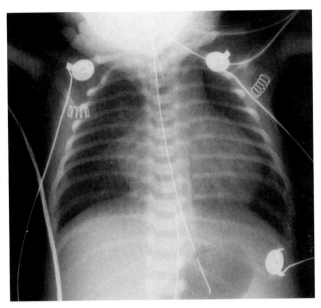

FIG. 7-24. This very cyanotic patient has a chest radiograph showing a large heart, narrow superior mediastinum, and pulmonary vascularity that is slightly, but not dramatically, increased. The patient is a 3-day-old infant with transposition of the great vessels and the vascularity is going through the transition between the very high vascular resistance in utero and the lower vascular resistance of an air-breathing baby. Over the course of subsequent days, the vascular resistance will drop further and the lungs will become flooded.

ray of a newborn with congenital heart disease. First, see if the heart is enlarged and if you can determine which chamber is enlarged. Next, determine if the vascularity is normal or increased, keeping in mind that the younger the baby, the less confident you can be to find increased vascularity. Finally, you need to talk to your clinical colleagues and find out if the baby is truly cyanotic, as defined by arterial oxygen saturation of under 80% with a normal arterial CO_2 saturation. With those pieces of information you can look at Figures 7-25 and 7-26 and make a rough estimate as to what type of congenital heart disease the baby may have (Figs. 7-27 to 7-29).

MEDIASTINAL MASSES

The remainder of the structures in the pediatric mediastinum are relatively inconspicuous, unless abnormal. The exception to this rule is the thymus, discussed earlier in this chapter. Pediatric mediastinal abnormalities conform to a compartmental scheme. If you can accurately identify the compartment where a mass is located, you can provide an intelligent differential diagnosis. The anterior mediastinum is defined as part of the mediastinum, visible in front of the airway on lateral view and the posterior mediastinum is defined as that portion of

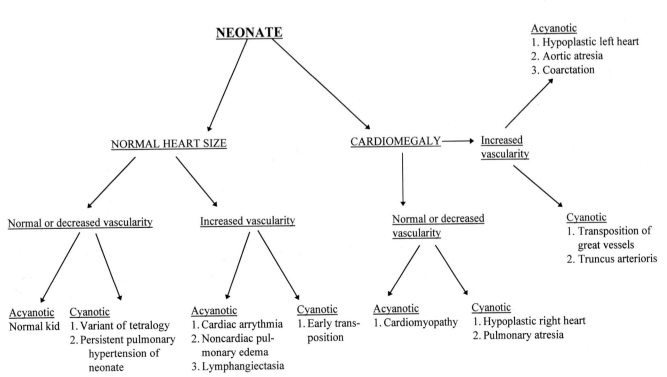

FIG. 7-25. Flow diagram for neonates suspect for heart disease.

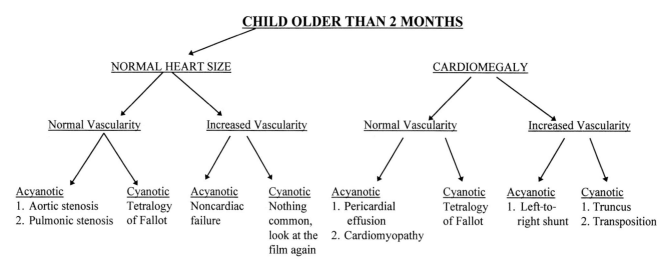

CHILD OLDER THAN 2 MONTHS

NORMAL HEART SIZE

Normal Vascularity

Acyanotic
1. Aortic stenosis
2. Pulmonic stenosis

Cyanotic
Tetralogy
of Fallot

Increased Vascularity

Acyanotic
Noncardiac
failure

Cyanotic
Nothing
common,
look at the
film again

CARDIOMEGALY

Normal Vascularity

Acyanotic
1. Pericardial
effusion
2. Cardiomyopathy

Cyanotic
Tetralogy
of Fallot

Increased Vascularity

Acyanotic
1. Left-to-
right shunt

Cyanotic
1. Truncus
2. Transposition

FIG. 7-26. Flow diagram for older children suspect for heart disease.

the mediastinum just posterior to the anterior edge of the vertebral bodies on lateral view. Everything else is the middle mediastinal compartment (Fig. 7-30). The whole trick is telling these compartments apart, and there are a few rules:

1. *Clavicle cutoff sign:* The anterior chest is anatomically lower than the posterior chest, so if a mass stops at the inferior margin of the clavicle on the PA chest radiograph, it has to be in the anterior mediastinum (Fig. 7-31).
2. *Hilum overlay sign:* Structures in the far anterior mediastinum overlie the vessels at the lung hilum;

therefore, the vessels are usually seen through these structures (Fig. 7-32).
3. *Posterior rib effacement:* Posterior mediastinal masses frequently spread the posterior ribs; therefore, distortion or asymmetry of the posterior ribs is a good sign that the mass is posterior (Fig. 7-33).
4. *Airway distortion sign:* Masses that distort the esophagus or compress the airways are almost surely middle mediastinum (Fig. 7-34).

Once you have applied these rules and decided in which compartment to look, the pathologic processes tend to categorize themselves fairly easily. Anterior

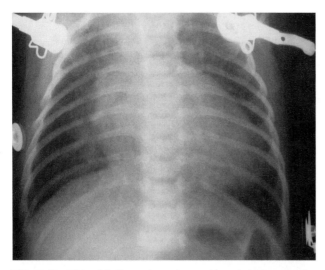

FIG. 7-27. This child has a huge heart. Note that the superior mediastinum has a large shadow to the right of the trachea, a right aortic arch. The vessels are large, flooding the lung. If we add the information that the child was cyanotic, then this becomes a characteristic truncus arteriosis. Approximately 40% of truncus patients have a right arch.

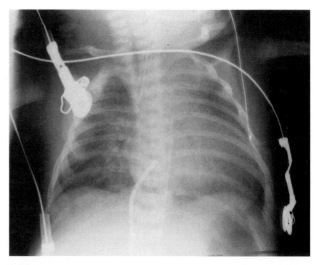

FIG. 7-28. A large heart and increased vascularity; however, this time the child is not cyanotic. This usually means either a left heart obstructive lesion or failure for some other reason. The child has a hypoplastic left heart.

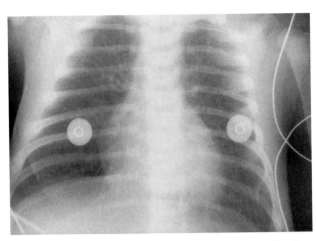

FIG. 7-29. A large heart and increased vascularity in a 2-week-old baby—findings typical for transposition of the great vessels. Note the very thin mediastinum because the pulmonary artery is directly in front of the aorta as opposed to being slightly to the left of it. This is characteristic of the transposition of the great vessels.

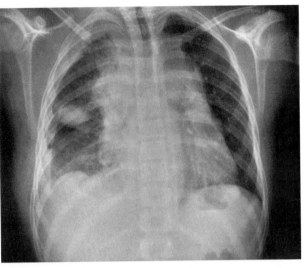

FIG. 7-31. This anterior mediastinal lymphoma stops right at the undersurface of the clavicles. Remember that the anterior portion of the chest is physically lower than the posterior portion of the chest; therefore, any mass that has the clavicle as its superior margin must be an anterior mediastinal mass.

mediastinal masses are almost always lymphoma- or thymus-related with the occasional thyroid mass or teratoma. An Aunt Minnie applies here: If the anterior mediastinal mass contains calcium, always go for teratoma (Fig. 7-35). Middle mediastinal masses are generally either lymph nodes or anomalous vessels related to the aortic arch. Esophageal and bronchial duplications are less frequent, but also occur in the middle mediasti-

num. Posterior mediastinum masses are neurogenic in origin, usually a neuroblastoma or ganglioneuroblastoma. When confronted with a suspected pediatric mediastinal mass, the first rule is to place it in the proper compartment; thereafter, it is a matter of pursuing the differential diagnosis.

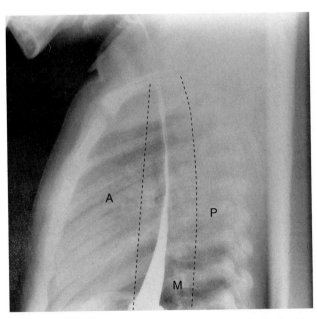

FIG. 7-30. A normal lateral view of the chest with barium in the esophagus, delineates the boundaries of the anterior middle and posterior mediastinum. When you consider mediastinal masses, it is important to divide in your mind the mediastinum into these components as it helps you to localize the likely diagnosis for the cause of the mass.

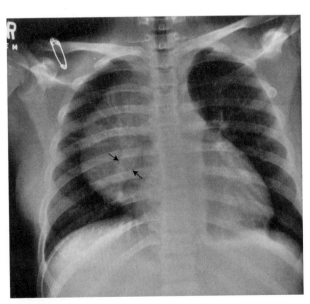

FIG. 7-32. This teenager has an anterior mediastinal mass. Note that the descending branch of the right pulmonary artery *(arrows)* is visible through the mass, documenting that the tumor is not in the same plane as the vessel; otherwise, the silhouette sign would prevent the vessel from being visible. This is called the hilum overlay sign where masses out of plane of the hilum (usually anterior mediastinal masses) allow hilar structures to be visualized.

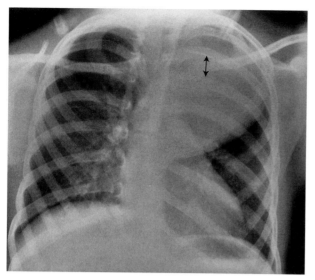

FIG. 7-33. This child has a huge posterior mediastinal mass on the left. Note how the mass has spread the ribs posteriorly. Masses that distort the posterior ribs are almost always neural crest in origin, in this case a ganglioneuroblastoma.

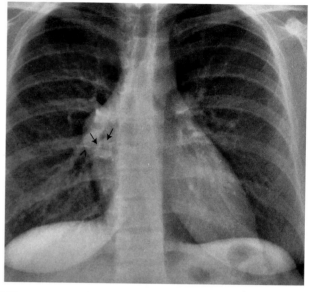

FIG. 7-35. The mass lying anterior to the right hilum *(arrowheads)* contains a large glob of high-density calcium. Remember that anterior mediastinal mass plus calcium equals teratoma.

SUMMARY

In this chapter, we have discussed the chest radiographs of children with particular emphasis on those conditions that are unique to pediatric chest. You should always remember the thymus as a deceiver in evaluating chest x-rays in children, particularly younger children. Neonatal medical and surgical disease can be easily differentiated in the vast majority of cases by remembering the rules of mediastinal shift and unilateral abnormality. If you apply carefully the rules of looking at congenital heart disease and mediastinal masses, you should be able to get into the ballpark about 80% of the time for making an accurate diagnosis of the correct lesion. That's a lot better than Babe Ruth did at batting, and look at how famous he is. Good luck!

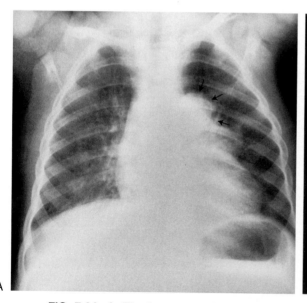

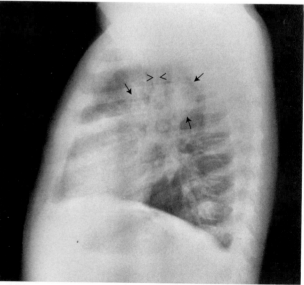

A

B

FIG. 7-34. A: The large mass *(arrows)* near the mediastinum is displacing the upper lobe bronchus on the left. Note that the left lung is blacker than the right because the mass is causing partial obstruction of the left main stem bronchus, allowing air to get in but not to escape easily. The effect on the bronchus or blood vessels is characteristic of a middle mediastinum mass, in this case, a bronchogenic cyst. **B:** Lateral view shows the rounded mass *(arrows)* of the bronchogenic cyst in the same plane as the airway *(arrows)*.

Key Points

- In some babies, in utero lung fluid takes more than a few minutes to clear, resulting in trasient tachypnea of the newborn. This appears on radiographs as pleural effusions and streaky densities. TTN should resolve within the first 24 hours after birth.
- TTN is indistinguishable on radiographs from early neonatal pneumonia.
- The best clue to diagnosing congestive heart failure in babies is a radiograph displaying a streaky density pattern in the lungs and cardiomegaly. If the heart protrudes significantly beyond the visible airway on a lateral radiograph, the heart is generally enlarged.
- Hyaline membrane disease displays four characteristic radiographic features: diffuse granularity, uniform disease, air bronchograms, and a relatively small lung volume.
- Generally, surgical conditions are unilateral amd will displace the mediastinum away from the more abnormal side.
- Radiographic features of cystic fibrosis include hyperexpanded lungs, mucoid impactions, very prominent hili, and peribronchial cuffing.

SUGGESTED READINGS

Strife JL, Bissett GS, Burrows PE. Cardiovascular system. In: Kirks DR, Griscom NT, eds. *Practical Pediatric Imaging: Diagnostic Radiology of Infants and Children.* Philadelphia: Lippincott-Raven Publishers, 1998.

Hedlund GL, Griscom NT, Cleveland RH, Kirks DR. Respiratory system. In: Kirks DR, Griscom NT, eds. *Practical Pediatric Imaging: Diagnostic Radiology of Infants and Children.* Philadelphia: Lippincott-Raven Publishers, 1998.

CHAPTER 8

Abdomen

William E. Erkonen

As elsewhere, the history and physical are the most important primary diagnostic steps to evaluate most abdominal complaints. In fact, the majority of diagnoses can be made on the basis of history alone. When the diagnosis remains uncertain following the history and physical examinations, an abdominal radiograph is often the first diagnostic imaging procedure requested.

PLAIN FILM RADIOGRAPH TECHNIQUE

The anteroposterior (AP) radiograph is the most frequently requested imaging study of the abdomen, and it is usually performed with the patient supine (Fig. 8-1). Occasionally, an AP upright radiograph (Fig. 8-2) is useful when searching for free intraperitoneal air and intestinal air–fluid levels. If the patient cannot tolerate the upright position, a decubitus radiograph can be substituted. Decubitus radiographs are obtained with the patient lying on either the right or, preferably, the left side (Fig. 8-3).

HOW TO VIEW AP ABDOMINAL RADIOGRAPHS

Step 1 is to position the radiograph correctly on the viewbox with the film R (right side) marker opposite the viewer's left side and the patient's head toward the top of the film. This is the same format as used for a chest radiograph. On the AP upright radiograph there should be an arrow near the R or L marker pointing toward the patient's head, indicating that it is an upright view. Similarly, decubitus radiographs should be clearly labeled decubitus with some indication as to which side is up or down.

Step 2 is to glance at the entire radiograph in a relaxed manner to allow an obvious abnormality to jump out at you (Fig. 8-4). When you do find an obvious abnormality on your first casual glance, do not allow it to interrupt your systematic search.

Step 3 is to systematically evaluate the radiograph. Any system or checklist will suffice, but the one listed in Table 8-1 will work until you develop your own.

TABLE 8-1. *Systematic checklist for evaluating abdominal radiographs*

1. Once-over glance
2. Liver and spleen sizes
3. Psoas shadows
4. Renal shadows size and position
5. Calcifications overlying kidneys, ureters, urinary bladder, and gallbladder
6. Intestinal gas pattern
7. Bones

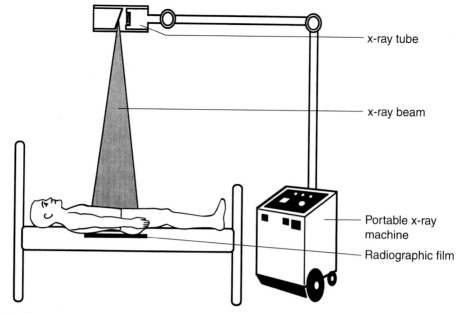

FIG. 8-1. Patient positioning for an AP supine abdomen radiograph. This examination is performed with the patient supine on a radiographic table or supine in bed using a portable x-ray unit.

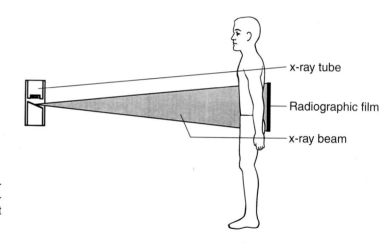

FIG. 8-2. Patient positioning for an AP upright abdomen radiograph. The examination is usually accomplished in the radiology department with the patient standing.

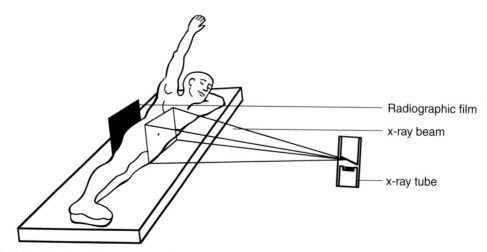

FIG. 8-3. Patient positioning for a left lateral decubitus abdomen radiograph. The patient's arms are positioned comfortably out of the way.

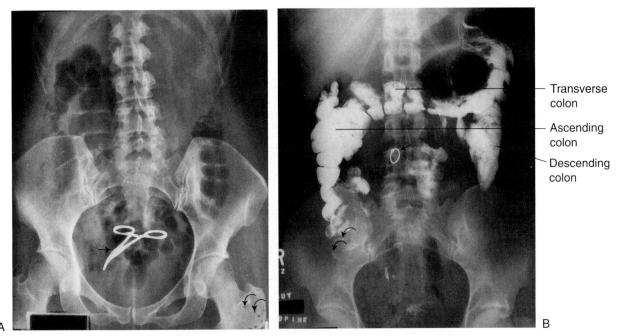

FIG. 8-4. A: Abdomen AP supine radiograph. Intraabdominal hemostat. This hemostat *(straight arrow)* was inadvertently left in the abdomen during abdominal surgery. Incidentally, note the black marks *(curved arrows)* on the film caused by static electricity. Static electricity artefacts are usually created during removal of the radiographic film from the radiographic cassette. **B:** Abdomen AP supine radiograph. Umbilical metallic ring. The metallic ring *(straight arrow)* was placed in the umbilicus for cosmetic reasons similar to an earring. There is residual barium in the appendix *(curved arrows)* and in the colon secondary to a previous upper GI study.

First, locate the water density liver and spleen silhouettes (Fig. 8-5). Occasionally it is difficult to determine the outline of the liver and spleen borders, but one clue to locating liver and spleen edges is the presence of bowel gas or air in the right and left upper abdominal quadrants. Bowel gas permits an indirect estimate of the location of the hepatic and splenic borders because where there is bowel gas there usually is not liver or spleen.

With a little experience you will automatically recognize a normal-sized liver. When the liver shadow hangs down to the iliac crest, it is usually enlarged (Fig. 8-6). Also, with more experience you will readily detect an enlarged spleen or splenomegaly (Fig. 8-7). After all, medicine is an apprenticeship and requires practice and repetition. Hence the phrase, the practice of medicine.

Next, identify the water density psoas muscles and kidneys (Fig. 8-8). The psoas muscle margins are usually visible. A nonvisible psoas margin should alert you to a possible abnormality, but an absent or partially absent psoas muscle margin can be normal. As your eyes drift toward the renal shadows, evaluate their size, shape, and position. Identifying renal outlines is about as easy for the rookie as visualizing the bottom of the muddy Mississippi River. Renal shadows are visible because they are water density structures (gray) surrounded by variable amounts of fat (black). You should attempt to locate the upper and lower renal poles as well as their medial and lateral borders. If the renal long axis is not parallel to the psoas muscle margin, you should beware of a mass or other water density abnormality in the kidney or the retroperitoneum. Always look for calcifications (white) and calcified calculi in the abdomen, especially in the region of the kidneys, ureters, urinary bladder, and the gallbladder.

Now, evaluate the bowel gas pattern which will be discussed in the next section. Last but not least, look at the bones systematically beginning with the lower ribs and the lower dorsal spine (Fig. 8-9). Always attempt to visualize the pedicles of the lower dorsal and lumbar spine proceeding from head to foot. The vertebral pedicles resemble automobile headlights on an AP radiograph, and a missing pedicle strongly suggests a destructive process such as metastatic disease. Always routinely evaluate all visible bones including the pelvis, hips, and

text continues on page 151

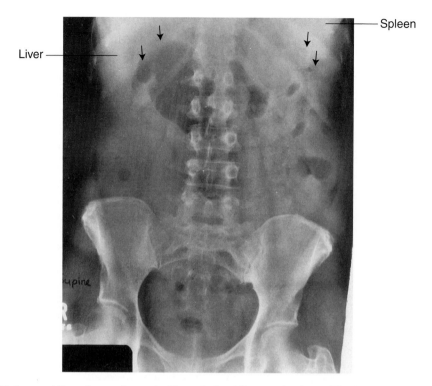

FIG. 8-5. Abdomen AP supine radiograph. Normal-sized liver and spleen. The intestinal gas *(straight arrows)* demarcates the inferior liver and spleen margins.

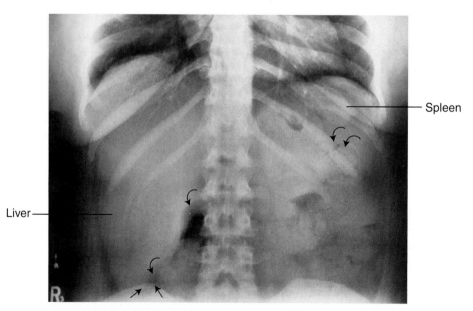

FIG. 8-6. Abdomen AP supine radiograph. Hepatomegaly. The water density liver is enlarged and the inferior margin projects over the iliac crest *(straight arrows)*. The spleen is normal in size. The lower edges of the liver and spleen are demarcated by intestinal air *(curved arrows)*.

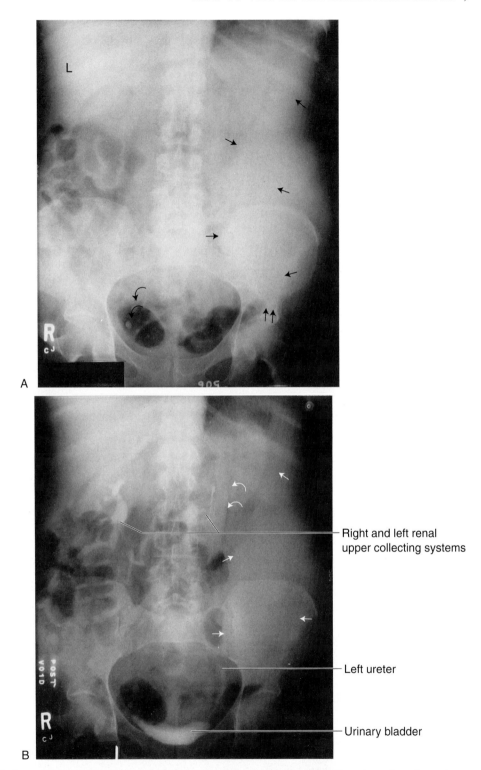

FIG. 8-7. A: Abdomen AP supine radiograph. Splenomegaly. The water density spleen is enlarged *(straight arrows)* and the inferior margin projects just above the left hip *(double straight arrows)*. The large spleen has displaced the intestinal gas into the right abdomen. The liver size is normal (L, liver). Incidentally noted are phleboliths *(curved arrows)* that are small stones in veins usually secondary to calcified thrombi. **B:** Abdomen AP supine postvoid radiograph from a subsequent excretory urogram in the same patient as A. The very large spleen is again outlined by straight arrows, and the spleen is displacing the left kidney medially *(curved arrows)* as they are both posterior structures.

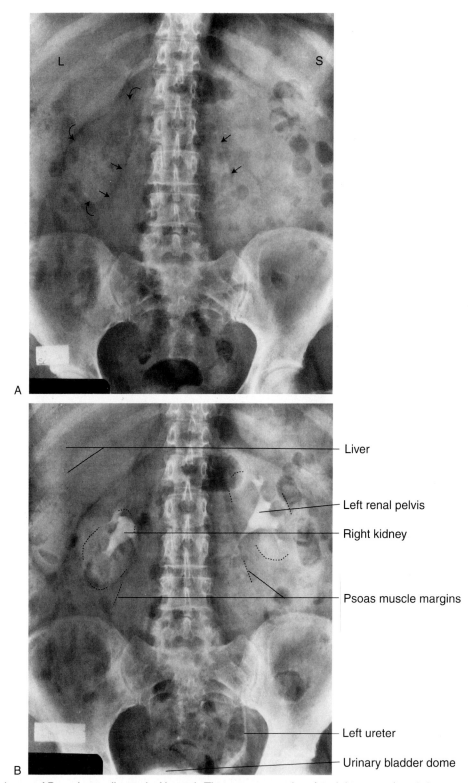

Liver

Left renal pelvis

Right kidney

Psoas muscle margins

Left ureter

Urinary bladder dome

FIG. 8-8. A: Abdomen AP supine radiograph. Normal. The psoas muscles *(straight arrows)* and the right kidney *(curved arrows)* are visible. The left renal silhouette is obliterated by intestinal gas, and it is not uncommon to have intestinal gas and contents obliterating the renal shadows. L, liver; S, spleen. **B:** Abdomen AP supine radiograph. Normal excretory urogram. Contrast media has been injected intravenously and confirms the renal sizes and locations. Notice that the renal long axes lie parallel to the psoas muscle margins.

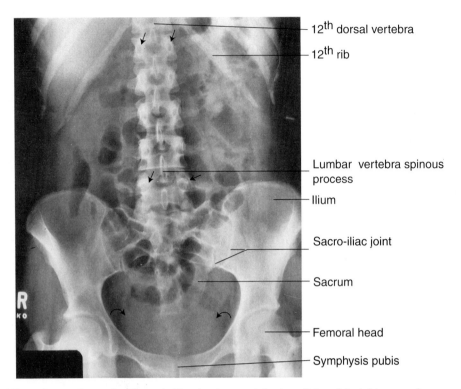

— 12th dorsal vertebra

— 12th rib

Lumbar vertebra spinous process

— Ilium

Sacro-iliac joint

— Sacrum

— Femoral head

— Symphysis pubis

FIG. 8-9. Abdomen AP supine radiograph. Normal. The lumbar vertebral pedicles *(straight arrows)* have the appearance of automobile headlights projecting over the vertebral bodies. The water density urinary bladder *(curved arrows)* is often visible on abdominal radiographs.

femurs for fractures, metastases, and their overall density.

Use a similar search system for the AP upright abdomen radiograph while being especially alert for free air beneath the diaphragms. In some clinical situations, free intraperitoneal air may be visualized only on an upright radiograph because this position often allows free air to rise to the subdiaphragmatic regions.

"AUNT MINNIES," OR UNFORGETTABLE IMAGES

The term "Aunt Minnie" was coined by the late Dr. Ben Felson, and it refers to the unmistakable and unforgettable appearance of your Aunt Minnie, or Uncle Al, or any other family character. Every family has such a character. A radiologic Aunt Minnie describes an image appearance so classic that once you see it you never forget it. It is something unique and distinctive just like your Aunt Minnie. The following are commonly encountered abdominal radiographic Aunt Minnies (Figs. 8-10 to 8-18). File them away in your visual-cerebral computer, and your ability to recognize them will make you a star in the eyes of your colleagues, teachers, and patients.

EVALUATING THE INTESTINAL AIR OR GAS PATTERN

Intestinal gas (black) provides a natural contrast media that can be useful for detecting abdominal disease. When evaluating the intestinal gas pattern, you should ask yourself several important questions. Is the bowel gas pattern normal? Remember that there is normally some air or gas in the stomach, small intestine, colon, and rectum. With experience you will begin to automatically recognize normal and abnormal amounts of air in the gastrointestinal (GI) tract. This is similar to recognizing a normal heart shadow on a chest radiograph. If the gas pattern is not normal, then ask some more questions. Is there too much or too little air? Is the air in the wrong place?

Too Much Bowel Gas

When there is too much gas, the differential diagnosis includes adynamic ileus and bowel obstruction. Again, we need a systematic approach to this situation to arrive at the correct diagnosis. Adynamic ileus is also referred to as paralytic ileus, or just ileus. In adynamic ileus, there simply is too much bowel gas distributed throughout the

text continues on page 155

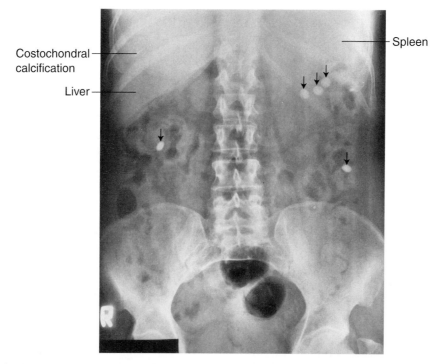

Costochondral
calcification

Liver

Spleen

FIG. 8-10. Abdomen AP supine radiograph. Classic appearance of tablets or pills *(straight arrows)* in the GI tract. All the tablets are the same size and shape with homogeneous density. Not all tablets or pills can be visualized on a radiograph.

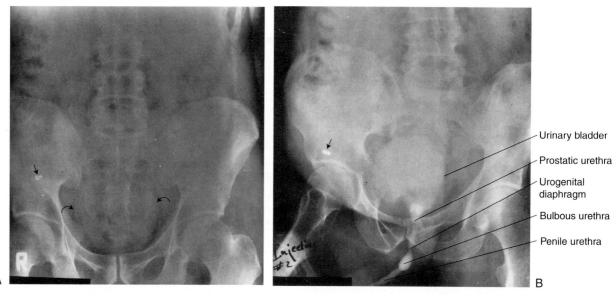

Urinary bladder

Prostatic urethra

Urogenital
diaphragm

Bulbous urethra

Penile urethra

A

B

FIG. 8-11. A: Abdomen AP supine radiograph. Buckshot in the appendix. There are rounded metallic densities projecting over the right lower quadrant of the abdomen consistent with buckshot in the appendix *(straight arrow)*. This is not an unusual finding in people who eat wild game. If the accidentally ingested buckshot does not break a tooth, they may occasionally lodge in the appendix. This is not an indication for appendectomy. Note the water density urine filled urinary bladder *(curved arrows)*. **B:** Abdomen AP oblique radiograph in the same patient as A. Buckshot in the appendix. This selected film from a retrograde urethrogram nicely demonstrates the linear alignment of the three metallic buckshot *(straight arrow)* that are lodged within the appendiceal lumen.

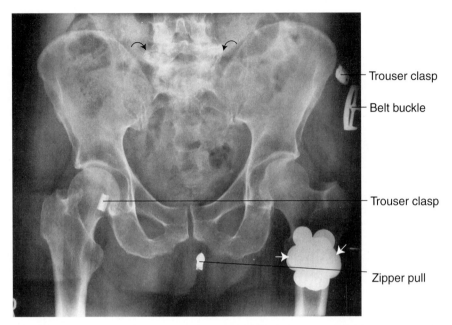

Trouser clasp

Belt buckle

Trouser clasp

Zipper pull

FIG. 8-12. Abdomen AP supine radiograph. Metal coins *(straight arrows)* in the left trouser pocket. Occasionally, the patient is not completely disrobed prior to obtaining the radiographs, and foreign bodies in and on the clothing might appear on the radiograph. Note the degenerative or osteoarthritic changes in the lower lumbar spine *(curved arrows)*.

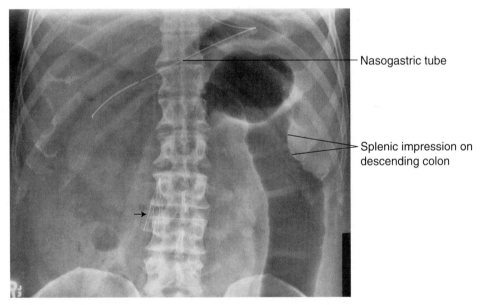

Nasogastric tube

Splenic impression on descending colon

FIG. 8-13. Abdomen AP supine radiograph. Inferior vena cava filter. The umbrella-shaped filter *(straight arrow)* is placed in the inferior vena cava by angiographic technique, and it is designed to entrap venous thromboemboli originating in the lower extremities and pelvis.

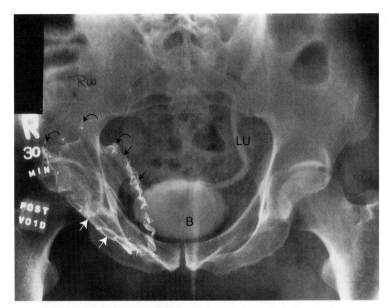

FIG. 8-14. Lower abdomen AP supine radiograph selected from an excretory urogram (EU). Herniorrhaphy mesh placed during a hernia repair. The mesh *(straight arrows)* projects over the right inguinal region, and the anchoring sutures *(curved arrows)* can be seen. B, urinary bladder; LU, left ureter.

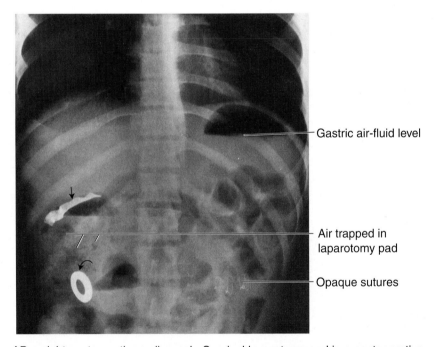

Gastric air-fluid level

Air trapped in laparotomy pad

Opaque sutures

FIG. 8-15. Abdomen AP upright postoperative radiograph, Surgical laparotomy pad in a postoperative abdomen. The radiograph was obtained when the patient experienced severe postoperative abdominal pain and distention. The straight arrow indicates the opaque strip in the laparotomy pad and the curved arrow indicates the metallic ring attached to the lap pad. Note the mottled black appearance of the air trapped in the laparotomy pad. The air–fluid level in the gastric fundus gives a clue to the upright position of the patient.

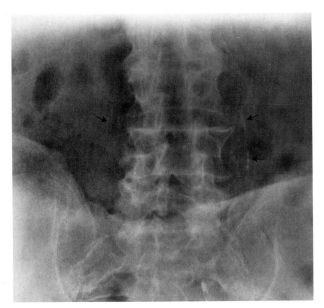

FIG. 8-16. Abdomen AP supine radiograph. Peripherally calcified aneurysm of the distal abdominal aorta. The straight arrows outline a large partially calcified aneurysm in the distal abdominal aorta.

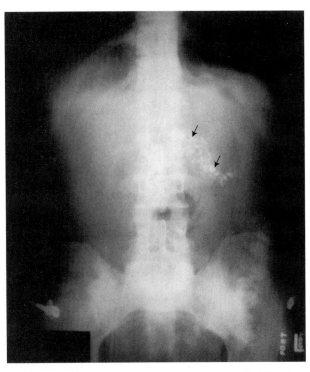

FIG. 8-18. Abdomen AP supine radiograph. Calcifications *(straight arrows)* in the pancreas body and tail secondary to chronic pancreatitis.

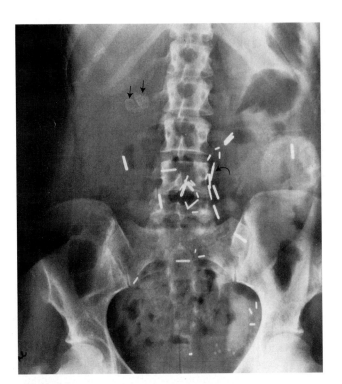

FIG. 8-17. Abdomen AP supine radiograph. Cholelithiasis or gallstones. The calcified calculi *(straight arrows)* are faceted. Approximately 5% to 15% of gallstones are calcified and visible on an abdominal radiograph. Surgical metallic clips *(curved arrow)* are secondary to previous abdominal surgery.

entire gastrointestinal GI tract including the small and large intestine and the rectum (Fig. 8-19). The multiple etiologies of adynamic ileus are listed in Table 8-2. If you can identify air in the small and large intestine and in the rectum, this generally indicates adynamic ileus and not obstruction. Air in the rectum is a key differential point. However, be careful as air can be introduced into the rectum by a rectal thermometer, enema, or digital rectal exam. Air introduced in this manner and subsequently visualized on a radiograph can easily mislead the unwary away from an obstruction.

Intestinal obstruction is another reason for too much bowel air. In intestinal obstruction there is usually air-filled, dilated intestine proximal to the point of obstruc-

TABLE 8-2. *Etiologies for adynamic ileus*

1. Postoperative
2. Posttraumatic
3. Medication
4. Infections
5. Inflammatory processes
    a. Pancreatitis
    b. Regional enteritis
    c. Ulcerative colitis
6. Uremia
7. Electrolyte imbalance
4. Prolonged bed rest

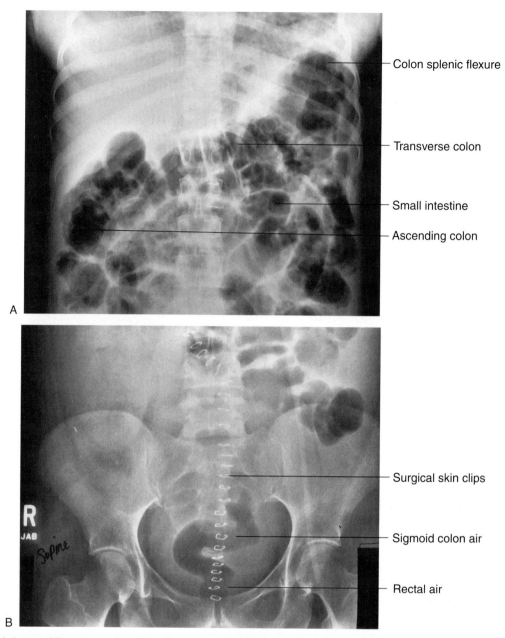

Colon splenic flexure

Transverse colon

Small intestine

Ascending colon

Surgical skin clips

Sigmoid colon air

Rectal air

FIG. 8-19. A: Abdomen AP supine radiograph. Postoperative adynamic ileus. Air is present throughout the entire GI tract including the rectum (not shown). **B:** Lower abdomen AP supine radiograph 24 hours later in the same patient. Adynamic ileus. A considerable amount of intestinal air has moved into the rectum and sigmoid colon, and this makes adynamic ileus a logical diagnosis.

tion and little or no air distal to the obstruction. No air distally or in the rectum should make you very suspicious for bowel obstruction. Often the dilated small and large bowel containing too much air will have air–fluid levels that are best appreciated on upright and decubitus radiographs.

If a diagnosis of obstruction or adynamic ileus is not readily apparent, it may be necessary to obtain follow up abdominal radiographs to arrive at the correct diagnosis.

Once you have diagnosed obstruction, you next need to determine the precise location of the obstruction. Is the obstruction in the small or large intestine? This is best accomplished by determining what parts of the GI tract are dilated. In small bowel obstruction there are multiple loops of dilated small bowel proximal to the obstruction site and little or no air distally and no air in the rectum. In large bowel obstruction, there is dilated colon proximal to the obstruction site, but little or no air distally and no air in the rectum.

Sometimes it is extremely difficult and even impossible to differentiate dilated small bowel from dilated large bowel, and the best way is to identify the *valvulae conniventes* and *colon septa*. Valvulae conniventes are regularly spaced thin transverse lines or mucosal folds that extend across the entire small bowel lumen (Fig. 8-20). On the other hand, the colon can usually be identified by the somewhat irregularly spaced transverse bands, called colon septa or haustra folds, that do not extend completely across the colon lumen (Fig. 8-21A, B).

Sigmoid volvulus is a dramatic clinical and radiologic finding that often occurs in elderly adults who have a long history of constipation. The chronic constipation results in a redundant sigmoid mesentery that has the potential to twist on itself like a garden hose. This sigmoid colon twisting mechanism can result in a complete or partial obstruction at the site of the twist, and then an AP radiograph often shows a dramatically dilated sigmoid colon (Fig. 8-21C). The diagnosis can be confirmed by barium enema that reveals a complete obstruction to the retrograde flow of barium at the site of the twist (Fig. 8-21D). The obstruction can often be relieved by gently passing a sigmoidoscope past the point of the obstruction or twist.

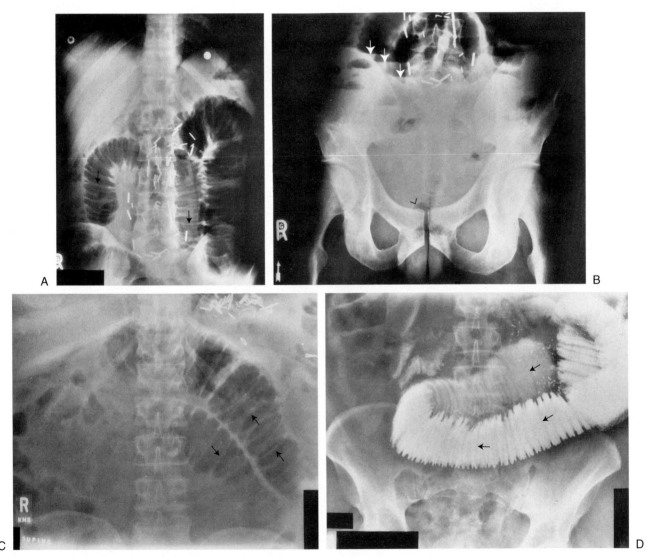

FIG. 8-20. A: Abdomen AP supine radiograph. Small bowel obstruction. The obstruction was secondary to adhesions caused by previous abdominal surgery, and the metallic densities are surgical clips from that surgery. The intestinal air is confined to dilated small intestine, wherein you identify the prominent valvulae conniventes *(straight arrows)*. There is no definite air in the colon. **B:** Abdomen AP upright radiograph in the same patient as in A. There are air–fluid levels in the small intestine *(arrows)* with little or no distal bowel gas. The small amount of rectal gas *(arrowhead)* was introduced during a rectal examination just prior to this study. **C, D:** Abdomen AP supine radiographs in a different patient. Small bowel obstruction. This is another demonstration of the valvulae conniventes in dilated and obstructed small intestine on a plain film (C) and during enteroclysis (D).

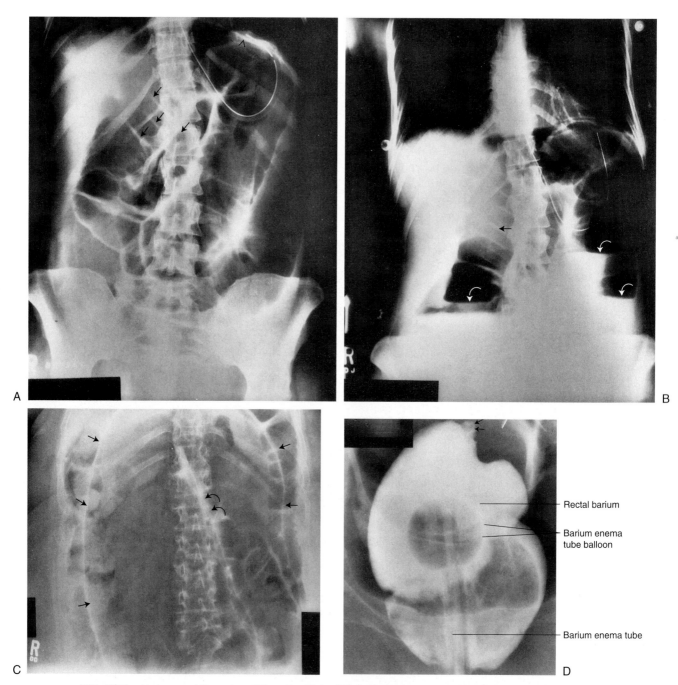

A

B

C

Rectal barium

Barium enema tube balloon

Barium enema tube

D

FIG. 8-21. Abdomen AP supine **(A)** and upright **(B)** radiographs. Large bowel or colon obstruction. Note the dilated air filled proximal colon with absence of air in the distal colon. The presence of colon septa in both views *(straight arrows)* indicate that the obstruction site is in the colon. On the upright radiograph (B) there are multiple colon air–fluid levels *(curved arrows)*. The tip of the nasogastric tube *(arrowhead)* projects over the gastric fundus. **C, D:** Abdomen AP supine radiograph (C) and radiograph from a barium enema (D). Sigmoid volvulus. On the AP radiograph the sigmoid colon is massively dilated *(straight arrows)* proximal to the point of the twist and obstruction. Where the dilated loops of sigmoid colon abut, they often form a white line *(curved arrows)* pointing toward the right upper quadrant of the abdomen. The barium enema radiograph shows the point of the twist or obstruction *(straight arrows)* called a beak sign.

TABLE 8-3. *Etiologies of too little intestinal gas on abdomen radiographs*

1. Large abdominal mass
2. Enlarged abdominal organs (Figs. 8-6, 8-7)
3. Fluid-filled loops of bowel with no air
4. Gastroenteritis

TABLE 8-4. *Abdominal air or gas in the wrong place*

1. Free intraperitoneal air due to perforation of bowel wall
   a. Peptic ulcer
   b. Blunt and penetrating trauma
   c. Cancer
   d. Appendicitis, diverticulitis
   e. Inflammatory bowel disease
2. Abscess
3. Pneumatosis intestinalis

Too Little Bowel Gas

When the abdominal radiographs show a marked paucity or absence of bowel gas, the differential diagnosis listed in Table 8-3 should be entertained.

Air or Gas in the Wrong Places

There are several situations where air is found outside of the intestinal lumen or in the wrong place (Table 8-4). Air in the wrong place might be free air in the peritoneal cavity that can result from any process that perforates the intestinal tract. These patients generally experience severe abdominal pain and usually exhibit rigid abdominal muscles, hence the term "board-like rigidity." AP supine and upright abdominal radiographs should be requested to confirm the clinical suspicion or impression of free intraperitoneal air.

The upright position allows free intraperitoneal air to rise to the subdiaphragmatic regions of the abdomen (Fig. 8-22). The upright view may not be possible due to severe abdominal pain and/or weakness. In this situation, the radiology technologist will usually proceed with a decubitus radiograph. On a decubitus radiograph, the air rises to the nondependent portion of the peritoneal cavity (Fig. 8-23). Either technique has the potential to identify just a few cubic centimeters of free intraperitoneal air as long as the patient is in the upright or decubitus position approximately 10 minutes prior to the radiograph.

Another cause of air in the wrong place is pneumatosis intestinalis (Fig. 8-24), and additional etiologies of pneumatosis intestinalis are listed in Table 8-5. Ab-

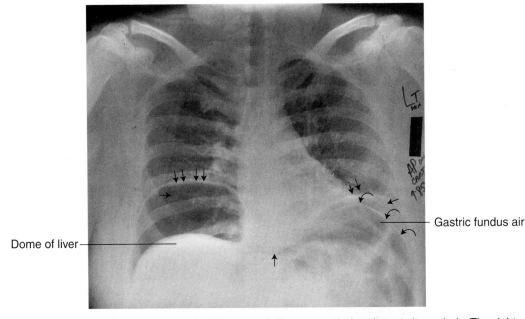

Dome of liver—

Gastric fundus air

FIG. 8-22. Chest AP upright radiograph. Bilateral subdiaphragmatic free intraperitoneal air. The right and left hemidiaphragms *(double arrows)* are elevated secondary to bilateral subdiaphragmatic air *(single straight arrows)*. The black zone between the right hemidiaphragm and the dome of the liver represents free intraperitoneal air. There is air in the gastric fundus as well as free air surrounding the gastric fundus, and this allows clear visualization of both sides of the gastric fundal wall *(curved arrows)*. When you see both sides of an intestinal wall, this most likely represents free intraperitoneal air or Rigler's sign (1).

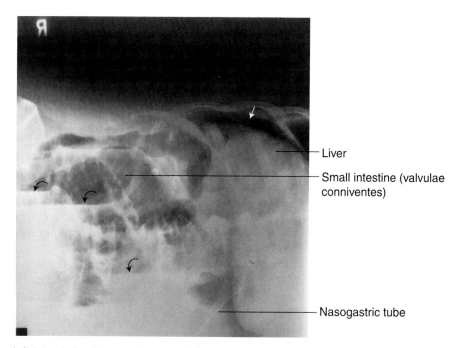

Liver

Small intestine (valvulae
conniventes)

Nasogastric tube

FIG. 8-23. Abdomen left lateral decubitus radiograph *(left side down)*. Free intraperitoneal air. This patient was found to have a small bowel obstruction with perforation. The free intraperitoneal air *(straight arrow)* can be seen between the right rib cage and the liver. The small bowel is markedly dilated and contains multiple air–fluid levels *(curved arrows)*.

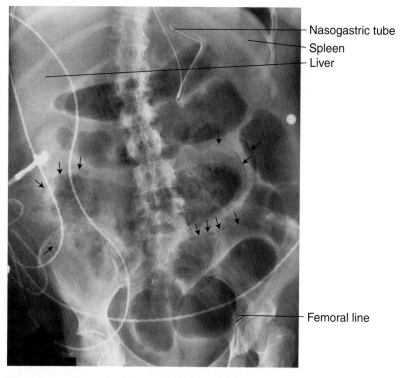

Nasogastric tube
Spleen
Liver

Femoral line

FIG. 8-24. Abdomen AP supine radiograph. Pneumatosis intestinalis or air in the bowel wall. There is widespread air within the small intestine walls *(arrows)*, and the etiology was unknown in this patient. See Table 8-5 for pneumatosis intestinalis etiologies. This process resolved spontaneously without therapy.

TABLE 8-5. *Pneumatosis intestinalis etiologies*

1. Ulcerative colitis
2. Regional enteritis
3. Gastroenteritis
4. Ischemia
5. Collagen disorders
6. Steroids
7. Immunosuppressive therapy
8. Necrotizing enterocolitis in the neonate (2)

scesses can be found at any location and the abdomen is no exception (Fig. 8-25).

GI CONTRAST STUDIES

Radiologic GI contrast studies have been around for many years. They are accurate, safe, much less expensive than the newer endoscopic studies and enjoy excellent patient acceptance. These studies consist of radiographs obtained following the introduction of barium sulfate (metallic density or white) and/or air (black) into the GI tract.

Upper GI Series

An upper GI series is accomplished by having the patient swallow gas-producing crystals and liquid barium under fluoroscopy to visualize the esophagus, stomach, and small intestine (Figs. 8-26 to 8-30). When both barium and air are used, it is referred to as a double-contrast study. When barium is used alone, it is a single-contrast study. Preparation for an upper GI series simply consists of fasting or nothing by mouth (NPO) for 8–12 hours prior to the study. When perforation of the upper GI tract is suspected, a water-soluble contrast media is employed. These studies enjoy excellent patience acceptance.

Enteroclysis

Enteroclysis is a focused examination of the small intestine, wherein air and barium sulfate are introduced directly into the small intestine via a nasointestinal tube with the tip placed just beyond the duodenal-jejunal junction under fluoroscopy (Fig. 8-31). This is an excellent diagnostic study to uncover a wide range of small intestine diseases. The advantage of this procedure is that the stomach, duodenum, and colon do not obstruct the visualization of the small intestine. The main disadvantages are the discomfort associated with a nasal tube and the fluoroscopic radiation exposure.

Barium Enema

Introduction of barium sulfate and/or air into the colon via a rectal tube is called a lower GI series, or barium enema. For this study, it is extremely important

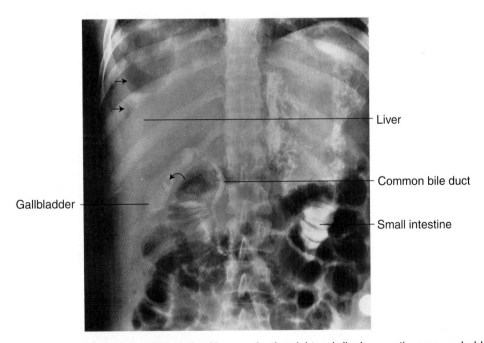

FIG. 8-25. Abdomen AP supine radiograph. Abscess in the right subdiaphragmatic area probably secondary to cholecystitis and cholelithiasis. The black areas along the right lateral aspect of the liver represent air in the abscess cavity *(straight arrows)*. Incidentally noted is contrast media in the common bile duct and gallbladder that was injected during an ERCP. Some of the contrast spilled into the small intestine. The filling defect in the gallbladder probably is a calculus *(curved arrow)*.

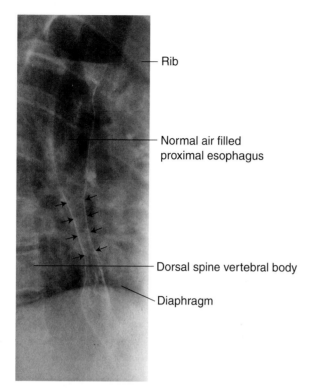

FIG. 8-26. Double-contrast esophagram. Distal esophageal stricture. The smooth long tapered appearance of the narrowed or strictured distal esophagus *(straight arrows)* is typical of a benign stricture. This stricture was caused by chronic reflux of the gastric contents into the distal esophagus.

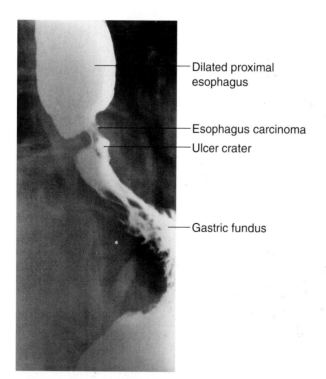

FIG. 8-27. Barium contrast esophagram. Carcinoma of the distal esophagus. The cancer resulted in a short narrowed segment with irregular mucosa and ulceration. The proximal esophagus is dilated but otherwise normal.

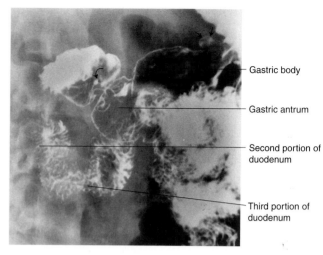

FIG. 8-28. Double-contrast upper GI series. Duodenal bulb ulcer and gastric ulcer. A moderate-sized gastric ulcer crater *(straight arrows)* is located along the lesser curvature of the gastric body. Incidentally noted is the duodenal ulcer crater *(curved arrow)* in the duodenal bulb base. Both ulcer craters healed completely with medical management.

to have a clean colon, and this is best accomplished with laxatives and large amounts of orally ingested fluids. The barium-, air-, and water-soluble contrast agents are administered via a rectal tube under fluoroscopic observation. When both air and barium are used, it is called a double-contrast study whereas barium alone is a single-contrast study. The double-contrast study is especially preferred when searching for small ulcers and polyps. Again, when perforation is suspected, a water-soluble contrast media may be employed. These studies may have a mild to moderate amount of associated discomfort, but usually a properly performed barium study of the colon has little or no discomfort associated.

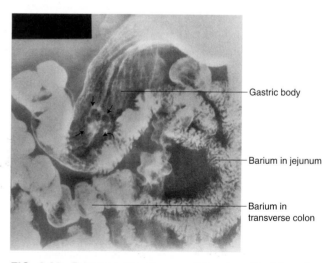

FIG. 8-29. Double-contrast upper GI series. Gastric polyp *(straight arrows)*. The stalk of the benign polyp *(curved arrow)* is clearly visible.

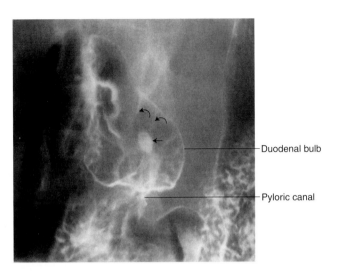

FIG. 8-30. Double-contrast upper GI series. Central duodenal bulb ulcer crater *(arrow)*. The duodenal mucosal folds radiate toward the ulcer crater *(curved arrows)*.

An alternative to colon barium studies is colonoscopy, but this is considerably more expensive and often more uncomfortable. The main advantage of colonoscopy is the ability to directly visualize the mucosa.

Barium colon studies or barium enemas or lower GI studies are useful in the workup of colon inflammatory diseases and neoplasms. Ulcerative colitis (Fig. 8-32) usually involves the rectum; shallow ulcers are typical findings. Granulomatous colitis (regional enteritis, Crohn's disease) often spares the rectum, and deep ulcer craters are more characteristic (Fig. 8-33). The radio-

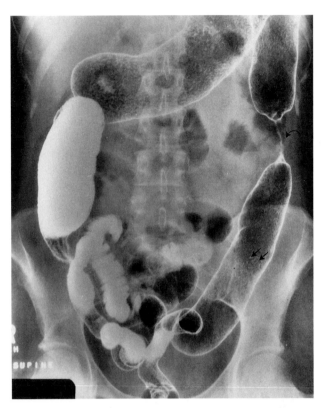

FIG. 8-32. Double-contrast colon study or lower GI series. Ulcerative colitis. Their is a fine network of small superficial ulcerations *(straight arrows)* throughout much of the colon. There is a benign stricture *(curved arrow)* in the proximal descending colon. The colon in general is foreshortened giving it a picture frame appearance.

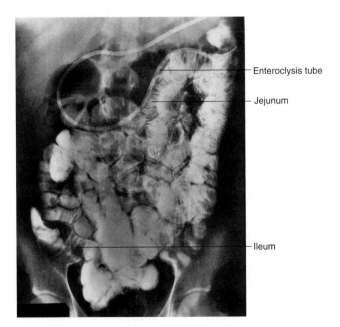

FIG. 8-31. Abdomen AP supine enteroclysis radiograph. Normal. Notice that the nasointestinal tube has been typically positioned just beyond the duodenal–jejunal junction.

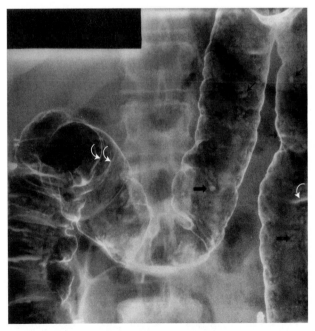

FIG. 8-33. Double-contrast colon study or lower GI series. Granulomatous colitis (regional enteritis, Crohn's disease). The straight arrows indicate the classic aphthous ulcers of regional enteritis that are deeper than those typically found in ulcerative colitis. Notice that the mucosal folds are thickened *(curved arrows)*.

TABLE 8-6. *Radiographic findings in ulcerative and granulomatous colitis*

Ulcerative Colitis
1. Frequently involves the rectum
2. Involves contiguous areas often in retrograde fashion
3. Bowel shortening (picture frame appearance to colon)
4. Superficial ulcers are typical

Granulomatous Colitis
1. Often spares rectum
2. Skip areas are characteristic
3. Deep ulcers are typical
4. Fistulas and sinus occur
5. Can involve all portions of the GI tract

graphic findings in these two important diseases are compared in Table 8-6. Figures 8-34 to 8-36 exhibit some of the common colon tumors detectable on a lower GI series. Adenomatous colon polyps (Fig. 8-34A) occur often, and they have the potential to become malignant. Thus, it is extremely important to detect and remove colon polyps. Familial colonic polyposis (Fig. 8-34B) is one of a number of syndromes characterized by multiple colonic polyps, and these polyps have the potential to become malignant. Adenocarcinoma of the colon (Figs. 8-35 and 8-36) is a common disease and must be considered whenever the patient complains of GI and abdominal symptoms, especially rectal bleeding and any change of bowel habits. There are approximately 150,000 new cases of carcinoma of the colon and rectum reported each year in the United States (3).

Oral Cholecystogram

The oral cholecystogram is a common diagnostic study that visualizes the gallbladder following the oral ingestion of special iodinated compounds. These compounds are metabolized by the liver, excreted into the biliary system, and subsequently concentrated in the gallbladder. The preparation for this study consists only of a small low-fat evening meal followed by the oral ingestion of iodine-containing tablets the night before the study. The following morning the gallbladder region is radiographed. This study is inexpensive, safe, and well tolerated by the patient (Fig. 8-37A). Ultrasound is especially useful in the workup of gallbladder and biliary duct diseases (Fig. 8-37B), and it is inexpensive, safe, and well tolerated by patients.

Endoscopic Retrograde Cholangiopancreatography

Another biliary tract study is endoscopic retrograde cholangiopancreatography (ERCP), wherein an endoscopist passes a fiberoptic scope retrograde under fluoroscopic control into the esophagus, stomach, duodenum, common and cystic bile ducts, and gallbladder. The pancreatic ducts can also be cannulated. Contrast media can be injected into any of these structures and the appropriate radiographs obtained (Fig. 8-38). ERCP is usually performed when the less invasive studies (computed tomography, ultrasound, magnetic resonance imaging, contrast studies) are indeterminate or not diagnostic.

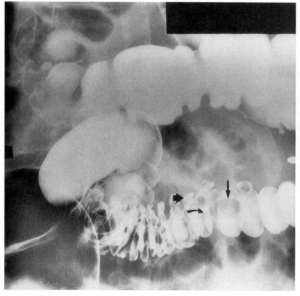
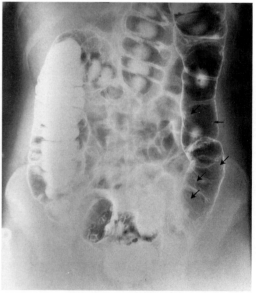

A   B

FIG. 8-34. A: Double-contrast colon examination. Sigmoid colon benign polyp. The body of the polyp is indicated by the long straight arrow, and the polyp stalk *(curved arrow)* is clearly visible. Multiple diverticula *(short straight arrowhead)* are present in the sigmoid colon. **B:** Double-contrast colon examination. Familial colonic polyposis. Multiple colonic polyps are indicated by the straight arrows.

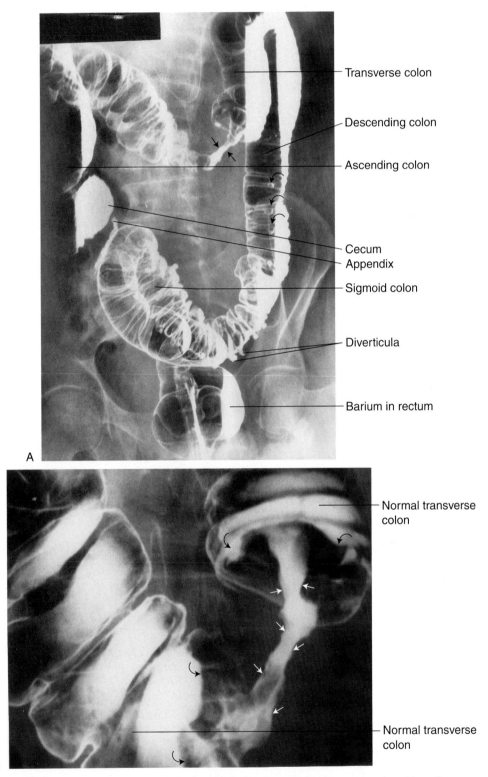

FIG. 8-35. A: Double-contrast colon examination. Adenocarcinoma of the transverse colon. Note the classic apple core appearance of the colon adenocarcinoma . The apple core represents the patent portion of the bowel lumen *(straight arrows)*. Descending colon diverticula *(curved arrows)* are seen en face. **B:** Double-contrast colon examination. Coned-down view of the tumor mass in A. Note the irregular mucosa along the narrowed lumen of the apple core lesion *(straight arrows)*. The cancer mass creates a shouldering *(curved arrows)* deformity in the neighboring transverse colon both proximal and distally.

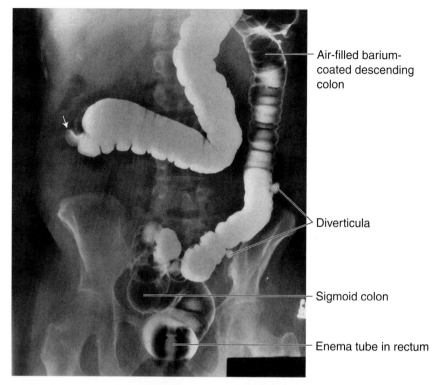

FIG. 8-36. Double-contrast colon examination. Carcinoma of the proximal transverse colon. The tumor mass in the proximal transverse colon *(straight arrow)* caused a complete retrograde obstruction to the flow of barium.

- Air-filled barium-coated descending colon
- Diverticula
- Sigmoid colon
- Enema tube in rectum

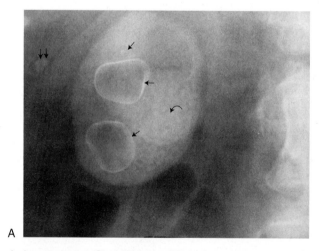

A

FIG. 8-37. A: Oral cholecystogram. Cholelithiasis. The contrast-media-filled functioning gallbladder contains two large partially calcified calculi (stones) in the gallbladder as well as multiple small stones. The multiple small stones gives a speckled appearance *(curved arrow)* to the gallbladder. Incidental costochondral calcification is indicated by double straight arrows.

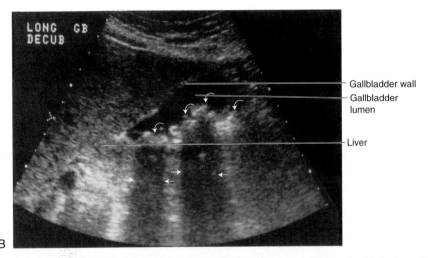

FIG. 8-37. *Continued.* **B:** Longitudinal decubitus cholecystosonogram. Cholelithiasis. Note how the dense gall stones or calculi *(curved arrows)* cast acoustic shadows *(between the straight arrows)* because the sound waves are unable to penetrate or traverse the dense calculi. This is similar to a shadow cast by a tree or building.

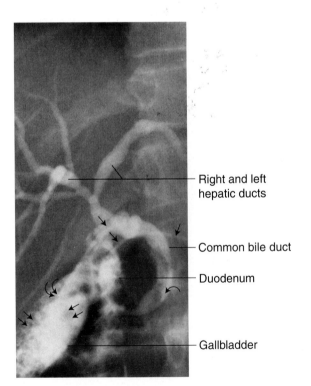

FIG. 8-38. Endoscopic retrograde cholangiopancreatography (ERCP). Cholelithiasis and choledocholithiasis. The gallbladder is full of calculi *(double straight arrows)*, and there is a large calculus in the distal common bile duct *(curved arrow)*. The endoscopist reported pus as well as calculi in the gallbladder and common bile duct. A nasobiliary drain *(straight single arrows)* was left in place with the tip *(double curved arrows)* in the gallbladder.

ULTRASONOGRAPHY

Ultrasonography has become a very effective and frequently used diagnostic tool in the abdomen (Table 8-7). Abdominal organs and pathologic processes have their own characteristic echo patterns as shown in Fig. 8-39. Ultrasonography is especially useful in the workup of diseases involving the liver and biliary tract, kidneys, abdominal aorta, and abdominal masses in general.

ANGIOGRAPHY

Nearly all of the abdominal vessels can be demonstrated by angiography, and abdominal aortography is commonly used to evaluate the abdominal aorta and its major branches (Fig. 8-40).

COMPUTED TOMOGRAPHY AND MAGNETIC RESONANCE IMAGING

Computed tomography (CT) and magnetic resonance imaging (MRI) are extremely useful in the diagnosis and management of abdominal disease. Both CT and MRI have the potential to differentiate between normal

TABLE 8-7. *Some indications for abdominal ultrasonography*

1. Evaluation of abdominal organ masses
2. Evaluation of abdominal masses
3. Evaluation of abdominal organ size, shape, and texture
4. Evaluation of the abdominal aorta and other vessels
5. Evaluation of the gallbladder and biliary ducts

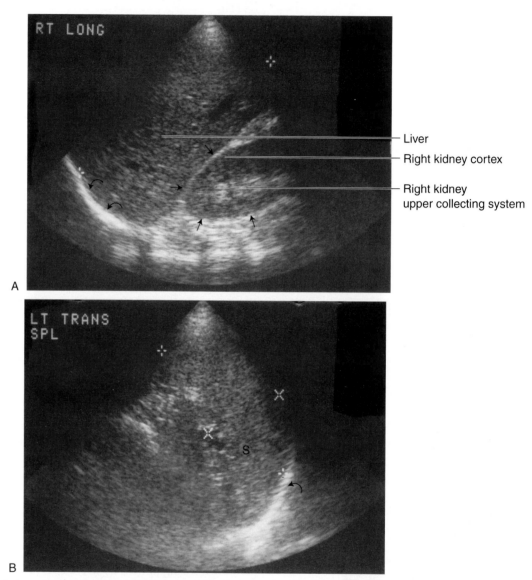

RT LONG

— Liver

— Right kidney cortex

— Right kidney
upper collecting system

A

LT TRANS
SPL

S

B

FIG. 8-39. A: Longitudinal or sagittal abdominal sonogram. Normal liver and right kidney echo patterns. The opaque markers indicate the longitudinal or sagittal liver dimension. The right kidney is demarcated by the straight arrows, and the right hemidiaphragm by the curved arrows. **B:** Transverse or axial abdominal sonogram. Normal spleen echo pattern. The side-to-side spleen dimension lies between the x marks, and the cephalocaudad dimension lies between the crosses. The left hemidiaphragm is indicated by the curved arrow. S, spleen.

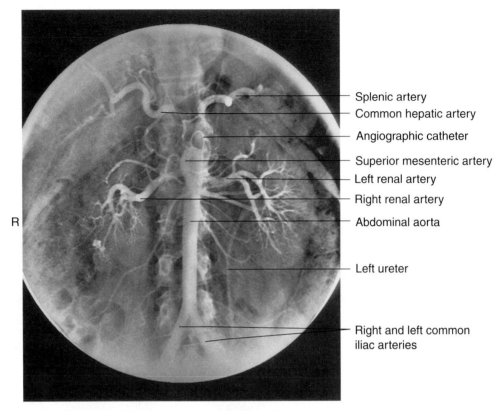

Splenic artery
Common hepatic artery
Angiographic catheter
Superior mesenteric artery
Left renal artery
Right renal artery
Abdominal aorta

Left ureter

Right and left common
iliac arteries

R

FIG. 8-40. Abdominal aorta angiogram. Normal.

and abnormal tissue and both accurately display sectional anatomy in multiple planes, but CT is used more frequently than MRI in the abdomen because of its superior capability for demonstrating the anatomy. Prior to an abdominal CT study the patient drinks a diluted iodinated solution (contrast media) or diluted barium to demarcate the GI tract, and intravenous contrast media is usually injected during the study to demonstrate vessels and organs.

Normal abdominal CT and MRI anatomy is illustrated in Figs. 8-41 to 8-45 (4), and some examples of abnormal CT images are demonstrated in Figs. 8-46 to 8-51.

(continued on page 178)

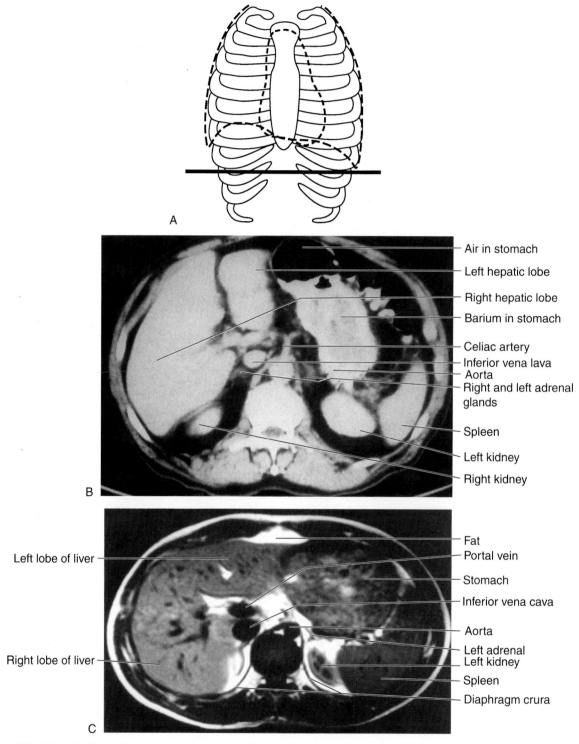

FIG. 8-41. A: Illustration of the approximate axial anatomic level through the liver and spleen for B and C. **B:** Abdomen axial CT image through the liver and spleen. Normal. **C:** Abdomen axial MR image through the liver and spleen. Normal.

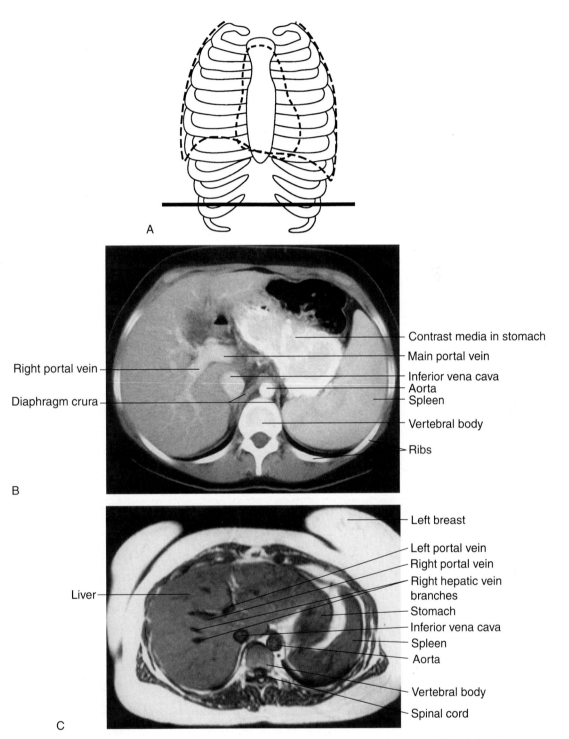

FIG. 8-42. A: Approximate axial anatomic level through the liver and spleen for B and C. This level is just caudad to the level in Fig. 41. **B:** Abdomen axial CT image through the liver and spleen. Normal. **C:** Abdomen axial MR image through the liver and spleen. Normal.

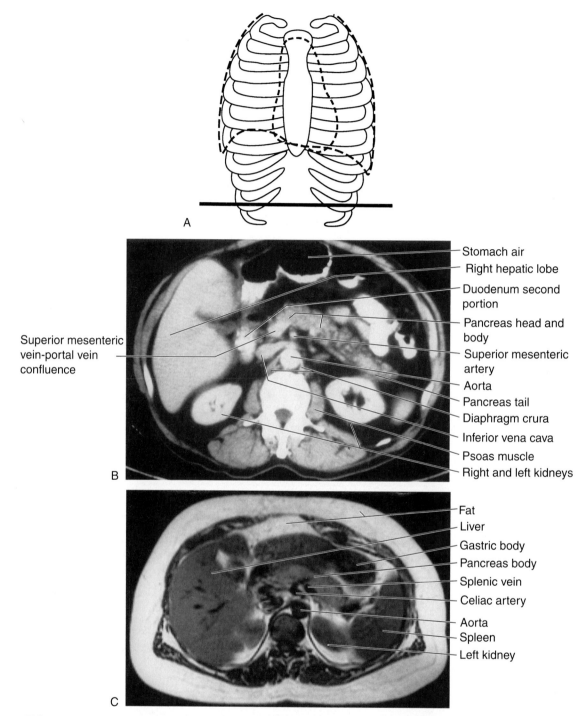

FIG. 8-43. A: Illustration of the approximate axial anatomic level through the pancreas for B and C. **B:** Abdomen axial CT image through the pancreas level. Normal. **C:** Abdomen axial MR image through the pancreas level. Normal.

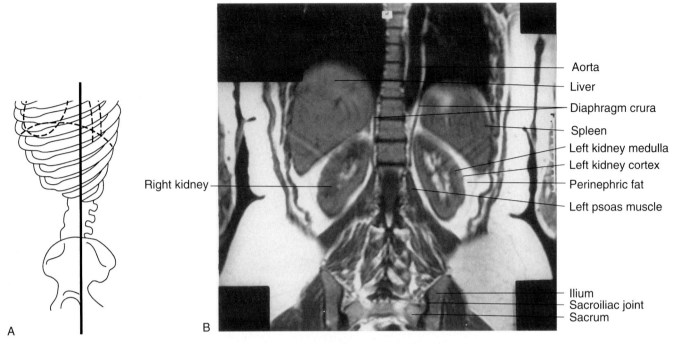

Right kidney

Aorta
Liver
Diaphragm crura
Spleen
Left kidney medulla
Left kidney cortex
Perinephric fat
Left psoas muscle

Ilium
Sacroiliac joint
Sacrum

A   B

FIG. 8-44. A: Illustration of the approximate coronal anatomic level through the kidneys for B. **B:** Abdomen coronal MR image through the kidneys. Normal.

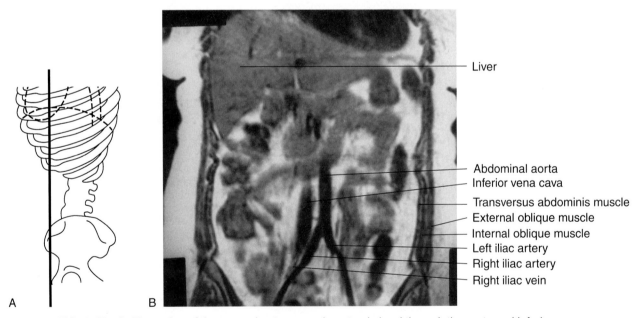

Liver

Abdominal aorta
Inferior vena cava
Transversus abdominis muscle
External oblique muscle
Internal oblique muscle
Left iliac artery
Right iliac artery
Right iliac vein

A   B

FIG. 8-45. A: Illustration of the approximate coronal anatomic level through the aorta and inferior vena cava for B. **B:** Abdomen coronal MR image through the abdominal aorta and inferior vena cava. Normal.

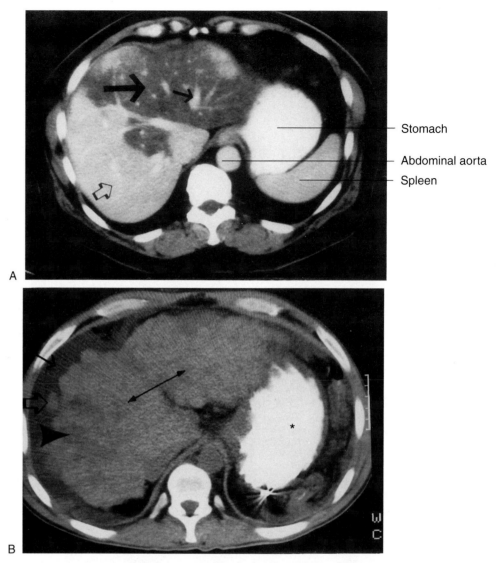

FIG. 8-46. A: Axial upper abdominal CT image. Fat deposition (fatty change or fatty metamorphosis) in the liver. This patient was a severe diabetic, but there are many other etiologies for this process (Table 8-8). The large black arrow indicates the fatty changes or deposition in the liver (black). The small black arrow indicates a vessel. If the black area had been tumor and not fat, the vessels usually would be displaced or stretched by the mass effect of tumor. The open arrow indicates normal enhanced liver. **B:** Axial upper abdominal CT image. Hepatic cirrhosis or Laennec's cirrhosis. This patient was a chronic alcoholic, and this type of cirrhosis is most commonly caused by alcohol in the United States. Note the classic contracted and nodular liver margin *(open arrow)*, fatty changes *(arrowhead)*, and ascites *(short black arrow)*. Both lobes of the liver are involved *(long two-headed arrow)*. *, gastric barium.

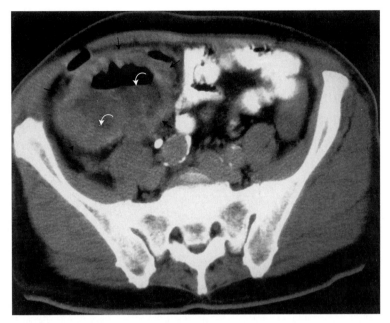

FIG. 8-47. Lower abdomen axial CT image. The straight arrows outline a large cecal neoplasm, and the curved arrows show an air–fluid level within the tumor mass secondary to necrosis.

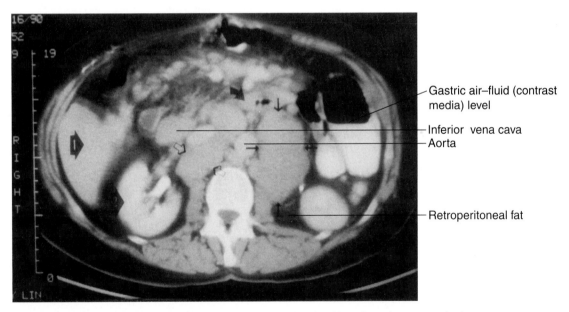

FIG. 8-48. Abdomen axial CT image. Lymphoma. The lymphoma involved lymph node masses in the retroperitoneum *(small black and short open arrows)* nearly hide the enhanced aorta and inferior vena cava. The arrow labeled 1 merely indicates the enhanced inferior aspect of the liver.

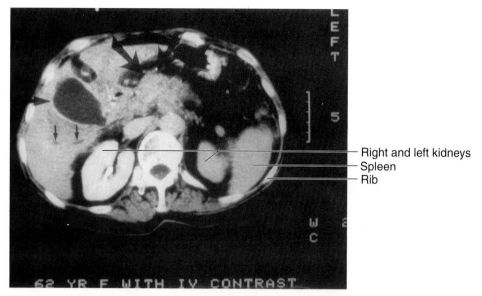

FIG. 8-49. Abdomen axial CT image through the liver and spleen level. Adenocarcinoma of the pancreas head. The following are visible: a tumor mass in the pancreas head *(large black arrow)*, a dilated gallbladder *(arrowhead)*, and dilated intrahepatic bile ducts *(small arrows)*. Note the printing below the image indicates the patient's age and intravenous contrast media information. Always read the printing on an image, as the information can be most helpful at times.

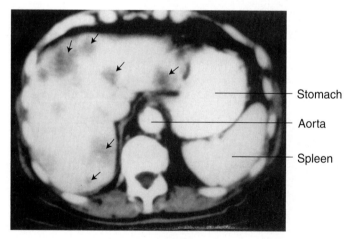

FIG. 8-50. Abdomen axial CT image through the liver and spleen. Right and left hepatic lobe metastases. The metastases *(straight arrows)* appear hypodense compared to the enhanced normal liver. Enhancement was accomplished by intravenous injection of contrast media.

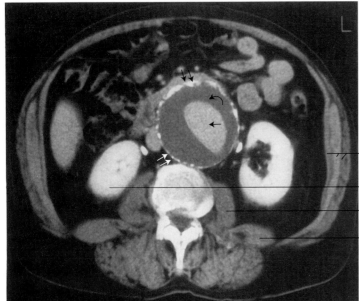

— Abdominal wall, three
   muscle layers

— Right and left kidneys

— Psoas muscle

— Quadratus lumborum
   muscle

A

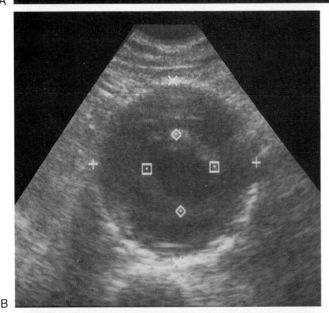

B

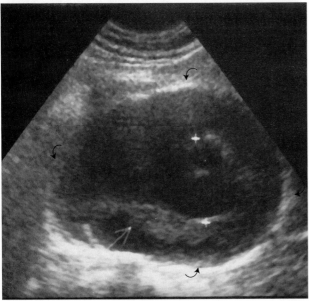

C

FIG. 8-51. A: Abdomen axial CT image through the kidneys. Abdominal aortic aneurysm. The patent lumen is the
contrast-filled area *(straight arrow)* and there is a large
thrombus *(curved arrow)* between the patent lumen and
the true aortic wall. The wall of the aorta is partially calcified
(double straight arrows). **B, C:** Transverse or axial (B) and
longitudinal or sagittal (C) abdominal sonograms. Abdominal aortic aneurysm. On the transverse image, the true
lumen lies between the boxes and diamonds, whereas the
aortic wall is indicated by the crosses. The straight arrow
indicates a thrombus between the patent lumen and the
true aortic wall. On the longitudinal sonogram©, the patent
lumen of the aorta lies between the cross marks, whereas
the straight arrow points to a thrombus or clot between the
patent lumen and the aortic wall *(curved arrows)*.

Key Points

- Radiologic evaluation of the abdomen usually begins with an AP supine abdominal radiograph.
- The presence or absence of rectal gas can be a key differential point between adynamic ileus versus intestinal obstruction.
- Adynamic ileus has intestinal gas throughout the small and large intestine and rectum.
- In general, large and small bowel obstructions have little or no bowel gas beyond the obstruction site and *usually there is no air in the rectum.*
- Once the diagnosis of obstruction is made you should attempt to accurately locate the exact site. In small bowel obstruction, there are loops of dilated small bowel proximal to the obstruction site with no air distally and no air in the rectum. In large bowel obstruction there is dilated colon proximal to the obstruction site with no air distally and no air in the rectum.
- Small bowel can be identified by the valvulae conniventes that extend completely across the small bowel lumen.
- Large bowel can be identified by the colonic septa that do not extend all the way across the bowel lumen.
- As little as a few cubic centimeters of free intraperitoneal air can be detected on properly performed upright and/or decubitus radiographs.
- Computed tomography, ultrasonography, and, to a lesser extent, magnetic resonance imaging are useful tools to evaluate for abdominal pathologic processes.

REFERENCES

1. Rigler LG. Spontaneous pneumoperitoneum: a roentgenologic sign found in the supine position. *Radiology* 1941, 37:604.
2. Chapman S, Nakielny R. *Aids to Radiological Differential Diagnosis,* 3rd ed. London: Saunders, 1995.
3. Juhl JH, Crummy AB. *Paul and Juhl's Essentials of Radiologic Imaging,* 6th ed. Philadelphia: JB Lippincott, 1993.
4. El-Khoury GY, Bergman RA, Montgomery WJ. *Sectional Anatomy by MRI,* 2nd ed. New York: Churchill Livingstone, 1995.

CHAPTER 9

Pediatric Abdomen

Wilbur L. Smith

Very much analogous to the situation with the chest x-ray, the abdominal radiographs of neonates are very different from those of adults, whereas radiographs of older children and teenagers begin to have a lot of similarities with adults. Abdominal films of neonates are especially discrepant due to a number of physiologic factors. First and foremost, neonates swallow a tremendous amount of air during their relatively inefficient breathing and eating. It is, therefore, not at all unusual to find many loops of small bowel in the plain film of a normal neonate (Fig. 9-1), whereas in an adult or older child it is unusual to see so much small bowel gas (Fig. 9-2). In fact, it is abnormal to see a gasless abdomen in a neonate! Such a finding usually means that the infant is so obtunded that it cannot swallow air, that there is a discontinuity of the gastrointestinal (GI) tract preventing air from entering the bowel, or that the infant is septic or otherwise critically ill (Fig. 9-3). All of this air in the small bowel makes the interpretation of the x-rays difficult as far as determining bowel distention. The best rule to remember is that the bowel loops of a normal neonate are thin-walled and lie in close proximity to each other. The appearance of thick-walled bowel or marked separation of the bowel loops suggest an abnormal intraabdominal process (Fig. 9-4). Comparison of Figs. 9-1 and 9-4 illustrates this point.

The haustra of the colon are notoriously variable in their development and do not become prominent until about 6 months of age. Due to this fact, it is fraught with difficulty to try to differentiate large from small bowel on the plain radiographs of a neonate's abdomen. Occasionally, you can get lucky and be reasonably certain in differentiation; however, most of the time it isn't even worth guessing. This makes the determination of whether there is rectal gas or not even more critical. The vast majority of newborns will have gas all the way through their GI tract by 24 hours after birth. If there is any doubt as to whether a child has rectal gas or has obstruction, the prone cross-table lateral film is invaluable in making this distinction (Fig. 9-5). Remember: if you are looking for distal gas in an infant in whom you are considering bowel obstruction, go right for the rectum! (Table 9-1).

Another big difference between neonates and older children or adults is the presence of the belly button. This necessary structure and the appurtenances appended to it make for some weird shadows on abdominal films of babies. Many an unsuspecting physician has called an umbilical clamp a bone or a foreign

TABLE 9-1. *Causes of bowel obstruction in the neonate*

Atresia
Malrotation
Hernia
Meconium ileus
Hirschsprung's disease
Bowel duplications

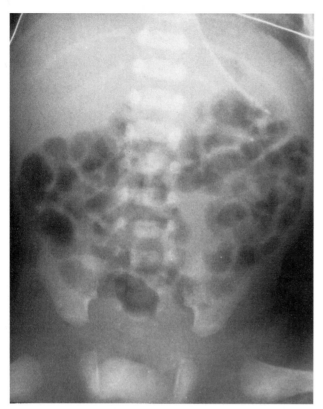

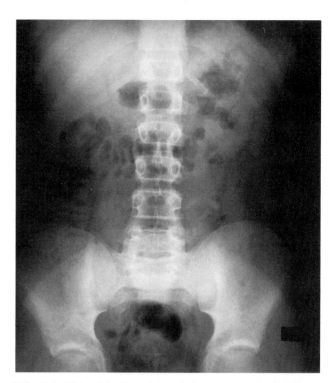

FIG. 9-1. This abdominal film shows the bowel gas pattern of a normal newborn baby. Notice there are a number of nondistended bowel loops with considerable small bowel gas. The loops lie next to each other and are thin-walled. This is a good visual picture to remember for the normal bowel gas appearance of a neonate. Older children do not have this much gas and adults have very little small bowel gas visible on plain films. Contrast this with Fig. 9-4, a baby with sepsis and some bowel wall edema.

FIG. 9-2. This plain film of the abdomen was obtained on a normal child with constipation. There is gas in the colon and stomach but very little gas in the small bowel. Contrast this to the appearance of Fig. 9-1, the neonate, where there is normally considerable small bowel gas.

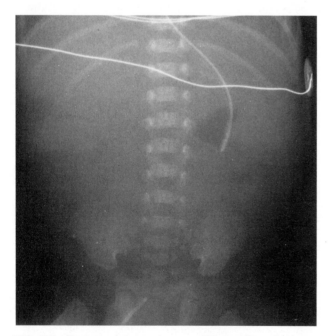

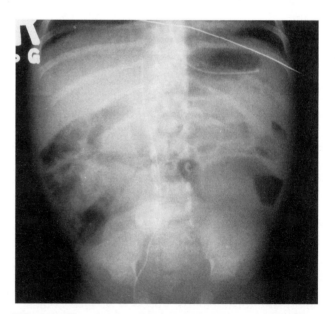

FIG. 9-3. Gasless abdomen in a very ill baby. There is almost always some gas in the stomach but very little gas distal. This is abnormal and can occur as a result of the baby being too ill to swallow or a systemic illness. In this case the baby was immobilized so that he would not fight the ventilator and this gasless abdomen resulted. Normally babies should have gas in both large and small bowel.

FIG. 9-4. Contrast the abdominal plain film in this critically ill and septic neonate with the normal bubbly pattern of bowel gas shown in Fig. 9-1. The loops of bowel are separated and some of the bowel shows evidence of a moderate degree of dilation. These findings are nonspecific and can be seen in any severely ill infant. In this case sepsis caused abnormal bowel motility in this abnormal appearing x-ray.

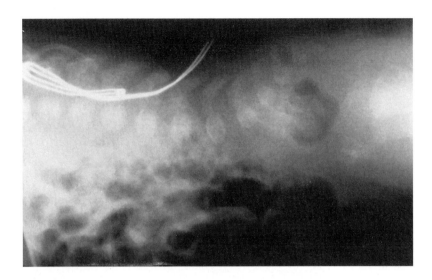

FIG. 9-5. A prone cross-lateral of the abdomen can often be helpful in showing whether or not gas is present in the rectum. Remember that because you cannot tell large bowel from small bowel in neonates it is important to identify the rectum when you are trying to look for distal gas. Rectal gas usually is identified in the hollow of the sacrum, as in this infant.

body (Fig. 9-6). The umbilicus itself protrudes much further in a neonate than in an adult. Any coin-shaped lesion in the lower midabdomen of a neonate should be considered the umbilical remnant until proven otherwise. A good clue is that, owing to the air surrounding the protruding umbilical stump, the edges of the umbilicus are very sharply defined, particularly the inferior edge (Fig. 9-7).

In summary, remember that it is normal for neonates to have considerable gas in their small bowel. As long as the walls are thin and the bowel loops are approximating each other, don't worry. Remember also that up to 6 months of age it is extremely difficult to tell large bowel from small bowel, and guesses as to whether a loop

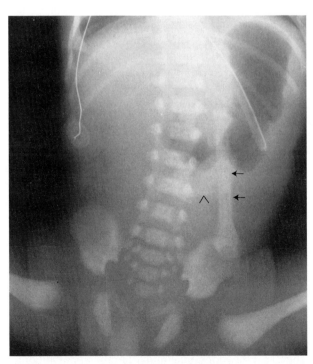

FIG. 9-6. A newborn infant who has just begun to swallow air. Notice the nasogastric tube marking the stomach. The oblong structure to the left of the spine *(arrows)* almost looks like a bone of some sort, however, it is clearly attached to the umbilical stump *(arrowhead)* and in fact represents an umbilical cord clamp superimposed on the abdominal film.

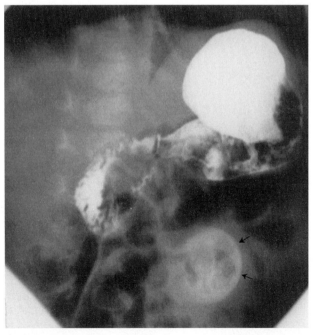

FIG. 9-7. This baby undergoing an upper GI has a circular, bowel-filled mass in the lower midabdomen. The mass projects slightly to the left because the baby is in an oblique position *(arrows)*. Note the very sharp margin indicating that the mass protrudes off the abdominal wall. Anytime you see an extremely sharp border on a plain film of the abdomen, there has to be either air or fat surrounding that structure. In this case air surrounds the structure because the umbilicus protrudes out from the abdominal wall. This is a typical umbilical hernia.

represents large or small bowel on plain film are exactly that, i.e., educated estimates.

CONGENITAL ABNORMALITIES

In general, congenital abnormalities are much more likely to present as clinical problems in neonates than they are in adults. Another way to look at it is if you got to adulthood without a congenital anomaly bothering you, it is likely that you will carry that anomaly to your grave. When you deal with an abnormal abdomen in a neonate, a congenital anomaly is extremely likely; in a 4-year-old it is somewhat likely; and in a 15-year-old it is less likely. If you play by the 99% rule in an 80-year-old, you probably shouldn't even think of congenital abnormalities as the cause of an acute abdomen. Having said this, I know that everyone will be able to find the unusual case of a congenital defect causing grief to an 80-year-old, but remember that's the zebra, not the horse!

Bowel Atresia

In babies, the commonest cause of bowel obstruction is atresia of the bowel. Atresia occurs owing to a number

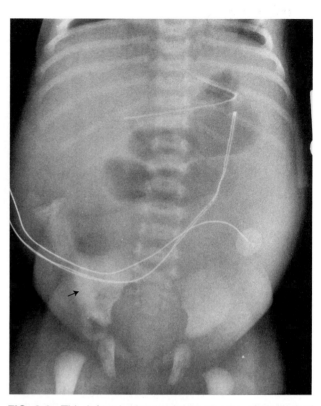

FIG. 9-9. This infant had a moderate degree of abdominal distention at birth, which progressed to a worrisome abdominal distention within 6 hours. Note that there is no gas in the rectum and that only two dilated loops of bowel are identified, predominantly in the upper abdomen and to the left of the spine. These films are most consistent with abdominal obstruction very high in the bowel but distal to the duodenum. This is an example of surgically proven jejunal atresia.

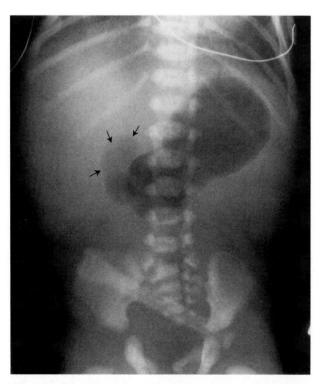

FIG. 9-8. A newborn infant with marked abdominal distention. Note that the gas goes no further than the very dilated duodenal bulb *(arrows)*. This is characteristic of the so-called double-bubble sign of duodenal atresia. Whenever you see a patient with duodenal atresia, think of the very frequent associations of Down's syndrome and congenital heart disease and the less frequent association of esophageal atresia.

of complex intrauterine processes most of which involve vascular supply to the wall of the bowel. Radiographs of the atresia vary tremendously according to the level at which the atresia occurs, however, they have common features. First, there is no gas distal to the level of the atresia and second, the bowel proximal to the atresia is disproportionately dilated. Beyond that, it is just a matter of looking at the radiograph to try to guess how far down the bowel you can go before you encounter the atresia (Figs. 9-8 to 9-10). As a general rule to help you establish the level, remember that the duodenal bulb is located in the right upper quadrant of the abdomen; therefore if you only have a dilated stomach and loop in the right upper quadrant, duodenal atresia is likely. The jejunum is predominantly in the upper abdomen and predominantly on the left side, whereas the ileum is in the right lower quadrant. If you see many dilated bowel loops and particularly large loops preponderantly to the right of the spine, it is probably an ileal atresia, whereas if the loops are confined to the upper abdomen and predominantly to the left, it is probably jejunal atresia. These are 70:30 rules, so don't get too preoccupied with them; on the other hand, they can be very helpful.

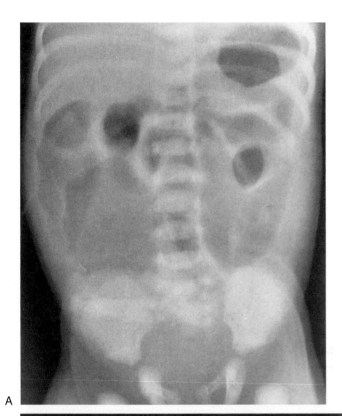

A

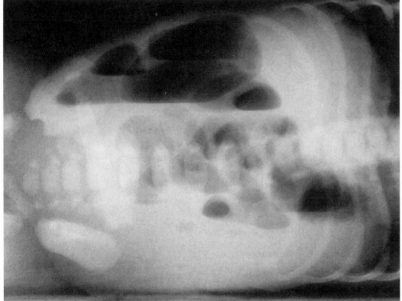

B

FIG. 9-10. A: Abdominal radiograph of a 1-day-old baby with abdominal distention shows evidence of multiple dilated bowel loops and no gas in the rectum. The findings are consistent with an ileal atresia. **B:** A decubitus view of the same infant illustrated in A shows multiple air–fluid levels. The presence of air–fluid levels is sometimes valuable in distinguishing ileal atresia from meconium ileus. Air-fluid levels favor ileal atresia. Incidentally, note our old friend, the cord clamp.

Meconium Ileus

Meconium ileus is a condition that mimics a distal bowel atresia and that deserves special note because of its prevalence in the Caucasian population. In meconium ileus, the contents of the bowel (meconium) are abnormal, becoming thick and viscous due to the lack of digestive enzymes. This material compacts in the ileum to cause a complete obstruction. One could think of it as analogous to filling a pipe with tar. Technically,

this is not an atresia, however, it mimics an atresia because the bowel is completely obstructed by intraluminal content. There are a few signs that can be used to distinguish meconium ileus from ileal atresia. The meconium ileus usually entraps some air, so that one sees a bubbly appearance at the level of the meconium-filled bowel (Fig. 9-11). Also, the meconium is so thick and tar-like that it does not form air–fluid levels with the swallowed intestinal gas. This is in contradistinction to an ileal atresia, whereby the fluid intraluminal con-

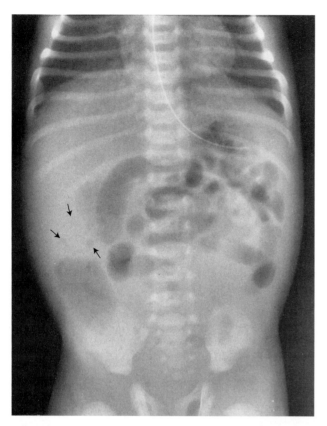

FIG. 9-11. A newborn infant with a very distended abdomen. Note the bubbly appearance *(arrows)* in the right lower quadrant of the abdomen. These bubbles coupled with a paucity of gas in the rectum are characteristic of meconium ileus. The vast majority of babies with meconium ileus will also have cystic fibrosis.

tents of the bowel interact with the swallowed gas to form multiple air–fluid levels.

No discussion of intestinal obstruction in neonates would be complete without mention of microcolon. Microcolon is another term for the small lumen colon that is encountered in babies with distal intestinal obstruction, usually either meconium ileus or ileal atresia. Babies' colons dilate because of the presence of intraluminal content, i.e., meconium. This meconium is formed in utero by sloughing of the cells and mucus from the GI tract. If there is enough downstream bowel from an obstruction (e.g., in the instance of duodenal atresia), there will be enough cells and mucus sloughed to form meconium and the colon will have this meconium content. If, however, the obstruction is low so that there is not enough bowel distal to the obstruction to form meconium, then one gets an unused or microcolon. Microcolon is therefore a common sign of distal bowel obstruction (Fig. 9-12). You can obviously get fooled, because diseases like Hirschsprung's disease, where the lumen is intact, but the colon does not transport meconium normally, occasionally give you a microcolon.

Again, the 99% rule prevails, microcolon means distal obstruction.

Hernias

Two other congenital anomalies merit discussion as the cause of abdominal catastrophes in neonates or in slightly older children. The first is the most common cause of bowel obstruction in children, the hernia. Hernias in children are usually congenital defects that allow the bowel to protrude into a space where it doesn't belong. The bowel then gets caught, swells, and complications ensue. The most common site of hernia is the inguinal area (Fig. 9-13), however, internal hernias, particularly in areas where the bowel goes from retroperitoneum to a intraperitoneal location, are also possible (Fig. 9-14). Hernias can go on for a long time if the bowel does not become compromised, but they can become very symptomatic very fast in instances where the bowel is compromised (Fig. 9-15). Some conditions of the neonate may enhance the possibility of a hernia, particularly conditions that involve chronic ascites, prematurity, or the presence of a ventricular peritoneal shunt for hydrocephalus (Fig. 9-16).

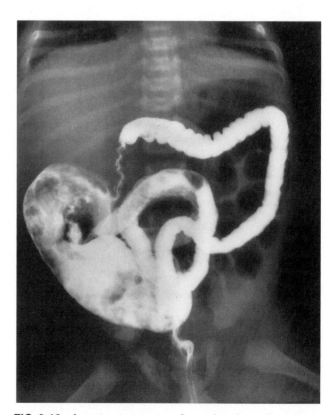

FIG. 9-12. A contrast enema performed on the patient shown in Fig. 9-11 shows a very small (micro-) colon leading to a very dilated ileum distended with multiple filling defects. The filling defects are the impacted meconium, which gives meconium ileus its name. Remember that a microcolon means a distal obstruction.

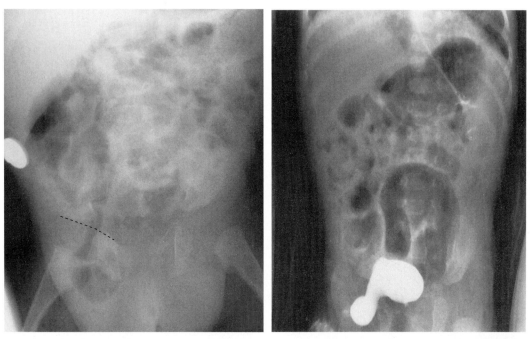

A

B

FIG. 9-13. A: Plain radiograph of the abdomen shows bowel lying below the inguinal ligament *(dotted line)*. On a plain radiograph the inguinal ligament is defined as the space between the symphysis pubis and the anterior superior iliac spine—in this case, the child had a large inguinal hernia filled with bowel. **B:** This baby, having a contrast study of the kidneys, had a protrusion of the lateral margin of his bladder into the right inguinal canal. A small protrusion can be normal, however, this large protrusion of bladder is associated with an inguinal hernia.

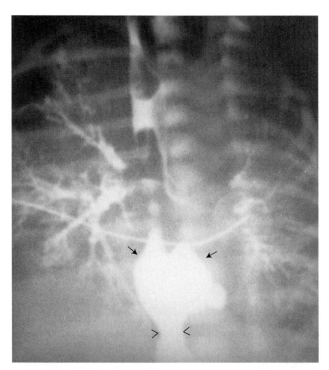

FIG. 9-14. This neonate has a large hiatus hernia or protrusion of stomach above the diaphragm. The hernia pouch *(arrows)* is shown in the chest, whereas the narrowing of the esophageal hiatus *(arrowheads)* shows the area where the stomach herniates through the periesophageal hiatus. Note that there is contrast in the lungs. This hernia was so large that it caused the baby to reflux contrast from his stomach to his esophagus and then aspirate. Unlike this one, most hiatus hernias are relatively benign.

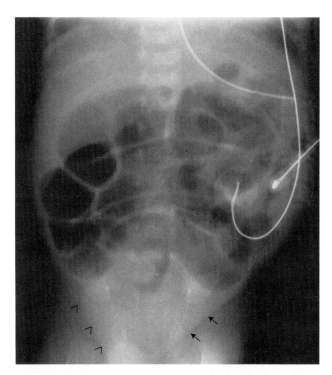

FIG. 9-15. This premature infant developed signs of a bowel obstruction. Note the very dilated loops of small bowel on the film. The most important finding is the asymmetry of the inguinal folds, the right bulging in a concave fashion *(arrowheads)* while the left is straight *(arrows)*. The bulge in the right groin is owing to an incarcerated inguinal hernia, a finding the clinician missed until they took off the patient's diaper.

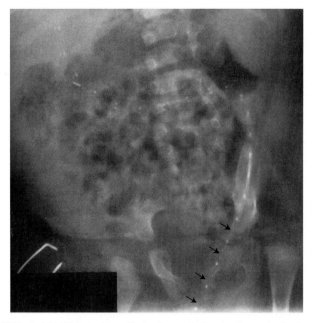

FIG. 9-16. This baby with hydrocephalus had a ventricular peritoneal shunt. The radiopaque markers *(arrows)* show the course of the shunt. Notice that the shunt extends into an inguinal hernia. Because these babies have chronic ascites from the drainage of the cerebrospinal fluid into the abdomen, they are more prone to have inguinal hernias. Approximately one-third of babies with ventricular peritoneal shunts develop inguinal hernias.

Malrotations

The other congenital abnormality worthy of special attention is that of malrotation. This condition occurs due to a congenital abnormality of fixation of the bowel. You will remember that the bowel forms about the axis of the superior mesenteric artery (I bet you never thought you'd ever need that bit of embryology) and that the bowel herniates out of the body through the omphalus, then returns to the abdominal cavity. If, upon return, the bowel does not rotate appropriately, it fixes in abnormal positions. This error in fixation of the bowel sets the scene for the bowel to twist and obstruct; the so-called midgut volvulus (Figs. 9-17 and 9-18). This is truly a surgical emergency and should be considered whenever you have an abnormal film suggesting obstruction, and the presence of bilious vomiting in a child. Since the bowel twists about the superior mesenteric artery and vein, the major complication is vascular compromise of the bowel. If the bowel is not untwisted, the gut will die leaving the child a nutritional cripple. While malrotation is discussed with the neonatal diseases, be aware that it can present at any time in life. The majority of malrotation patients who get in trouble do so before 2 years of age, however, older children and adults can occasionally have malrotation-related problems.

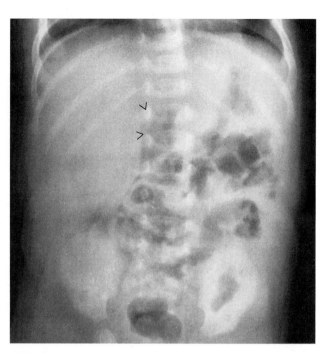

FIG. 9-17. This 36-day-old infant began vomiting bilious material and became acutely ill. The plain abdominal radiograph is not diagnostic; however, note the gas-filled duodenal bulb *(arrowheads)*. It is very unusual to see gas in a normal duodenal bulb. The subsequent upper GI proved that this patient had a midgut volvulus. The plain film findings in midgut volvulus range from normal to complete bowel obstruction. When in doubt with an infant with bilious vomiting, note that an upper GI is always indicated.

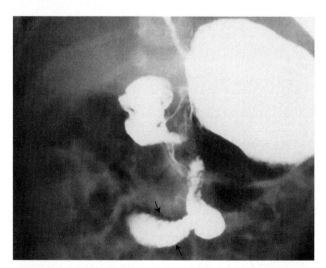

FIG. 9-18. Upper GI in a 27-day-old baby who suddenly developed bilious vomiting. Note that the duodenum descends in the midline, then passes off to the right at the duodenal–jejunal junction *(arrows)*, never coming to the left of the spine and behind the stomach as is normal. This is characteristic of malrotation, an anomaly that occurs due to malfixation of the gut in utero. The greatest danger with these infants is midgut volvulus and infarction of the small bowel because of twisting about the vascular pedicle at the root of the mesentery.

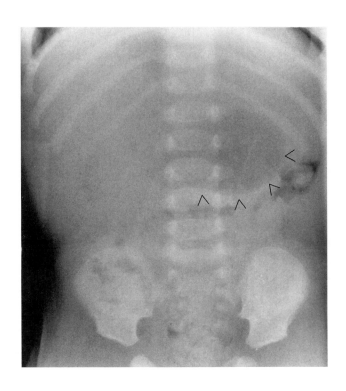

FIG. 9-19. This 6-week-old infant had severe and pernicious vomiting that had become progressively worse over the course of a week. The impact on his nutrition was so severe that he had actually lost weight. Note the distended stomach *(arrowheads)*. The presence of distal gas in his rectum shows that he was not completely obstructed, but the film is suggestive of a high-grade partial gastric outlet obstruction. About 90% of pyloric stenosis patients will have a plain film that looks like this.

PYLORIC STENOSIS

The final common intraabdominal condition worth discussion in babies—pyloric stenosis—is and isn't a congenital anomaly. Pyloric stenosis occurs due to hypertrophy of the pyloric muscle induced by a heritable error in metabolism. Because of the heritable nature of the disease, it is somewhat a congenital defect, but it does not usually present until about 6 weeks of age. It takes that long for the muscle with the abnormal metabolic activity to hypertrophy. The disease is male-preponderant and classically presents with nonbilious vomiting and weight loss in a 6-week-old. The plain abdominal radiograph suggests a partial obstruction with a very dilated stomach. Upper GI will show elongation of the pyloric channel and the narrowing of that channel. Ultrasound is the current favored method for the definitive diagnosis, showing the very large pyloric muscle tumor in exquisite detail (Figs. 9-19 to 9-21).

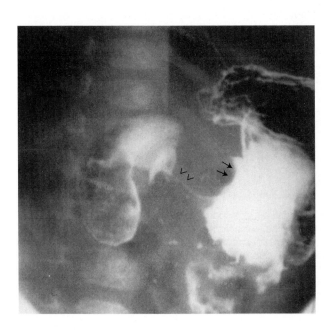

FIG. 9-20. The upper GI in this 6-week-old baby shows elongation and narrowing of the pyloric channel *(arrowheads)*. On the stomach side, notice the rounded indentation *(arrows)* caused by the very hypertrophied pyloric muscle. This is called the shoulder sign. Together this combination of signs is diagnostic for pyloric stenosis.

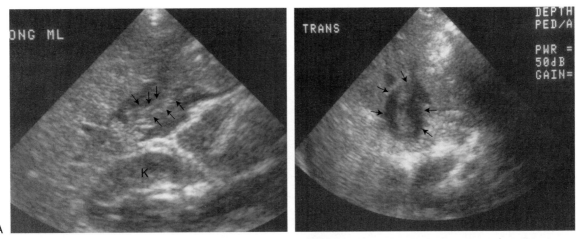

FIG. 9-21. A: A longitudinal ultrasound view of the pylorus in a 6-week-old boy with vomiting. The pyloric muscle appears black, while the mucosa of the central lumen appears white *(arrows)*. During the entire period of observation, the configuration of the pyloric muscle did not change and measurement of the pyloric muscle revealed a thickness of 6 mm (normal is <4 mm). This is diagnostic of pyloric stenosis. Note the intimate relationship of the pylorus to the right kidney (K). **B:** Transverse ultrasound view of the pylorus in the same infant as shown in A. Again the black or hypoechoic muscle surrounds the very echogenic mucosa. Arrows outline the transverse view of the pylorus. In pyloric stenosis the muscle is thick and unchanging throughout the examination.

COMMON DISEASES OF OLDER CHILDREN

As the child ages, the likelihood of various other diseases occurring increases. Two diseases in particular are prevalent and radiology plays a major role in their diagnosis. It seems fitting that they should get their own special sections of discussion here.

Intussusception

Intussusception, a disease in which one segment of bowel telescopes into another, has its maximum prevalence between the ages of 6 months and 2 years. The bowel is constantly in motion due to normal peristaltic activity. Theoretically, an inflamed intramural lymph node or some other structure alters this peristaltic activity, such that, one segment of bowel begins to be propelled at a differential rate leading to prolapse of one segment (intussusceptum) into the next contiguous portion of bowel (intussuscipiens). The intussusceptum becomes edematous because the blood supply of the prolapsed bowel is compromised and the intussusceptum begins to swell. This compounds the problem and leads to further extension of the intussusception. The ultimate extension is protrusion of the intussusceptum from the rectum! In fact, in nineteenth century textbooks, the differential diagnosis of intussusception was rectal prolapse. The most common anatomic area involved in intussusception is the terminal ileum and most intussusceptions are ileocecal.

Radiology plays a key role in the diagnosis as the child often presents with acute abdomen. Plain film shows

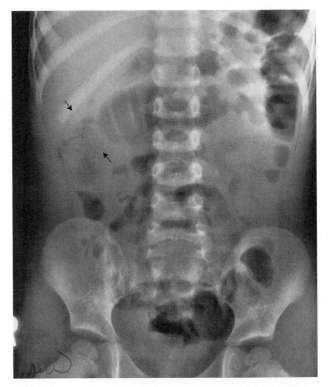

FIG. 9-22. Notice the rounded density and a spiral gas pattern located in the right upper quadrant in this 2-year-old child with recurrent cramping abdominal pain and hematochazia *(arrows)*. This plain film alone, if not diagnostic, is certainly very suspicious of intussusception. About 80% of the time you can make the diagnosis of intussusception on plain film by looking for a rounded mass and the spiral air pattern which is so characteristic.

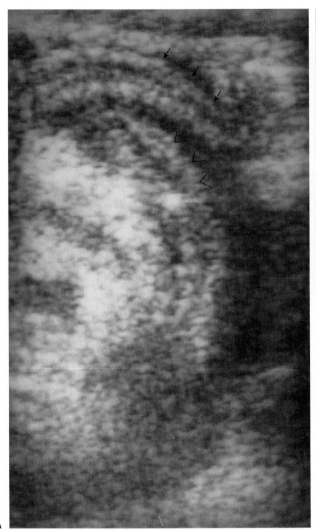

A

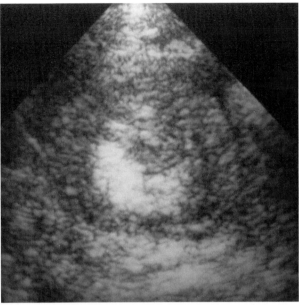

B

FIG. 9-23. A: A longitudinal ultrasound view of an intussusception. Notice the intussusceptum *(arrowheads)* telescoping into the intussuscipiens. With a little imagination you can almost see a coiled spring signal as the bowel wrinkles, with one loop of the bowel prolapsing into the other. **B:** A transverse view of an intussusception showing the target sign. The brightly echogenic material is the edematous mucosa, whereas the less echoic material is the wall of the intussusceptum.

evidence of partial bowel obstruction and the intussusceptum is frequently visible on the plain film as a rounded density near the point of obstruction (Fig. 9-22). Diagnosis is confirmed either by ultrasound or by barium enema (Figs. 9-23 and 9-24). Radiology often plays both a diagnostic and a therapeutic role in intussusception. Between 50% and 80% of intussusceptions can be nonoperatively reduced using either an air enema or a contrast enema. These techniques are very specialized and should be performed only by trained personnel. They are, however, part of the standard armamentarium of any Board-certified radiologist.

Appendicitis

Appendicitis is the most common abdominal surgical emergency of childhood. Appendicitis is one of the great mimics in that the symptoms can be fairly protean and the diagnosis in many instances is obscure (Table 9-2). There is an old adage that the clinical certainty

of appendicitis should be about 85%, meaning that 15% of the appendices that a surgeon removes should be normal or the surgeon is going to begin to miss some true-positive cases of appendicitis. Various radiology imaging techniques can narrow this false-positive rate somewhat, but really the value of imaging is in those cases where the diagnosis is at serious doubt. Look at it in another way. If imaging tests can give you 95% sensitivity, whereas clinical tests are 85% sensitive, the imaging doesn't add much in a situation where you are quite sure that appendicitis exists. On the other hand, in that case when you aren't sure or, let's

TABLE 9-2. *Classic signs of appendicitis*[a]

1. Right lower quadrant pain
2. Leukocytosis
3. Anorexia/vomiting

[a] Only half of appendicitis patients under age 5 or over age 50 exhibit these signs!

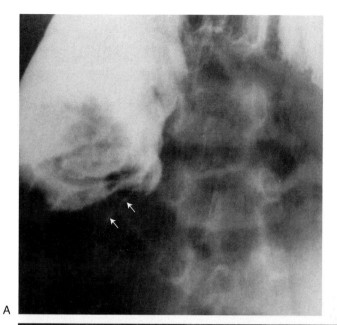

A

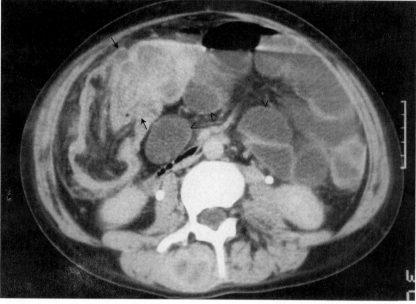

B

FIG. 9-24. A: The barium enema in this 2-year-old child shows a round defect in the area of the cecum. Notice how the barium infiltrates in a spiral pattern as it pushes its way between the intussusceptum and the intussuscipiens. This so-called coiled spring *(arrows)* is characteristic of intussusception. **B:** This is a CT scan of a child with known tumor affecting the bowel wall. The child presented with abdominal pain owing to an intussusception *(arrows)* caused by a metastasis to a lymph node near his ileocecal valve. Note on this CT how you can see the same signs: the blunt-headed intussusceptum and the stretched fat of the mesentery, as the intussusceptum is propelled forward into the intussuscipiens. Note also the multiple fluid filled bowel loops *(arrowheads)* from dilated small bowel secondary to the partial small bowel obstruction from the intussusception.

say, you are only 30% sure, a 95% sensitivity test is crucial in deciding appropriate patient management. At current hospital prices, it is cheaper to do the test than to put the patient in the hospital overnight for observation.

The plain film is of limited value in the diagnosis of appendicitis, being normal in about 50% of instances. In the majority of those instances where it is abnormal, the plain film shows evidence of adynamic ileus or possibly a mass in the right lower quadrant of the abdomen. Occasionally, you get lucky on plain film and detect a calcification in the right lower quadrant of the abdomen. This calcification is an appendolith or a concretion in the appendix. If you see this calcification in a child with

evidence of an acute abdomen, you can be 99% sure that the child has appendicitis. Be aware that only a small minority of patients with appendicitis have appendoliths that are visible by plain film. Ultrasound, on the other hand, adds a huge dimension to the diagnosis of appendicitis. Ultrasound is, in fact, an ideal way to find and define an inflamed appendix, appendiceal abscess, or an appendolith that is not visible by x-ray. In appropriate hands (those of an individual who has done many such studies) ultrasound is approximately 95% sensitive and specific for the diagnosis of appendicitis (Figs. 9-25 and 9-26). Remember to refer to the discussion of appropriateness when you decide which patient needs ultrasound.

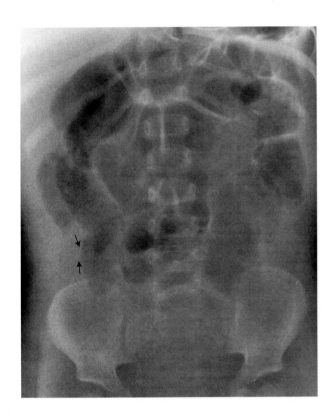

FIG. 9-25. This child had severe right lower quadrant abdominal pain showing signs of partial bowel obstruction. Note the faint calcification *(arrows)* in the right lower quadrant. This is a stone or appendolith within the appendix causing obstruction. This child had severe appendicitis and was very ill. Most appendicitis associated with a visible appendolith is the severe type, complicated either by gangrene of the appendix or appendiceal abscess.

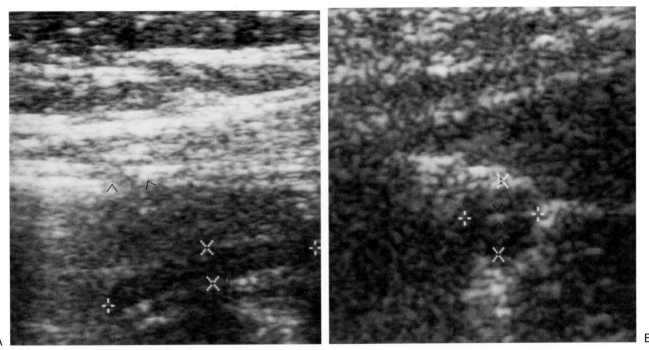

A   B

FIG. 9-26. A: The tubular structure, outlined by the x(s) of the ultrasound caliper, represents a longitudinal view of an inflamed appendix. If the appendix wall measures >6 mm, there is a 95% chance that the patient has appendicitis. For orientation purposes, notice that the arrowheads are showing the interior wall of the anterior abdominal muscles. The appendix actually lies very close to the ventral surface of the body. Ultrasound is most useful in those cases of appendicitis where you are suspicious but uncertain; there it adds great value to the diagnosis. **B:** Transverse view of an inflamed appendix. The linear bright spot *(arrowheads)* in the middle is the mucosa while the echolucent area is the inflamed muscularis and serosa.

Key Points

- In summary, the rules for evaluating an infant's abdomen are different from those used for adults.
- The younger the child, the more discrepant the rules. Babies have a lot of air, and it is difficult to differentiate large from small bowel by plain film.
- Young children usually have congenital anomalies or atresias; slightly older children have manifestations of either congenital anomalies or heritable anomalies such as pyloric stenosis and malrotation.
- In children beyond 6 months, intussusception and appendicitis are the major clinical entities.
- In looking at abdominal films of children, remember that your odds are much better in diagnosing an unusual manifestation of a common disease (such as appendicitis) than in diagnosing a common manifestation of a rare disease. If you stick with the diagnosis and rules from this chapter, you will be right more often than you will be wrong.
- With a little perseverance and applying the principles you learned in Chapter 8 to those outlined in Chapter 9, you should be able to do a reasonable job of radiographic evaluation.

REFERENCES

1. Silverman FN, Kuhn JP. *Caffey's Pediatric X-ray Diagnosis: An Integrated Imaging Approach,* 9th ed., Vols. 1 and 2. St. Louis: CV Mosby, 1993.

2. Franken EA Jr, Smith WL. *Gastrointestinal Imaging in Pediatrics,* 2nd ed. New York: Harper and Row, 1982.

CHAPTER 10

Genitourinary System

William E. Erkonen

For many years, the radiologic evaluation of the urinary tract was primarily limited to excretory urography (EU), retrograde pyelography, cystography, and angiography. Other names for the excretory urogram are the intravenous urogram (IVU) and the intravenous pyelogram (IVP). The term IVP has become less popular, whereas EU and IVU have become the preferred names. With the advent of ultrasonography (US), computed tomography (CT), and magnetic resonance imaging (MRI), we now have a multifaceted radiologic approach to genitourinary (GU) problems.

EXCRETORY UROGRAPHY

Indications and Contraindications

EU can be performed on almost all patients, but there are some clinical situations that require extreme caution. In these situations (Table 10-1), the risks versus the benefits must be seriously discussed by the radiologist and referring physician prior to the study.

If a pheochromocytoma is suspected, the clinician must be very careful. Pheochromocytomas secrete catecholamines that can precipitate a hypertensive crisis when there is a stress such as introduction of an intravenous contrast material. Also, be wary if you suspect multiple myeloma. Multiple myeloma patients often have abnormal serum proteins and proteinuria, and the combination of contrast media and these abnormal proteins has the potential to cause renal function impairment and even renal failure.

A previous serious reaction to contrast media is a worrisome situation, but usually EU can be performed. However, significant precautions should be employed, possibly including premedication (antihistamines and steroids), a crash cart nearby, as well as having an anesthetist and other expert help readily available.

When medically indicated, a pregnant or possibly pregnant patient can undergo modified EU that might consist of preliminary and 10-minute postcontrast radiographs. The pregnant patient, the referring physician, and the radiologist should always thoroughly discuss and understand the risks versus the benefits of the situation before proceeding, as this approach minimizes radiation exposure to the fetus and mother.

TABLE 10-1. *Excretory urogram high-risk situations*

Previous serious reaction to contrast media
Severe cardiovascular disease, especially with coexisting
  renal failure
Diabetes, associated with severe renal disease
Renal failure
Pheochromocytoma (known or suspected)
Multiple myeloma
Pregnancy (known or suspected)

Technique

EU does not require special patient preparation. It is helpful to cleanse the colon with a mild cathartic, especially when there is residual barium in the GI tract. Avoid enemas whenever possible, as enemas tend to introduce air into the colon which can potentially interfere with radiographic interpretation. Also, it is not necessary to dehydrate or overhydrate the patient prior to the procedure. Dehydration can lead to renal problems in some patients, especially renal vein thrombosis in infants.

The timing of EU radiographs varies depending on local practice, and a typical EU filming sequence is listed in Table 10-2. Additional radiographs are optional and usually tailored to the patient's clinical problem. Delayed films can be obtained for hours and days in situations such as obstruction, trauma, and renal failure.

How to View an Excretory Urogram

An EU study must always begin with a preliminary or scout radiograph that includes the entire abdomen, as it is sometimes possible to establish a diagnosis on the basis of this radiograph alone. The preliminary radiograph is sometimes referred to as a KUB, and this is an acronym for kidney, ureter, and bladder. You can evaluate this preliminary radiograph using the same system as described for the abdomen in Chapter 7. Allow your eyes to glance at the entire radiograph, the liver and spleen, psoas muscle margins, renal silhouettes, search for calcifications over the kidneys and ureters and bladder, the bony skeleton, and the bowel gas pattern (Fig. 10-1). Figures 10-2 to 10-4 demonstrate more Aunt Minnies that can be diagnosed on scout films.

TABLE 10-2. *Typical excretory urogram radiograph sequence*

Preliminary radiograph of the abdomen (always)
One or more radiographs during the 60 sec immediately following contrast injection
5- and 15-min radiographs post contrast injection
Pre- and postvoid radiographs of the urinary bladder

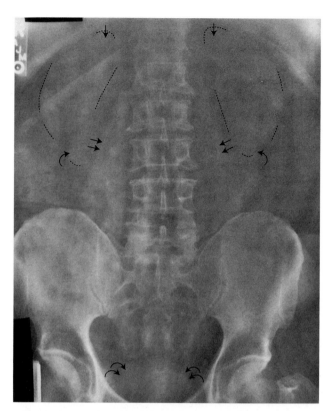

FIG. 10-1. Abdomen anteroposterior (AP) preliminary radiograph. Whenever possible, every effort should be made to identify the renal shadows *(dotted lines)*, renal upper poles *(single straight arrows)* and lower poles *(single curved arrows)*, psoas muscle margins *(double straight arrows)*, and the urinary bladder shadow *(double curved arrows)*. Also, there should be a careful search for radiopaque urinary calculi overlying the kidneys, ureters, and urinary bladder (Figs. 10-19 and 10-20).

Some of these Aunt Minnies were known in advance, whereas others came as a complete surprise.

Next, evaluate the radiographs obtained during the 60 seconds immediately following the intravenous bolus injection of contrast media. These radiographs are usually performed at 20, 40, and 60 seconds, and they demonstrate the *nephrogram phase*, wherein the contrast media is located in the capillaries, glomeruli, and proximal convoluted tubules (Fig. 10-5). Always compare the nephrograms for symmetry, as any asymmetry is suspicious for renal artery stenosis, ureteral obstruction, and impaired renal function.

Next, evaluate the 5- and 15-minute postcontrast injection radiographs at which times the contrast media is normally present in the calyces, infundibula, renal pelves, ureters, and the urinary bladder (Figs. 10-6 and 10-7). Begin evaluating the 5- and 15-minute radiographs with the calyces. Normal calyces should be sharp in outline, and their numbers and geometry are as vari-

text continues on page 198

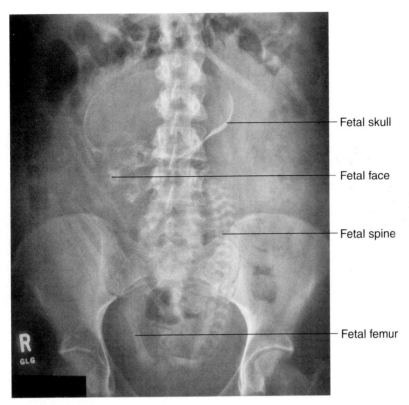

— Fetal skull

— Fetal face

— Fetal spine

— Fetal femur

FIG. 10-2. Abdomen AP preliminary radiograph. Third-trimester intrauterine pregnancy in a breech presentation.

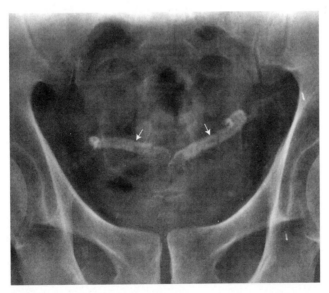

FIG. 10-3. Pelvis AP radiograph. Calcified vas deferens *(straight arrows)*. Diabetes mellitus and chronic infections must be considered as etiologic possibilities.

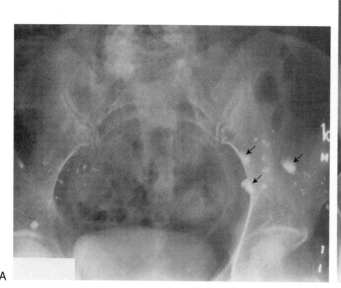
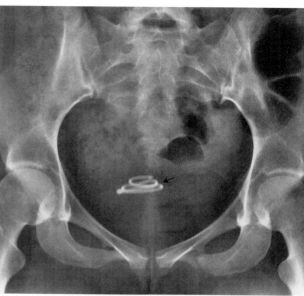

A

B

FIG. 10-4. A: Abdomen AP 10-minute EU. Bismuth deposits in the gluteal muscles. These metallic deposits *(straight arrows)* are secondary to prior intramuscular injections of a bismuth compound. In the past heavy metal salts were used therapeutically for some diseases such as syphilis. **B:** Pelvis AP radiograph. Intrauterine contraceptive device (IUD). The straight arrow indicates the normal position and appearance of the IUD.

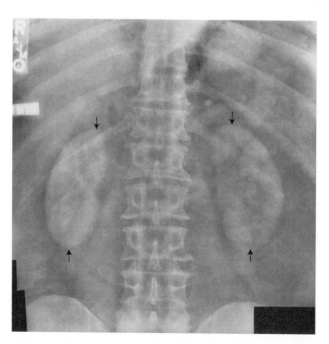

FIG. 10-5. Abdomen AP 1-minute EU. Normal. There are symmetric nephrograms one minute post injection of contrast media. The renal outlines *(straight arrows)* are now more clearly defined than on the preliminary radiograph (Fig. 10-1) due to the presence of the contrast media within the kidneys.

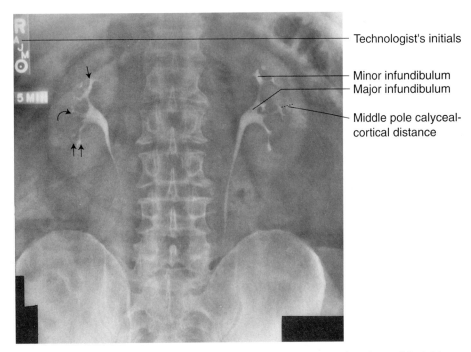

Technologist's initials

Minor infundibulum
Major infundibulum

Middle pole calyceal-
cortical distance

FIG. 10-6. Abdomen AP 5-minute EU. Normal. The calyces are now visible: upper pole calyces *(straight arrows)*, middle pole calyces *(curved arrows)*, and lower pole calyces *(double straight arrows)*.

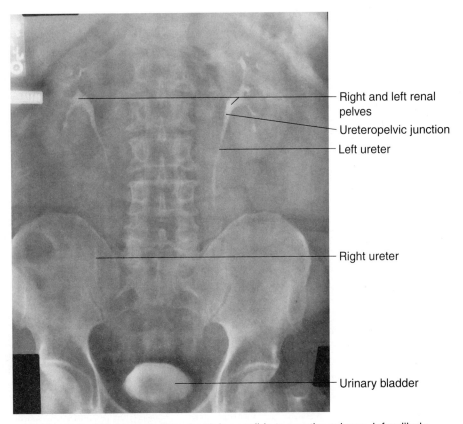

Right and left renal pelves

Ureteropelvic junction

Left ureter

Right ureter

Urinary bladder

FIG. 10-7. Abdomen AP 15-minute EU. Normal. Note that it is possible to see the calyces, infundibula, renal pelves, ureters, and urinary bladder on both the 5- and 15-minute radiographs.

able as the appearances of people. Calyces should be present in the upper, middle, and lower sections (poles) of each kidney. If calyces are absent from one of these areas, a significant problem must be suspected. The distance from the tip of the calyces to the renal border (calyceal–cortical distance) is a good indicator of renal cortex thickness. This distance usually measures 2.5–3 cm (Fig. 10-6) and should be approximately equal in both kidneys. This distance decreases with age as our renal cortex thins, so that by the time a person becomes a professor his or her renal (and cerebral) cortices may be much thinner than that of the students.

Renal pelves also vary greatly in their appearance, so you must program your cerebral computer to know when they are normal and abnormal. This takes time and experience so don't be discouraged if you feel inadequate at first. The position and size of the ureters should be noted. When the ureters are dilated, there may be distal obstruction. If a ureter is displaced from its normal course, then something must be displacing it.

Next evaluate the pre- and postvoid anteroposterior (AP) radiographs of the pelvis and bladder (Figs. 10-8 and 10-9). If the bladder empties poorly or incompletely, there may be some kind of obstruction at the bladder neck as seen with prostatic enlargement (Fig. 10-10). Also, there could be some neurologic reason for poor bladder emptying (Fig. 10-11). Always keep in mind that the patient may not have understood the voiding directions and just did not urinate. This, of course, would

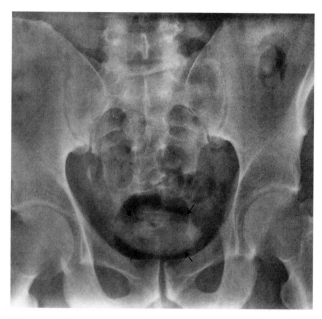

FIG. 10-9. Pelvis AP 15-minute postvoid EU. Normal. The urinary bladder *(straight arrows)* has emptied fairly well.

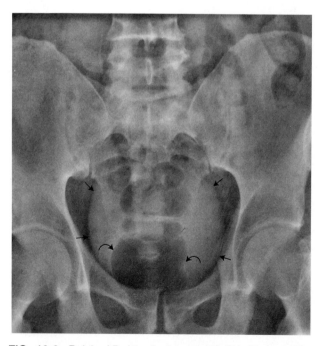

FIG. 10-8. Pelvis AP 15-minute prevoid EU. Normal. The contrast filled urinary bladder is outlined by the straight arrows. Rectal air *(curved arrows)* projects over the bladder.

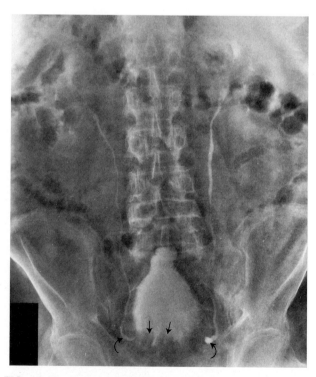

FIG. 10-10. Abdomen AP postvoid EU. Partial bladder neck obstruction secondary to benign prostatic hypertrophy. The enlarged prostate has created a filling defect in the floor of the bladder *(straight arrows)*, hooking of the distal ureters *(curved arrows)*, and incomplete emptying of the bladder.

give the false impression of bladder malfunction or obstruction. Your instructions to the patient must be precise and should communicate what it is that you want them to do.

Oblique, prone, and abdominal compression radiographs are occasionally obtained to better display kidneys, ureters, and bladder.

CONGENITAL ANOMALIES

Congenital anomalies occur in the urinary tract, and it is important to recognize them as such. One of the more common anomalies is the *bifid pelvis* (Fig. 10-12A), wherein there are two renal pelves. A bifid pelvis is considered a variant of normal (1). The renal pelvis can on a rare occasion be *trifid* (Fig. 10-12B). The bifid and trifid pelves rarely create problems for the patients. However, another anomaly that does have the potential to create clinical problems is a *complete duplication*. Complete duplication should not be confused with a bifid or trifid renal pelvis, as in complete duplication, there are two completely separate upper collecting systems in a kidney, and each collecting system has its own ureter that empties into the urinary bladder via separate ureteral orifices (Fig. 10-13A). Embryologically this is an abnormality of the ureteric bud. In a complete duplication the two ureteral orifices are usually in the bladder, and the cephalad upper collecting system ureter almost always inserts into the bladder

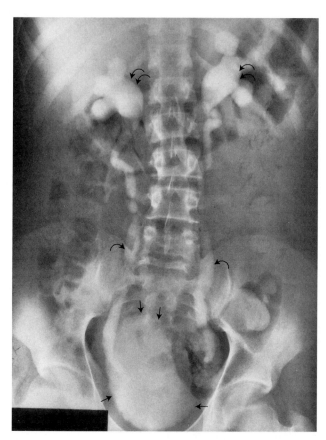

FIG. 10-11. Abdomen AP postvoid EU. Neurogenic bladder. The bladder has emptied incompletely and remains filled *(straight arrows)* on the postvoid film, and as a result the ureters *(curved arrows)* and upper collecting systems *(double curved arrows)* are dilated.

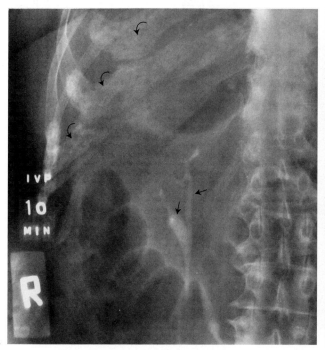
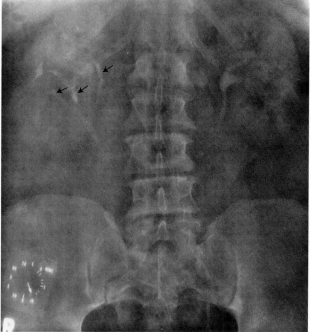

FIG. 10-12. A: Abdomen AP 10-minute EU. Bifid right renal pelvis *(straight arrows)*. Note the calcified costochondral structures *(curved arrows)*. **B:** Abdomen AP 10-minute EU. Trifid right renal pelvis *(straight arrows)*. If something can be bifid, it has the potential to be trifid.

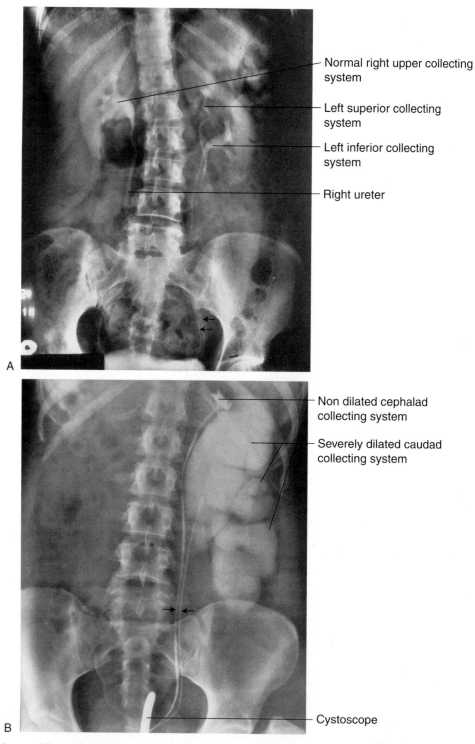

Normal right upper collecting system

Left superior collecting system

Left inferior collecting system

Right ureter

Non dilated cephalad collecting system

Severely dilated caudad collecting system

Cystoscope

A

B

FIG. 10-13. A: Abdomen AP 20-minute EU. Left-sided complete duplication. There are two separate nondilated left upper collecting systems and two separate nondilated left ureters *(straight arrows)* that extend into the urinary bladder. Note the mild scoliosis of the lumbar spine. **B:** Abdomen AP left retrograde pyelogram in a different patient. Left-sided duplication. There is a retrograde catheter in each of the two left ureters *(straight arrows)*, and both ureters extend into the urinary bladder. There are two left upper collecting systems. Note the severely dilated caudad upper collecting system that is secondary to chronic reflux while the cephalad upper collecting system is normal in size.

distal and medial to the ureter from the inferior collecting system. This distal insertion of the ureter from the cephalad system can occur at any site in the male and female GU tract including the prostate, base of penis, scrotum, uterus, vagina, and perineum. Of course, it is possible that the inferior collecting system ureter may also have an anomalous insertion, but it will always be proximal to the superior collecting system ureteral orifice. Reflux often occurs in complete duplications and usually it is into the more caudad upper collecting system (Fig. 10-13B).

An *incomplete duplication* is similar in that there are two separate upper collecting systems with two separate ureters, but the two ureters unite distally to form one ureter that enters the bladder via one ureteral orifice.

Another anomaly of the upper collecting system is *medullary sponge kidney* or tubular ectasia (Fig. 10-14A, B). In medullary sponge kidney, the distal collecting tubules are congenitally dilated, and these dilated tubules are a common place for calculus formation (Fig. 10-14A). These patients usually have normal renal function.

Embryologically, the kidneys develop in the pelvis and migrate cephalad into the abdomen. When the embryologic kidney reaches the abdomen, it normally rotates 90 degrees along the long renal axis toward the midline. If a kidney ascends into the abdomen, but does not rotate into a normal position or overrotates, it is called a *malrotation* (Fig. 10-15A). Ectopic kidneys end up in locations other than the renal fossa, and these ectopic kidneys exhibit increased susceptibility to infection and trauma. When the kidney fails to migrate cephalad into the abdomen and remains in the pelvis, it is called a *pelvic kidney, sacral kidney,* or *simple ectopia* (Fig. 10-15B). Occasionally, a kidney will migrate to the side opposite where it should normally reside, and this is called *crossed ectopia.* Crossed ectopic kidneys may or may not fuse to the normally located kidney (Fig. 10-15C).

A *horseshoe kidney* is shaped like a horseshoe because the lower poles of the right and left kidneys are connected by a bridge or isthmus of renal tissue (Fig. 10-16). This isthmus is situated anterior to the aorta and inferior vena cava. Horseshoe kidneys are always located low in the abdomen because the inferior mesenteric artery impedes the cephalad migration. In other words, the horseshoe kidney makes a ringer on the inferior mesenteric artery.

Another GU congenital abnormality is a *ureterocele* (Fig. 10-17). Ureterocele refers to a dilated intramural ureteral segment that protrudes into the bladder simulating a cobra's head. Ureteroceles result from either congenital or acquired stenosis at the ureteral orifice (1). A ureterocele can cause partial ureteral obstruction resulting in a dilated ureter. An intramural ureteral calculus or a bladder tumor may cause ureteral dilation that mimics a ureterocele.

Bladder diverticula (Fig. 10-18) generally are acquired but on rare occasions are congenital (1), and a single diverticulum is most likely congenital. Calculus formation can occur in a diverticulum.

text continues on page 205

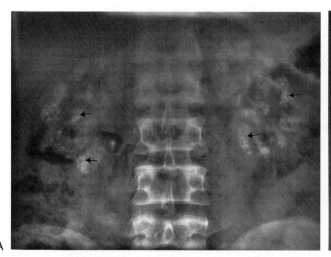 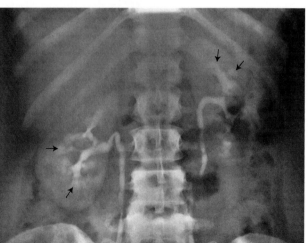

A   B

FIG. 10-14. A: Abdomen AP preliminary radiograph. Extensive bilateral calculi *(straight arrows)* in medullary sponge kidneys (MSK) or renal tubular ectasia. MSK patients have dilated collecting tubules, and intratubular calculi are present in approximately 50% of these patients (2). **B:** Abdomen AP EU. Medullary sponge kidneys. The classic appearance of MSK is this paint-brush-like appearance in the pyramids *(straight arrows)* secondary to contrast media in the dilated collecting tubules.

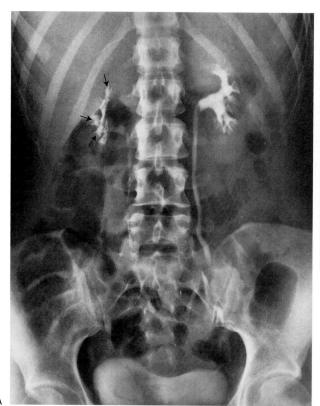

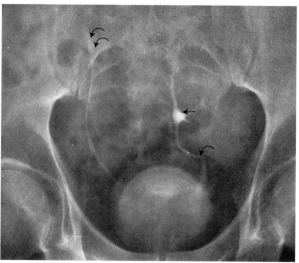

Right kidney (uncrossed)

Fused right and left kidneys

Left kidney (crossed)

Left ureter

Displaced right ureter

Urinary bladder

FIG. 10-15. A: Abdomen AP EU. Right renal malrotation. Because the kidney did not rotate along its long axis into a normal position, the calyces are seen on end *(straight arrows)*. The left kidney is normal. **B:** Pelvis AP EU. Pelvic kidney (sacral kidney) or simple ectopia. The left kidney is situated in the left pelvis just cephalad to the urinary bladder. The upper collecting system of the pelvic kidney is indicated by the straight arrow. A renal transplant will have this appearance, as it are usually placed in the pelvis. Note the foreshortened left ureter *(curved arrow)* and the normal right ureter *(double curved arrows)*. **C:** Abdomen AP 20-minute EU. Crossed fused ectopia. The crossed ectopic kidney may be fused (most common) or nonfused to the uncrossed kidney. When crossed fused ectopia does exist as in this patient, the upper pole of the crossed kidney is usually fused to the lower pole of the uncrossed kidney.

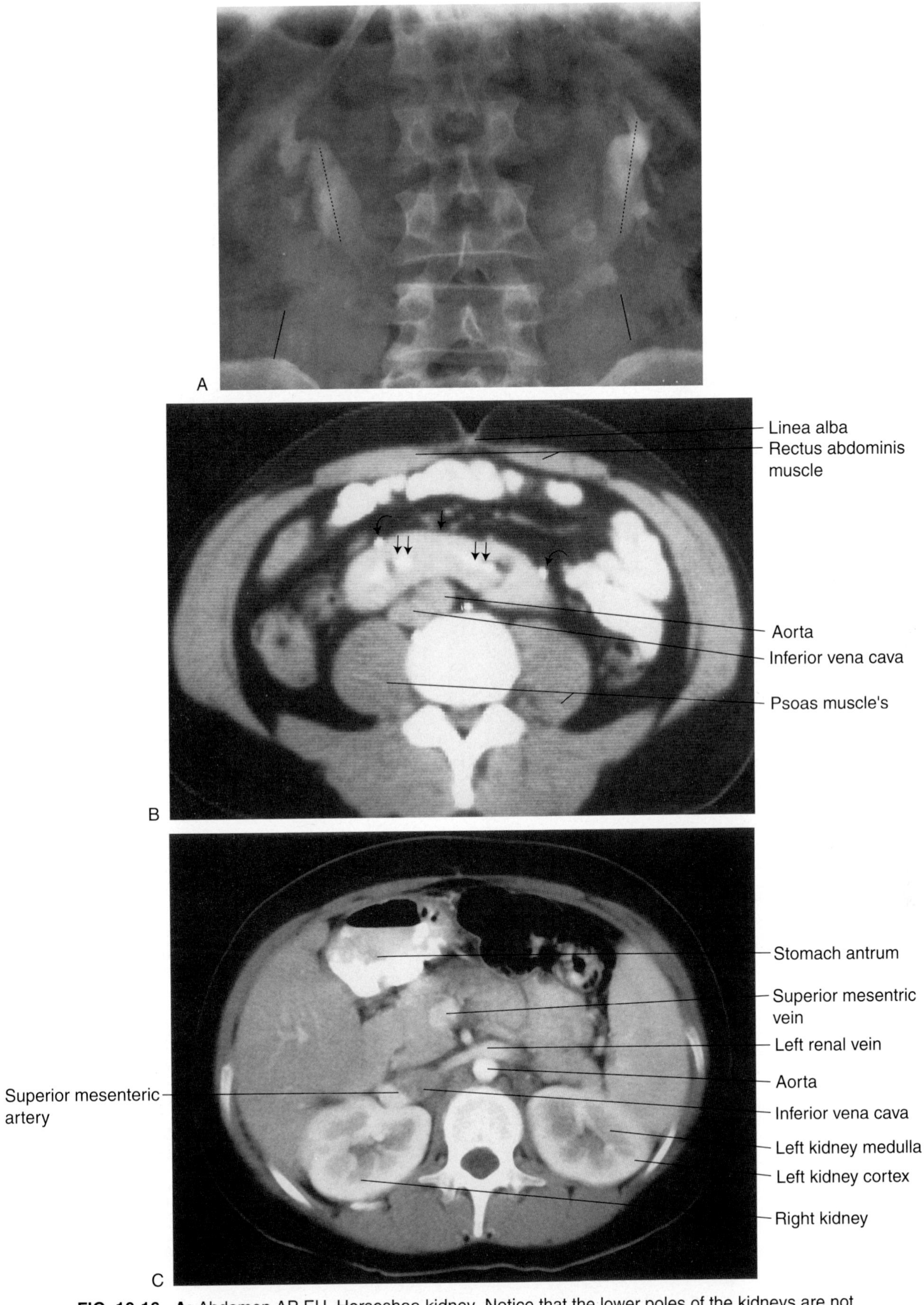
A
Linea alba
Rectus abdominis muscle
Aorta
Inferior vena cava
Psoas muscle's
B
Stomach antrum
Superior mesentric vein
Left renal vein
Aorta
Superior mesenteric artery
Inferior vena cava
Left kidney medulla
Left kidney cortex
Right kidney
C

FIG. 10-16. A: Abdomen AP EU. Horseshoe kidney. Notice that the lower poles of the kidneys are not visible, and the caudad aspect of the kidneys are oriented medially. The isthmus is not seen. A helpful clue to the diagnosis is that the renal long axes *(dotted lines)* are not parallel to the psoas muscle margins *(solid lines)*. **B:** Lower abdomen axial CT with intravenous contrast media. Horseshoe kidney. A bridge of renal tissue or isthmus *(straight arrow)* connects the renal lower poles, and this isthmus lies anterior to the aorta and inferior vena cava. The ureters cross the isthmus anteriorly *(curved arrows)*, and the upper collecting systems are indicated by the double straight arrows. **C:** Abdomen axial CT through normal kidneys for comparative purposes.

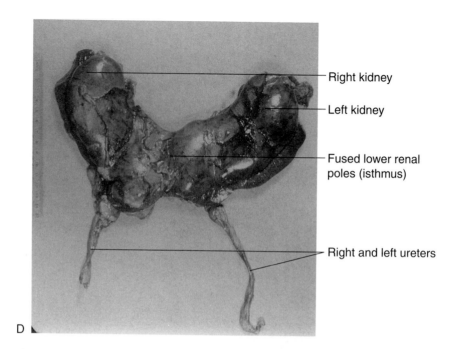

Right kidney

Left kidney

Fused lower renal poles (isthmus)

Right and left ureters

FIG. 10-16. *Continued.* **D:** Autopsy photograph of a horseshoe kidney.

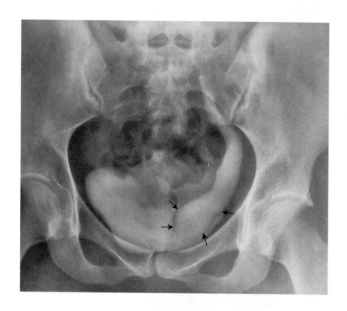

FIG. 10-17. Pelvis AP postvoid EU. Left ureterocele. Note the classical cobra head *(straight arrows)* appearance of the ureterocele. The left ureter is moderately dilated distally.

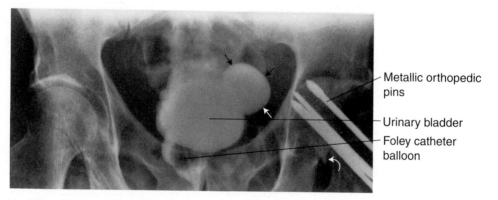

Metallic orthopedic pins

Urinary bladder

Foley catheter balloon

FIG. 10-18. Pelvis AP cystogram. Urinary bladder diverticulum. This patient sustained a fracture of the left femoral neck *(curved arrow)*, and a bladder injury was suspected. This cystogram revealed only an incidental bladder diverticulum *(straight arrows)* of unknown etiology.

UROLITHIASIS OR CALCULI

Urolithiasis is one of the most common urologic problems encountered in the everyday practice of medicine, and the calculi are often affectionately referred to as stones or rocks. They are encountered by nearly all physicians as they can cause renal and ureteral pain that is often severe. Ureteral colicky pain is especially severe as the ureter attempts to push the calculus distally. Just ask a friend who has passed a stone, and he or she will tell you that it brings tears to the eyes. Older and experienced physicians will tell you that when you make a house call, people with biliary colic are usually lying on the sofa, whereas patients with renal and ureteral pain are often on the floor with their heels dug into the rug. Renal and/or ureteral colicky pain usually begins in the lower back or flank and radiates to the inguinal-genital areas. This pain may be accompanied by frequent and painful urination, and there may be microscopic or even gross hematuria. Most ureteral stones are less than 1 cm in diameter, and approximately 75% are located in the distal third of the ureter. Approximately 90% of all GU calculi are radiopaque, and radiopaque calculi are best appreciated on the preliminary EU film.

Some radiopaque renal calculi actually fill all or part of an upper collecting system and resemble the horns

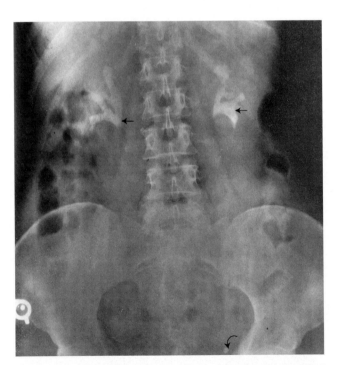

FIG. 10-19. Abdomen AP preliminary radiograph. Bilateral renal staghorn calculi. The staghorn calculi *(straight arrows)* closely resemble contrast media in upper collecting systems, and this demonstrates the importance of the preliminary radiograph. Incidentally noted is a left pelvis phlebolith *(curved arrow).*

TABLE 10-3. *A partial differential diagnosis for a renal pelvis filling defect*

Tumor (primary and secondary)
Calculus
Mycetoma (fungus ball)
Blood clot
Papillary necrosis tissue fragments
Air

of a stag, hence the name staghorn calculi (Fig. 10-19). When staghorn calculi are bilateral, their appearance should not be mistaken for contrast media in the upper collecting systems. Obviously, calculi can occur at any location in the urinary tract as demonstrated in this next case (Fig. 10-20).

Cystine and xanthine stones are usually not radiopaque, but occasionally they are faintly visible on radiographs. Uric acid stones occur in patients with gout, and these calculi are radiolucent except when they contain sufficient amounts of calcium (Figs. 10-21 and 10-22). A partial differential diagnosis for a renal pelvis filling defect is listed in Table 10-3.

Multiple unilateral or bilateral interstitial renal calcifications are referred to as nephrocalcinosis. Some common etiologies of nephrocalcinosis are listed in Table 10-4.

Ultrasound has become a useful tool not only for the diagnosis of renal disease, but for fragmenting or breaking up calculi. This fragmentation of a calculus with ultrasound is called extracorporeal sound wave lithotripsy, or ESWL (Fig. 10-23). Once the calculus is fragmented by ESWL, it has a chance to pass spontaneously without surgical intervention.

TRAUMA

GU tract injuries have multiple etiologies including motor vehicle accidents, falls, blunt injuries as in football and boxing, and penetrating injuries. The injuries range from contusions to lacerations and occur at any location in the GU tract. Renal and splenic injuries often are associated with lower thoracic injuries (Fig. 10-24), whereas bladder and urethral injuries occur with pelvis injuries and fractures (Fig. 10-25).

text continues on page 210

TABLE 10-4. *Some common causes of nephrocalcinosis*

Hyperparathyroidism
Anything causing hypercalcemia
Infections especially tuberculosis
Chronic glomerulonephritis
Chronic renal transplant rejection

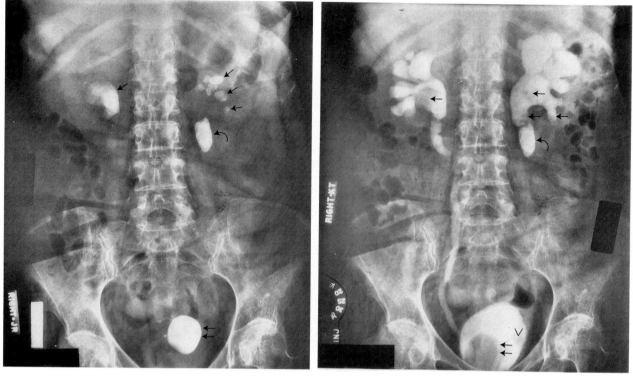

FIG. 10-20. A: Abdomen AP preliminary radiograph. Bilateral radiopaque renal calculi *(straight arrows)*, a large radiopaque calculus in the proximal left ureter *(curved arrow)*, and a large radiopaque calculus in the urinary bladder *(double straight arrows)*. This preliminary radiograph explained the patient's severe left flank colicky pain. **B:** Abdomen AP 5-minute EU in the same patient as A. Bilateral dilated upper collecting systems containing multiple filling defects secondary to calculi *(straight arrows)*. The proximal left ureter is totally obstructed by a large calculus *(curved arrow)*, and the entire right ureter is dilated suggesting a partially obstructing calculus in the distal right ureter at the ureteral vesicle junction. The opaque urinary bladder calculus *(double straight arrow)* now appears nonopaque relative to the more dense surrounding contrast media. Note bladder catheter *(arrowhead)*.

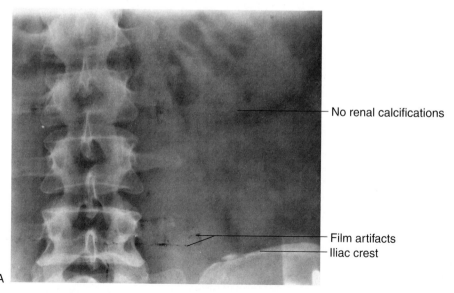

FIG. 10-21. A: Abdomen AP radiograph. Normal. This patient had symptoms suspicious for a left renal calculus, but there is no evidence of a radiopaque urinary calculus.

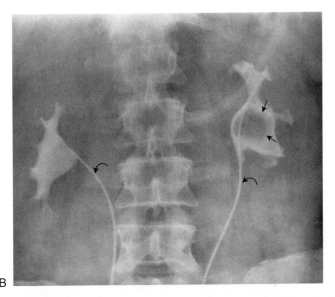

FIG. 10-21. *Continued.* **B:** Bilateral retrograde pyelogram in the same patient as A. Uric acid calculus. A bilateral retrograde pyelogram was accomplished by injecting contrast media into the ureteral catheters *(curved arrows)* that were passed retrograde through a cystoscope. There is a radiolucent or nonopaque filling defect in the left renal pelvis *(straight arrows)*. The filling defect proved to be a uric acid calculus, and typically they are not radiopaque on an abdominal radiograph. A patient's history is always invaluable, and this patient had gout or hyperuricemia.

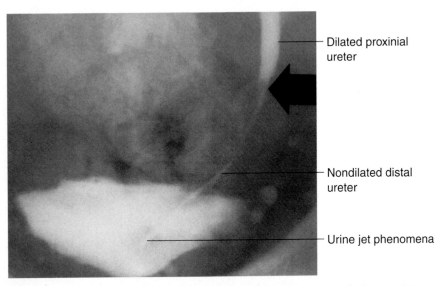

Dilated proxinial ureter

Nondilated distal ureter

Urine jet phenomena

FIG. 10-22. Pelvis AP prevoid EU. The large black arrow indicates a nonopaque calculus partially obstructing the distal left ureter. The urine jet phenomena is a normal finding and merely represents a stream of contrast media and urine entering the urinary bladder.

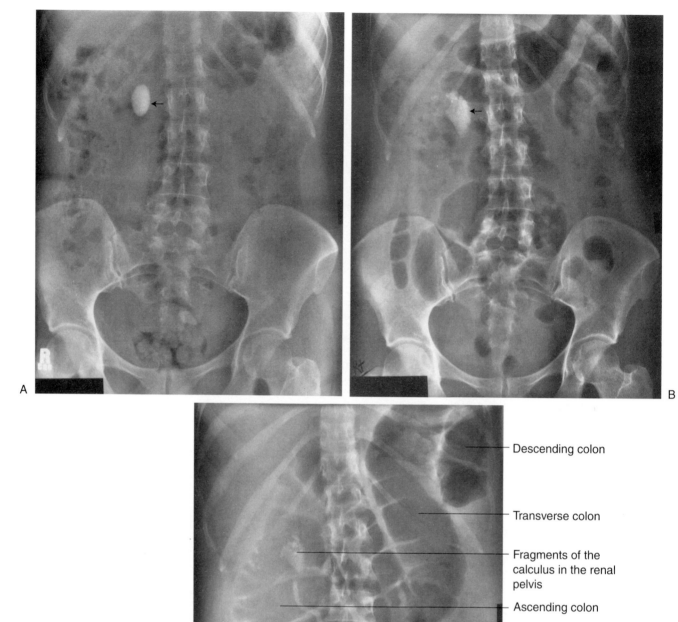

Descending colon

Transverse colon

Fragments of the calculus in the renal pelvis

Ascending colon

Fragments of the calculus in the ureter

Point of ureteral obstruction

FIG. 10-23. A: Abdomen AP radiograph. Solitary radiopaque calculus in the right renal pelvis *(straight arrow)*. **B:** Abdomen AP radiograph. Calculus fragmentation by extracorporeal sound wave lithotripsy (ESWL), or bombardment of the calculus with ultrasound. The calculus is now fragmented *(straight arrow)* into multiple small pieces. **C:** Abdomen AP radiograph 24 hours post-ESWL. Right ureteral obstruction secondary to multiple small calculus fragments. As you might expect, the patient presented with ureteral colic, hematuria, dysuria, and frequency. The ureter is filled with multiple small fragments of the calculus, and this appearance of the ureter is called "steinstrasse" (or "stone street"). This situation usually requires a retrograde catheter or stent to relieve the obstruction and to enable the calculi to pass. The colon is now significantly air-filled and dilated (adynamic ileus) secondary to the severe pain caused by the multiple ureteral calculi.

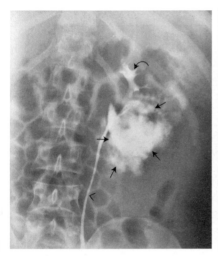
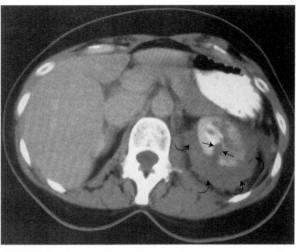

A   B

FIG. 10-24. A: Abdomen AP left retrograde pyelogram. Renal laceration secondary to a motor vehicle accident. The extravasated contrast media *(straight arrows)* originates from the left renal laceration, and the renal outline is indistinct due to perinephric blood. The upper pole collecting system is normal *(curved arrow)*. Note the left ureteral catheter in place *(arrowhead)*. **B:** Abdomen axial CT image through the left kidney. Left renal laceration. The laceration is the nonenhanced defect *(straight arrows)*, and the extent of the perinephric blood *(curved arrows)* is now clearly demonstrated.

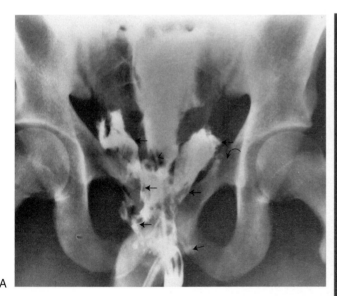
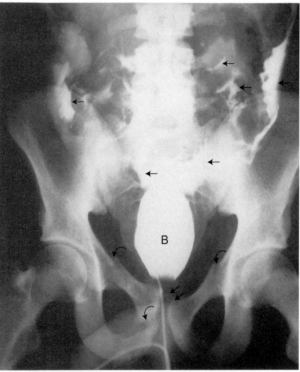

A   B

FIG. 10-25. A: Pelvis AP retrograde urethrogram and cystogram. Traumatic lacerations of the urethra and bladder secondary to multiple pelvic fractures. Contrast media injected into the urethra and the urinary bladder demonstrated extensive extraperitoneal extravasation *(straight arrows)* from lacerations of the urethra and bladder. A mildly distracted left superior pubic ramus fracture is indicated by the curved arrow, and there is overall asymmetry of the pelvis secondary to the fractures. Note the retention catheter in place *(arrowhead)*. **B:** Pelvis AP cystogram. Traumatic rupture of the urinary bladder in the same patient as in A. Contrast media was injected via a Foley or retention catheter to evaluate the bladder. The extravasated contrast material *(straight arrows)* clearly lies outside the bladder and is intraperitoneal. There are bilateral pubic rami fractures *(curved arrows)* along with dislocation at the pubic symphysis *(double straight arrows)*.

INFECTION

GU infections are a common occurrence in the practice of medicine, and usually they do not require diagnostic imaging procedures. Infections can reach the GU tract via the hematogenous route, ascend from the urethra and/or bladder, or be secondary to obstruction in the GU tract. The severity of these infections ranges from mild cystitis and/or pyelonephritis to a severe pyelonephritis (Fig. 10-26) or even a perinephric abscess (Fig. 10-27). The presenting symptoms of cystitis often include frequency of urination, dysuria, hematuria, and cloudy urine. Urinalysis in patients with cystitis almost always reveals the presence of white and red blood cells and bacteria.

TABLE 10-5. *Radiographic findings of pyelonephritis*

Renal enlargement in acute infections
Decreased renal size in chronic infections
Delayed function
Upper collecting system distortion and dilatation

The signs and symptoms for pyelonephritis may be similar to those found in cystitis, along with chills, fever, flank pain and tenderness. Patients with perinephric abscess usually are severely ill and may have any or all of the above symptoms. Some of the radiographic findings for pyelonephritis are listed in Table 10-5.

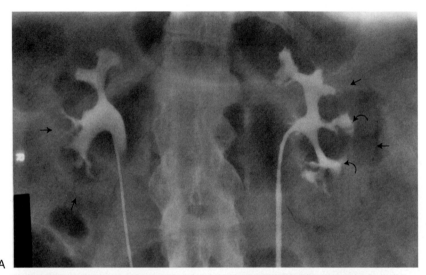

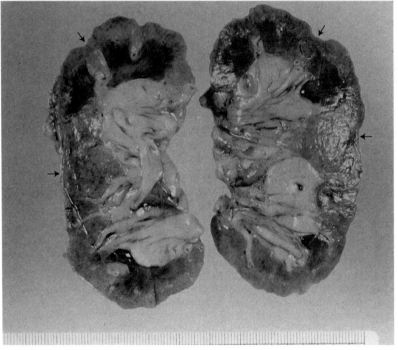

FIG. 10-26. A: Abdomen AP bilateral retrograde pyelogram. Chronic pyelonephritis. The renal contours are irregular *(straight arrows and dotted lines)* due to cortical damage caused by chronic infection. The calyces are blunted and ragged in appearance *(curved arrows)*, and the renal cortices are thinner than normal. **B:** Autopsy photograph of the kidneys in patient A. The irregular contour and thinned cortices *(straight arrows)* are more clearly visible on the autopsy specimen.

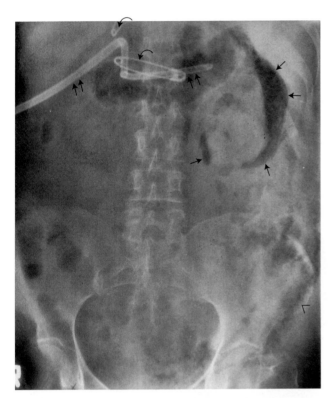

FIG. 10-27. Abdomen AP supine radiograph. Left perinephric abscess. There is air in the abscess surrounding the left kidney *(straight arrows)*. An abscess drain *(double straight arrows)* is in place, and common safety pins *(curved arrows)* project over the abdomen. There is left abdominal subcutaneous air *(arrowhead)* secondary to extension of the infection into these tissues.

Always consider GU tract infections in your differential diagnosis for a fever of undetermined origin, especially in children and infants.

TUMORS

Benign

The diagnosis of some benign GU tumors can be made merely by their classic appearance on an AP radiograph of the abdomen or pelvis. One such tumor is the leiomyoma (myoma or fibromyoma), which is more commonly referred to as a fibroid. Fibroids are the most common GU tumor in women, and these benign tumors of smooth muscle origin arise in the myometrium. Fi-

broids (Fig. 10-28) can partially or completely calcify, and these calcifications typically appear curvilinear and mottled on a radiograph and are another Aunt Minnie. They usually require no treatment unless their size creates problems.

Another GU tumor that can present with a striking radiographic appearance is an ovarian teratoma. Teratomas of the ovaries are either cystic (dermoids) or solid tumors derived from all three germ layers, and they may contain any or all of the structures derived from these layers including hair, teeth, skin, cartilage, and bone. They are usually smaller than other ovarian tumors and account for approximately 10% to 15% of all ovarian neoplasms. Their radiographic appearance depends on the tissue content of the tumor. If a tooth is visualized on a radiograph, this often leads to the diagnosis of teratoma (Fig. 10-29). Teratomas do have the potential for malignant transformation, especially in solid lesions.

Renal cysts (Fig. 10-30) are important as they can be confused with a malignant renal tumor. They may be single, multiple, unilateral or bilateral, and their radiologic characteristics are listed in Table 10-6. These lesions are usually silent or asymptomatic and often are an incidental finding on EU.

text continues on page 214

TABLE 10-6. *Radiologic features of a benign renal cyst (2)*

Radiography:
    Variable locations
    Mass lesion with calyceal distortion
    Thin and smooth wall
    Sharply delineated from surrounding parenchyma
    Radiolucent mass
    Avascular at angiography
    "Beak" sign or "claw" sign
Computed tomography:
    Thin and smooth wall
    Clear demarcation between cyst and surrounding parenchyma
    Water density
    No contrast enhancement
    Slightly ovoid shape
Sonography:
    Posterior enhancement
    No internal echoes

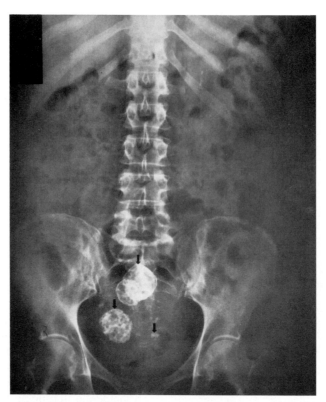

FIG. 10-28. AP abdomen radiograph. Multiple calcified uterine fibroids (leiomyomatosis). The black arrows indicate uterine fibroids with their classic-appearing calcifications.

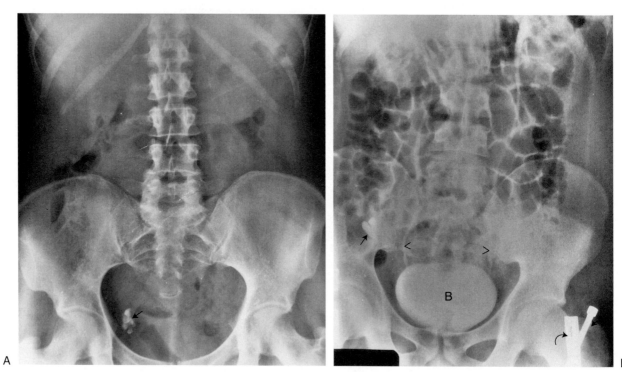

FIG. 10-29. A: Abdomen AP radiograph. Teratoma of the right ovary containing teeth and calcifications *(straight arrow)*. **B:** Abdomen AP excretory urogram. Tooth in a right ovary teratoma in a different patient. A large tooth *(straight arrow)* is clearly visible in the lower abdomen giving a high degree of suspicion for an ovarian teratoma. Orthopedic appliances are present in the proximal left femur *(curved arrows)*. Ureters are indicated by arrowheads. B, urinary bladder.

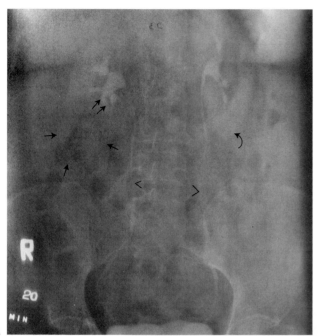

FIG. 10-30. A: Abdomen AP 20-minute EU. Mass lesion involving the right renal lower pole. The right kidney lower pole is poorly defined, especially when compared to the more clearly defined lower pole in the normal left kidney *(curved arrow)*, and the right kidney lower pole calyces are displaced cephalad *(double straight arrows)*. These findings are consistent with a right renal soft tissue mass *(straight arrows)*, and the differential diagnosis should essentially be renal cyst versus renal tumor. Ureters are indicated by arrowheads. **B:** Abdomen axial CT image through the right kidney with intravenous contrast media in the same patient as in A. Right renal cyst. Note that the cyst has sharp smooth margins *(straight arrows)*, and it has a low tissue density when compared to the remaining normal right kidney *(curved arrow)*. **C:** Abdomen AP selective right renal arteriogram in the same patient as in A and B. Right renal cyst. The renal cyst is avascular with sharp smooth margins *(straight arrows)*, and a classic beak sign *(curved arrow)* is present. The right renal arterial selective catheter can be seen *(double straight arrows)*.

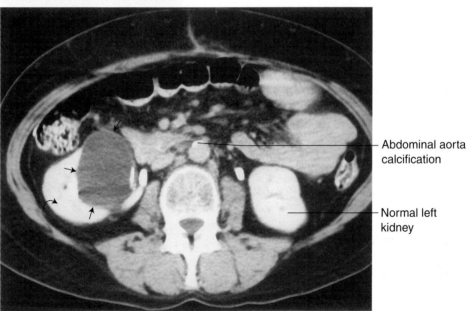

Abdominal aorta calcification

Normal left kidney

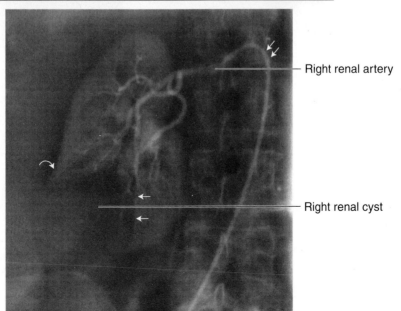

Right renal artery

Right renal cyst

TABLE 10-7. *Differential diagnosis for a renal mass (3)*

    Benign neoplasm:
        Hamartoma
        Hemangioma
        Adenoma
        Lipoma
    Malignant neoplasm:
        Renal cell carcinoma
        Transitional cell carcinoma
        Lymphoma
        Metastases
        Wilms' tumor (children)
    Renal cyst
    Abscess
    Hydronephrosis
    Multicystic and polycystic kidneys

Renal cysts are usually of no clinical significance, but occasionally they become large enough to cause obstruction and even renal damage.

When a renal mass is discovered, further workup with US, CT, or MRI is often used to assist in arriving at an accurate diagnosis (Table 10-7). CT is especially helpful for the staging of a malignant lesion, and US helps to distinguish between a solid and a cystic lesion.

Malignant

Approximately 90% of all adult renal malignant tumors are renal cell carcinomas. A differential diagnosis for adult malignant renal neoplasms is listed in Table 10-7. Patients with renal cell carcinomas may present with gross or microscopic hematuria as well as a wide range of other presenting symptoms, including pain. The radiologic features of primary renal malignancies are

TABLE 10-8. *Radiologic features of primary renal cell carcinoma (2)*

Radiography:
    General renal enlargement
    Localized mass
    Tumor calcification (curvilinear or rim-like)
    Renal displacement
    Calyceal displacement or cutoff
    Density on excretory urogram varies from hypo- to
        hyperdense
    Angiographic hypervascularity and AV communications
Computed tomography:
    Solid mass
    Postcontrast enhances more than cyst and less than
        normal parenchyma
    Good for staging
        Extension outside the kidney
        Involving lymph nodes
        Invading the renal vein and inferior vena cava

shown in Table 10-8, and some examples of these tumors are shown in Figs. 10-31 and 10-32.

Primary and secondary malignancies can involve the ureters by displacing or obstructing them (Fig. 10-33 to 10-35). Primary and secondary neoplasms can also involve the urinary bladder (Fig. 10-36).

ANGIOGRAPHY

Renal arteriography may be indicated for a renal mass workup (see Figs. 10-30C and 10-31B), or when searching for renal artery disease (Fig. 10-37). This subject has been discussed in greater detail in Chapter 2.

FEMALE PELVIS

Ultrasonography

US has become a powerful tool for evaluating the female pelvis and serves as an extremely valuable adjunct to the bimanual pelvic examination. Both transabdominal and transvaginal US techniques are used, but transvaginal imaging is now considered the gold standard. The transabdominal (Fig. 10-38) and transvaginal (Fig. 10-39) sonograms

text continues on page 214

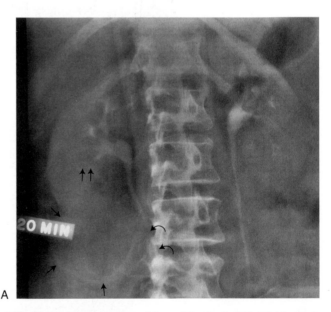

FIG. 10-31. A: Abdomen oblique 20-minute EU. Right renal cell carcinoma. Note the bulbous appearance of the right renal lower pole *(straight arrows)*, and the lower pole calyces are indistinct and displaced *(double straight arrows)*. Also, something is displacing the right ureter medially *(curved arrows)*. These findings indicate the presence of a right renal lower pole mass lesion, and again the differential diagnosis primarily involves renal cyst versus tumor. The left kidney is normal.

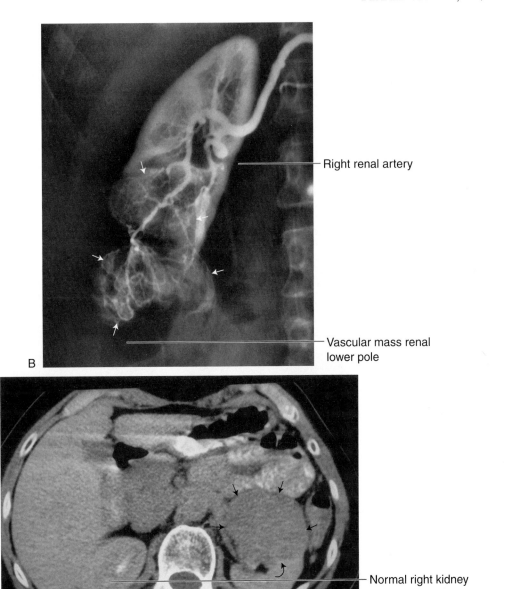

Right renal artery

Vascular mass renal
lower pole

Normal right kidney

Normal portion left kidney

B

C

FIG. 10-31. *Continued.* **B:** AP selective right renal arteriogram. Right kidney lower pole renal cell carcinoma in the same patient as A. This highly vascular mass in the right renal lower pole *(straight arrows)* is the typical appearance of a renal cell carcinoma. The increased vascularity of the tumor mass is secondary to new vessels (neovascularity) and arteriovenous connections within the tumor. Overall, this appearance is dramatically different from the avascular benign renal cyst in Fig. 10-30C. **C:** Abdomen axial renal CT in a different patient. Large left renal cell carcinoma *(straight arrows)*. The mass lesion is solid appearing, and the border between the mass and the normal kidney *(curved arrow)* is poorly defined.

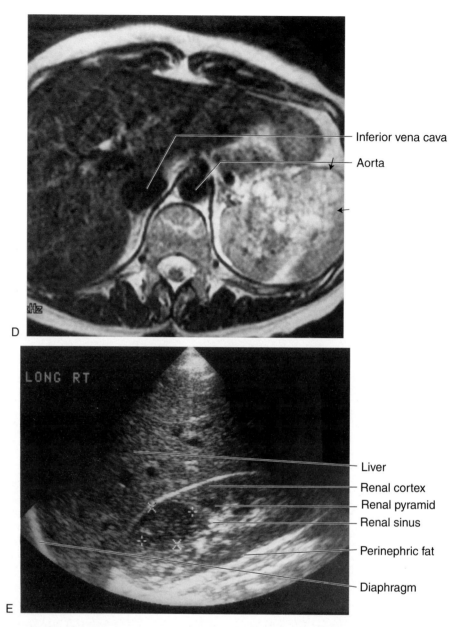

Inferior vena cava

Aorta

Liver

Renal cortex

Renal pyramid

Renal sinus

Perinephric fat

Diaphragm

D

E

FIG. 10-31. *Continued.* **D:** Abdomen axial T-2 MR image through the left kidney in a different patient. Large left renal cell carcinoma *(arrows)*. **E:** Right renal longitudinal sonogram in another patient. Renal cell carcinoma. The electronic caliper x's and crosses delineate a right kidney upper pole renal cell carcinoma. The numerous internal echoes (hyperechoic) within the mass indicate that the mass is solid.

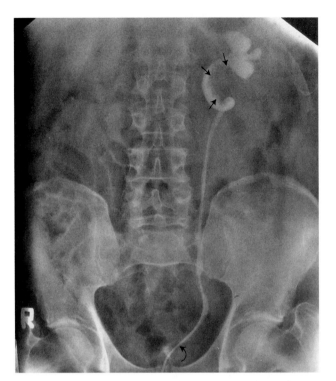

FIG. 10-32. Left retrograde pyelogram. Transitional cell carcinoma of the left renal pelvis *(straight arrows)*. A left ureter retrograde catheter *(curved arrow)* is in place.

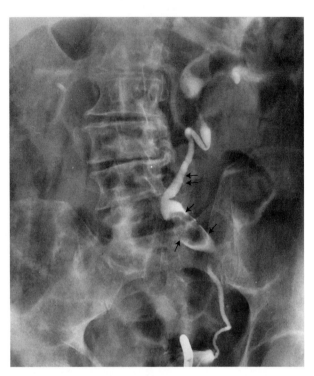

FIG. 10-33. Abdomen left retrograde pyelogram. Carcinoma of the left midureter. The partially obstructing ureteral carcinoma *(straight arrows)* has resulted in a dilated proximal ureter *(double straight arrows)*. A cystoscope is in the bladder.

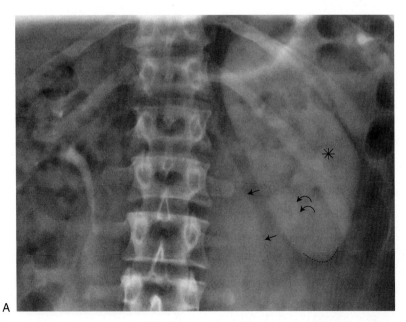

A

FIG. 10-34. A: Abdomen AP 5-minute EU. Retroperitoneal lymphoma. There is a delayed left renal nephrogram (*) that proved to be secondary to partial obstruction of the left ureter. The left renal lower pole *(dotted line)* is mildly displaced laterally by the retroperitoneal lymphomatous mass. The mass *(curved arrows)* can be distinguished from the left psoas muscle margin *(straight arrows)*.

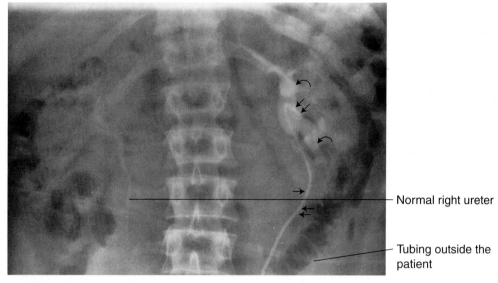

— Normal right ureter

— Tubing outside the patient

B

FIG. 10-34. *Continued.* **B:** Abdomen AP left retrograde pyelogram in the same patient as A. A stent *(double straight arrows)* in the left ureter is displaced laterally *(straight arrow)* by the lymphomatous mass. When the ureter is displaced in this manner, the mass is generally retroperitoneal. The ureteral displacement becomes more apparent when the course of the left ureter is compared to the course of the normal right ureter. The left upper collecting system is mildly dilated *(curved arrows).*

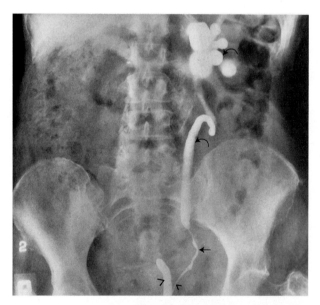

FIG. 10-35. Abdomen AP left retrograde pyelogram. Encasement of the distal left ureter by cancer of the cervix. The encasement has resulted in stricture and partial obstruction of the distal left ureter *(straight arrow).* As a result of the partial obstruction, the left ureter proximal to the stricture and the left upper collecting system are mildly dilated *(curved arrows).* The cystoscope and retrograde catheter *(arrowheads)* can be seen radiographically.

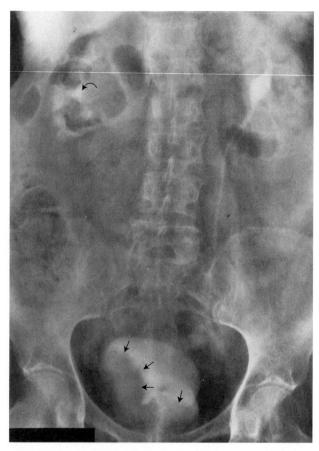

FIG. 10-36. Abdomen AP EU. Transitional cell carcinoma of the bladder. The bladder mass *(straight arrows)* is partially obstructing the right ureteral orifice resulting in a dilated right upper collecting system *(curved arrow).* The left kidney and ureter are normal.

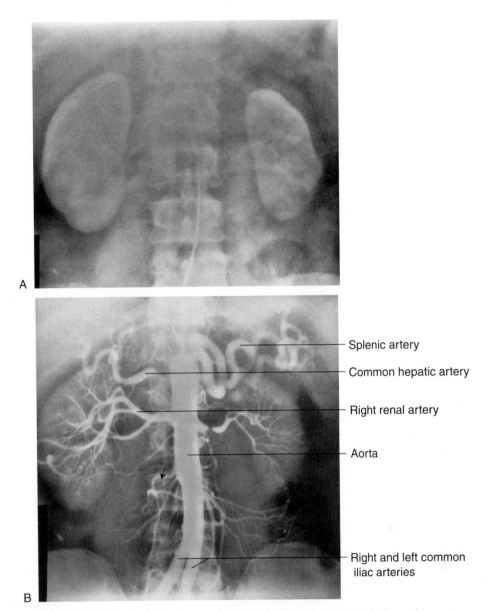

Splenic artery

Common hepatic artery

Right renal artery

Aorta

Right and left common
iliac arteries

FIG. 10-37. Selected abdominal AP radiographs from an abdominal aorta angiogram. Left renal artery stenosis in a patient with hypertension. The radiograph obtained early during the injection of contrast media **(A)** shows a small left kidney with an irregular contour, and this is similar to the appearance of the left kidney on the one minute EU. On the radiograph obtained later during the injection **(B)** there is a significant stenosis demonstrated in the left renal artery *(straight arrow)*. The stenosis required surgical correction, and the patient's hypertension improved following the renal artery stenosis repair. Note in A the angiographic catheter in the aorta overlying the spine.

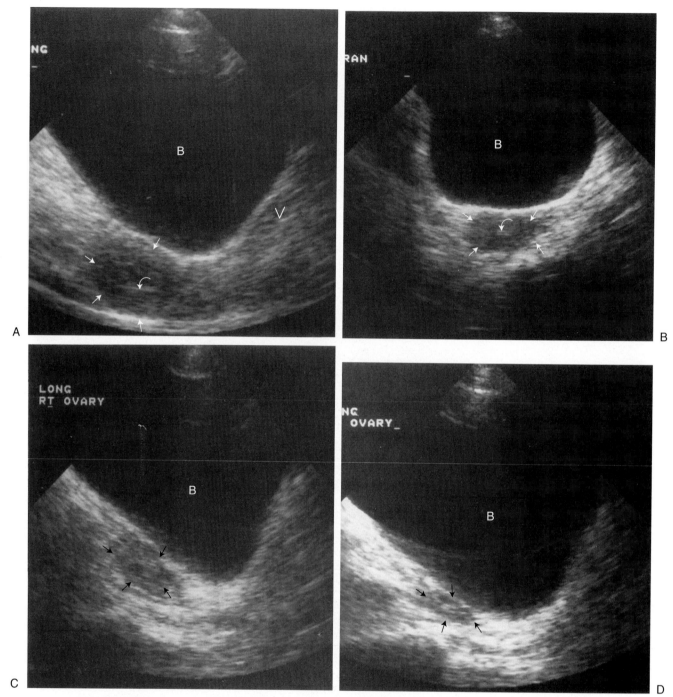

FIG. 10-38. A: Transabdominal midline longitudinal or sagittal sonogram. Normal uterus *(straight arrows).* The urine-filled urinary bladder is essentially echo-free, and thus it serves as an acoustic window to the pelvis. Notice the characteristic homogeneous echo pattern found in the normal uterus. The endometrial stripe *(curved arrow)* results from the endometrial layers that line the endometrial cavity being in close proximity. The presence of the endometrial stripe indicates that there is not an intrauterine pregnancy or other intrauterine mass. V, vagina. **B:** Transabdominal transverse or axial sonogram. Normal uterus. The uterine fundus is outlined by the straight arrows, and the endometrial stripe *(curved arrow)* appears smaller on the transverse image. **C:** Transabdominal right longitudinal or sagittal sonogram. Normal right ovary *(straight arrows).* **D:** Transabdominal left longitudinal or sagittal sonogram. Normal left ovary *(straight arrows).* B, urinary bladder.

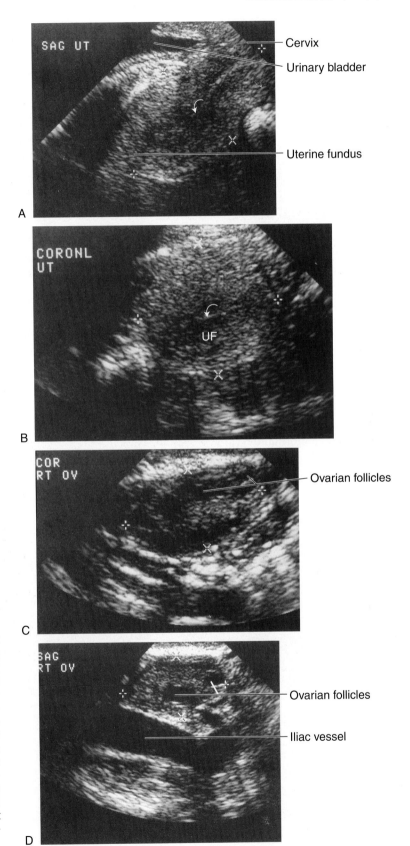

FIG. 10-39. A: Transvaginal longitudinal or sagittal sonogram. Normal uterus. The uterine borders are delineated by the electronic caliper x's and crosses, and the endometrial stripe by the curved arrow. Notice that the uterine images are similar on both the transabdominal and transvaginal techniques. **B:** Transvaginal coronal sonogram. Normal uterus. The uterine borders are delineated by the electronic caliper x's and crosses, and the endometrial stripe by the curved arrow. UF, uterine fundus. **C:** Transvaginal coronal sonogram. Normal right ovary. The borders of the right ovary are delineated by x's and crosses. **D:** Transvaginal longitudinal or sagittal sonogram. Normal right ovary. The borders of the right ovary are delineated by the electronic caliper x's and crosses.

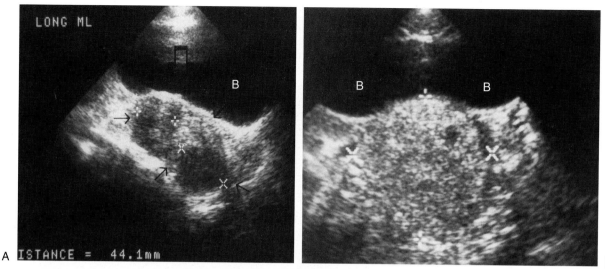

FIG. 10-40. A: Transabdominal longitudinal or sagittal sonogram. Multiple uterine fibroids or uterine leiomyomatosis. The enlarged fibroid uterus is outlined by the black straight arrows. The electronic caliper x's and crosses outline two large fibroids. The electronic calipers are used primarily to measure the size of lesions and structures. The many internal echoes within the fibroid masses indicate that they are solid. **B:** Transabdominal transverse or axial sonogram. Ovarian teratoma. Again, the numerous internal echoes indicate that this is a solid mass lesion. The mass is outlined by the caliper x's and crosses. B, urinary bladder.

demonstrate normal female pelvic anatomy. Some gynecologic abnormalities are shown in Figs. 10-40 and 10-41.

An extremely important indication for GU sonogra-

phy is for the diagnosis and management of pregnancies (Fig. 10-42) and their complications (Fig. 10-43). As a result, sonography has become an invaluable tool for the obstetrician.

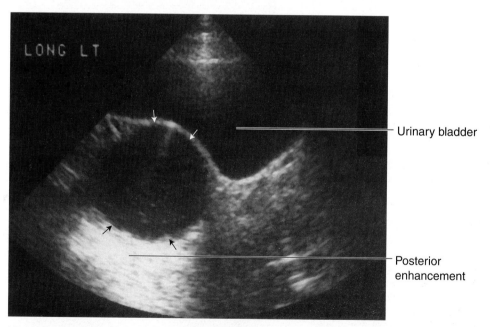

FIG. 10-41. Transabdominal longitudinal or sagittal sonogram. Left ovary benign mucinous cystadenoma. This left ovarian mass *(straight arrows)* demonstrates posterior enhancement and only a few internal echoes. When sound waves encounter an acoustic interface (where tissues of differing densities abut), the result is a reflection of the sound waves or enhancement. The marked posterior enhancement is typical for a cystic structure. Note the markedly different appearance of this cystic mass compared to the solid masses in Fig. 10-40A and B.

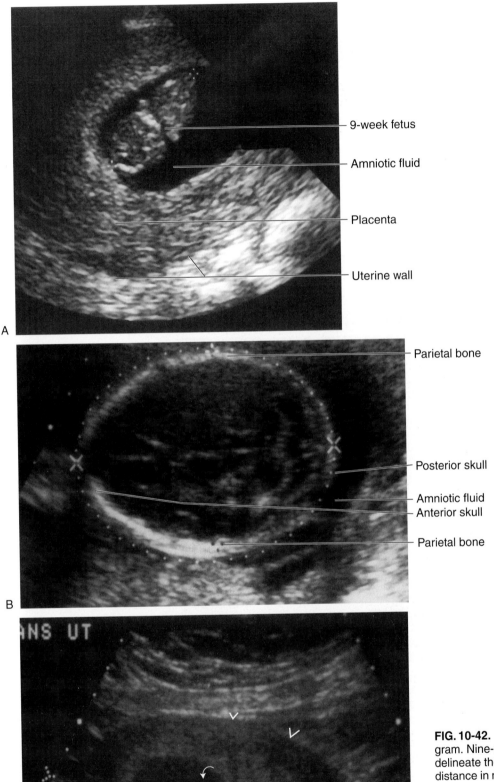

— 9-week fetus

— Amniotic fluid

— Placenta

— Uterine wall

A

— Parietal bone

— Posterior skull

— Amniotic fluid
— Anterior skull

— Parietal bone

B

C

FIG. 10-42. A: Transvaginal obstetric sonogram. Nine-week fetus. The caliper crosses delineate the crown rump distance, and this distance in millimeters translates accurately on tables to a gestational age of 9 weeks. **B:** Transabdominal obstetric sonogram. Fetal skull of a near-term fetus. The white dotted lines outline the fetal skull. The biparietal distance measured in millimeters translates on tables to a gestational age that is accurate to within a few days. **C:** Transabdominal transverse obstetrical sonogram. Twin pregnancy. The twin fetuses *(straight arrows)* are located in separate sacs and are surrounded by amniotic fluid *(curved arrows)*. The uterine wall is indicated by arrowheads.

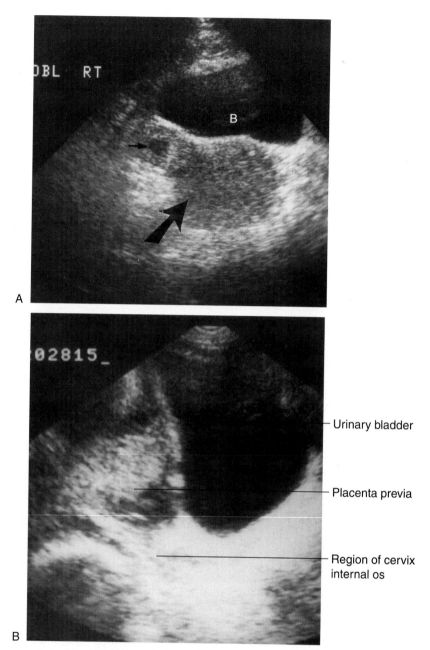

Urinary bladder

Placenta previa

Region of cervix internal os

FIG. 10-43. A: Transabdominal oblique sonogram. Ectopic pregnancy. The patient had experienced vaginal bleeding, severe right pelvic pain, and was amenorrheic for 3 months. The large arrow indicates a hyperechoic blood-filled uterus. The small arrow indicates the gestational sac in the right fallopian tube. B, urinary bladder. **B:** Transabdominal longitudinal or sagittal sonogram. Placenta previa. The patient experienced painless vaginal bleeding during her pregnancy. The sonogram shows the placenta to be covering the internal cervical os, thus precluding a vaginal delivery.

Computed Tomography and Magnetic Resonance Imaging

CT and MRI are also used to evaluate the female pelvis (Figs. 10-44 and 10-45).

Hysterosalpingography

The uterus and fallopian tubes can be demonstrated by the direct injection of contrast media into the uterine cavity via a uterine cervical cannula (Fig. 10-46A). One abnormality that can be nicely demonstrated by hysterosalpingography is the bicornuate uterus (Fig. 10-46B).

MALE PELVIS

Both CT and MRI are useful for evaluation of the male pelvis, and MR images of the male pelvis are shown in Figs. 10-47 to 10-51.

text continues on page 231

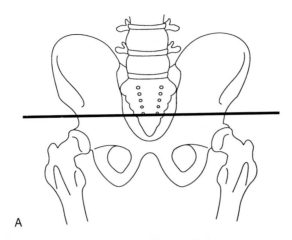

A

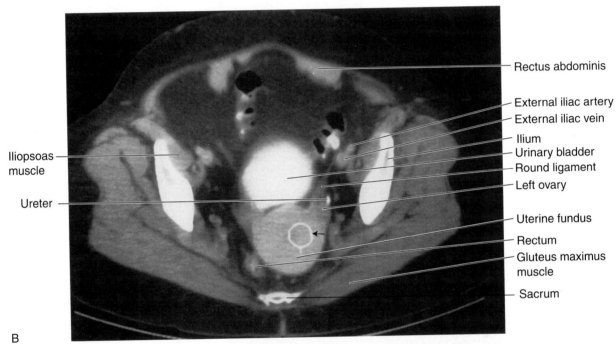

Iliopsoas
muscle

Ureter

Rectus abdominis

External iliac artery
External iliac vein
Ilium
Urinary bladder
Round ligament
Left ovary

Uterine fundus

Rectum
Gluteus maximus
muscle

Sacrum

B

FIG. 10-44. A: Illustration of the approximate axial anatomic level for B. **B:** Female pelvis axial CT image through the uterus with intravenous contrast media. Normal. The white metallic density ring *(straight arrow)* that projects over the uterus is merely a region of interest (ROI) cursor for measuring tissue density.

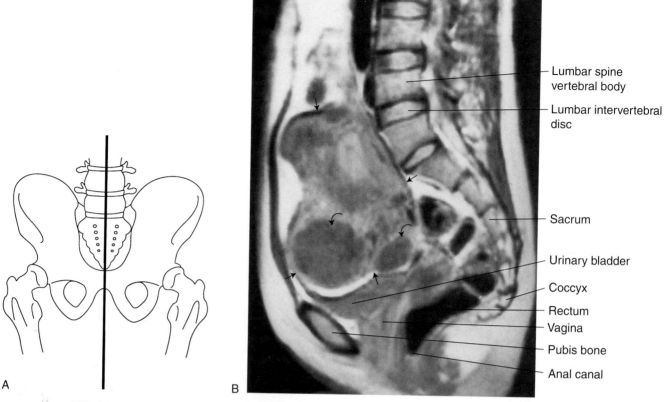

— Lumbar spine vertebral body

— Lumbar intervertebral disc

— Sacrum

— Urinary bladder

— Coccyx

— Rectum

— Vagina

— Pubis bone

— Anal canal

A

B

FIG. 10-45. A: Illustration of approximate midline sagittal anatomic level for the image in B. **B:** Female pelvis midline sagittal T1 MR image. Uterine leiomyomatosis or fibroid uterus. The moderately enlarged fibroid uterus is outlined by straight arrows. Two large fibroids are indicated by the curved arrows.

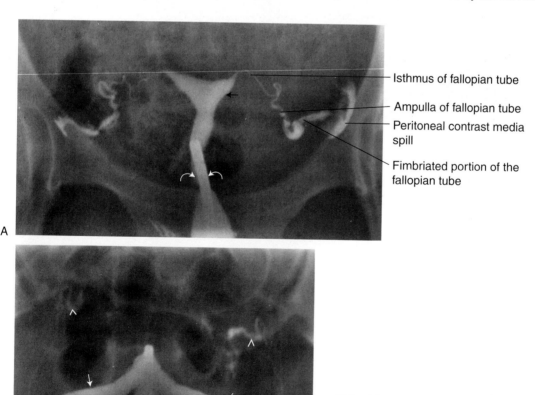

— Isthmus of fallopian tube

— Ampulla of fallopian tube

— Peritoneal contrast media spill

— Fimbriated portion of the fallopian tube

A

B

FIG. 10-46. A: Pelvis AP hysterosalpingogram. Normal uterus *(straight arrow)* and fallopian tubes. Contrast media was injected into the uterus via a cervical cannula *(curved arrows)*, and the spill of contrast media into the peritoneal space indicates fallopian tube patency. **B:** Pelvis AP hysterosalpingogram. Bicornuate uterus. This is a congenital anomaly where there are two uterine fundi *(straight arrows)* and one cervix. Note the fallopian tubes, indicated by arrowheads.

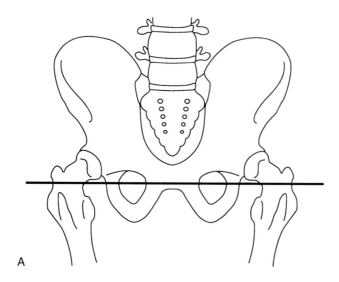

A

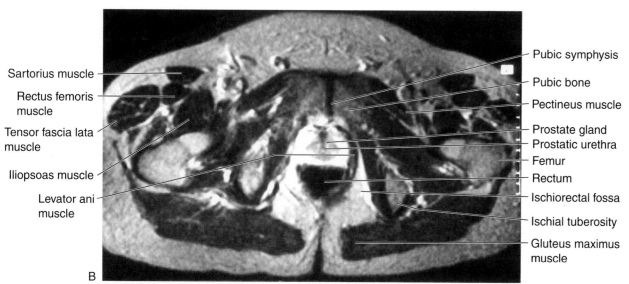

Sartorius muscle

Rectus femoris
muscle

Tensor fascia lata
muscle

Iliopsoas muscle

Levator ani
muscle

B

Pubic symphysis

Pubic bone

Pectineus muscle

Prostate gland

Prostatic urethra

Femur

Rectum

Ischiorectal fossa

Ischial tuberosity

Gluteus maximus
muscle

FIG. 10-47. A: Illustration of the approximate axial anatomic level for B. **B:** Male pelvis axial T2 MR image at the level of the pubic symphysis and prostate. Normal.

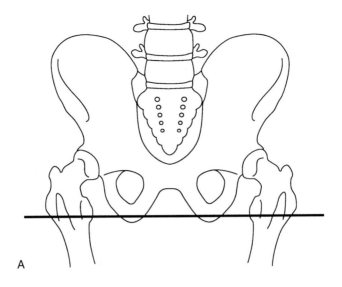

A

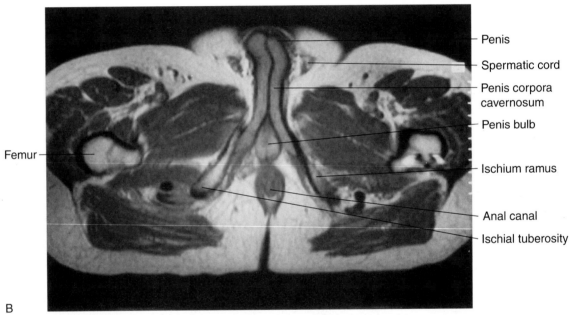

B

FIG. 10-48. A: Illustration of the approximate axial anatomic level for B. **B:** Male pelvis axial T2 MR image at the level of the penile structures. Normal.

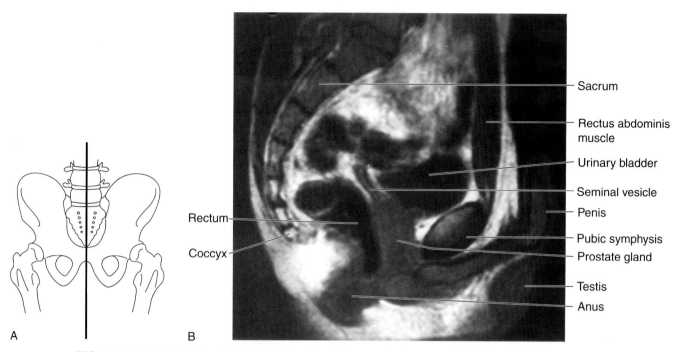

FIG. 10-49. **A:** Illustration of the approximate midline sagittal anatomic level for B. **B:** Male pelvis midline sagittal T2 MR image at level of the urinary bladder and the pubic symphysis. Normal.

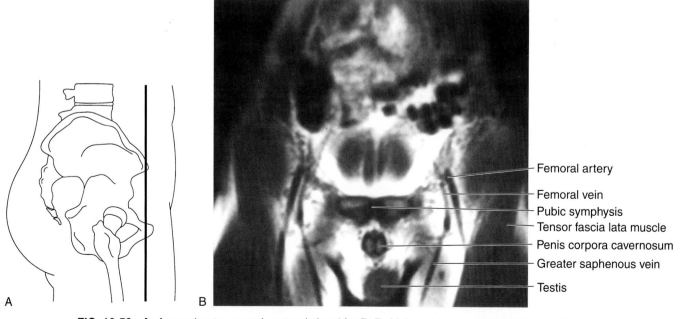

FIG. 10-50. **A:** Approximate coronal anatomic level for B. **B:** Male pelvis coronal T1 MR image through the pubic symphysis. Normal.

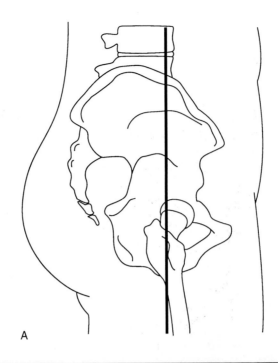

A

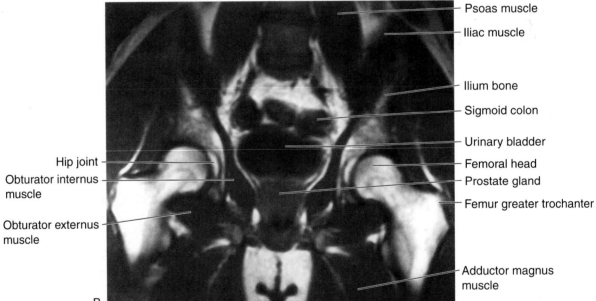

Psoas muscle

Iliac muscle

Ilium bone

Sigmoid colon

Urinary bladder

Femoral head

Prostate gland

Femur greater trochanter

Hip joint

Obturator internus muscle

Obturator externus muscle

Adductor magnus muscle

B

FIG. 10-51. A: Approximate coronal anatomic level for B. **B:** Male pelvis coronal T1 MR image through the prostate gland level. Normal.

Key Points

- EU can be performed on almost all patients, but radiologic consultation should be sought when the following are present or suspected: (a) pregnancy, (b) multiple myeloma, (c) pheochromocytoma, (d) severe renal disease especially when associated with diabetes and/or heart disease, (e) renal failure, and (f) previous severe reaction to contrast media.
- EU requires no preparation, although a mild cathartic improves interpretation. Enemas may introduce air into the colon and so should be avoided.
- EU is especially helpful for working up known or suspected urolithiasis. Approximately 90% of renal calculi are radiopaque. Uric acid calculi are usually radiolucent. Cystine and xanthine are radiolucent, but can be faintly visible especially if they contain calcium. Nearly all ureteral calculi are less than 1 cm in diameter.
- Ureteral dilation can result from partial or complete obstruction due to calculus or tumor, bladder neck obstruction due to prostatic enlargement, or neurogenic bladder.
- Fibroids are a common type of benign tumor that can partially or completely calcify; these calcifications typically appear curvilinear and mottled on a radiograph.
- On CT, primary renal cell carcinoma presents as a solid mass that postcontrast enhances more than a cyst and less than normal parenchyma.

REFERENCES

1. Barbaric ZL. *Principles of Genitourinary Radiology.* New York: Thieme, 1991.
2. Juhl JH, Crummy AB. *Paul and Juhl's Essentials of Radiologic Imaging,* 6th ed. Philadelphia: JB Lippincott, 1993.
3. Chapman S, Nakielny R. *Aids to Radiological Differential Diagnosis,* 3rd ed. London: WB Saunders, 1995.

SUGGESTED READING

El-Khoury GY, Bergman RA, Montgomery WJ. *Sectional Anatomy by MRI,* 2nd ed. New York: Churchill Livingstone, 1995.

CHAPTER 11

Musculoskeletal System

William E. Erkonen

NORMAL EXTREMITY IMAGES

When you think about it, bones are visible on nearly all radiographs. Therefore, radiologic anatomy of the musculoskeletal system is extremely important, but it is time consuming to learn. Entire textbooks are dedicated to this subject, and there are just no shortcuts to mastering this detailed material. As always, a solid knowledge of normal image anatomy is a prerequisite for intelligent image evaluation. Let us begin with normal image anatomy of the hand and move systematically cephalad to the shoulder girdle. This will be followed by normal image anatomy of the lower extremity from the foot to the hip.

Upper Extremity

People commonly injure their extremities because we actively encounter the environment with our arms, legs, and lungs. Consequently, you will probably order many radiographs of the extremities in your clinical practice. Thus, we need a system to evaluate upper and lower extremity images (Table 11-1). Each bone in an image must be carefully evaluated for density, variations of normal, and fracture. Also, each joint must be evaluated for width, smoothness of the articular surfaces, dislocation, arthritis, fracture, and foreign body. Next, the soft tissues should be evaluated for edema, hemorrhage, masses, calcifications, and foreign bodies.

The hand is so complex as to be a subspecialty in orthopedics, so don't expect to conquer the anatomy overnight. When you request radiographs of the hand, the standard study usually consists of posteroanterior (PA), oblique, and lateral views (Fig. 11-1). *Remember that one of the most difficult aspects of medicine is to learn the jargon and routines, so we need to get the hand terminology correct from the beginning.* Each digit of the hand must be properly named to accurately communicate and document information. The proper terminology for each digit and the numbering system for the metacarpals are displayed in Fig. 11-1A. Simply numbering the digits does not suffice, especially in situations

TABLE 11-1. *Observation checklist for bone radiographs*

Each bone should be evaluated for
  Density
  Anomaly
  Fracture
  Tumor
  Foreign body
  Infection
Each joint should be evaluated for
  Articular surface smoothness
  Fracture
  Dislocation
  Arthritis
  Foreign body
Soft tissues should be evaluated for
  Edema
  Hemorrhage
  Calcifications
  Masses
  Foreign bodies

where digits are missing. Would you refer to the index finger as the 1st or 2nd finger when the thumb is missing? So, beginning on the radial side of the hand, the thumb is always the thumb and not the first finger. Next is the index finger (not the 2nd finger). Then the long finger (not the 3rd or middle finger), the ring finger (not the 4th), and the short or little finger (not the 5th). Metacarpals (see Fig. 11-1A) are numbered logically with the thumb articulating with the 1st metacarpal and the index finger with the 2nd metacarpal, and so on. As a general

rule, each hand digit has three phalanges except the thumb, which has only two. The phalanges are named proximal, middle, and distal. The joint between the proximal phalanx and the metacarpal is called the metacarpal phalangeal, or MP, joint (see Fig. 11-1A). The joint between the proximal and middle phalanges is the proximal interphalangeal, or PIP, joint. The joint between the distal and middle phalanges is called the distal interphalangeal, or DIP, joint. The distalmost aspect of the metacarpals and phalanges is the heads, whereas the proximal portions are the bases. The central aspects of these bones are the shafts.

Commonly used bone terms such as physis, epiphysis, metaphysis, and diaphysis can be confusing to the novice, but actually they are very simple. The locations of these entities are demonstrated in Fig. 11-1C. The physis (physeal or epiphyseal plate) is the growth plate as bone formation occurs on both sides (epiphysis and metaphysis) of the physis. The physis is the weakest part of a growing bone. The epiphysis is a secondary ossification center at the end of the bone, the metaphysis is just proximal to the physis, and the diaphysis (bone shaft) is proximal to the metaphysis. Eventually, the epiphysis and metaphysis fuse as the physis closes. The term apophysis is confusing and merely refers to an epiphysis that does not articulate with another bone and does not contribute to bone length growth.

The wrist and forearm are common fracture sites, especially in children. If we are to intelligently under-

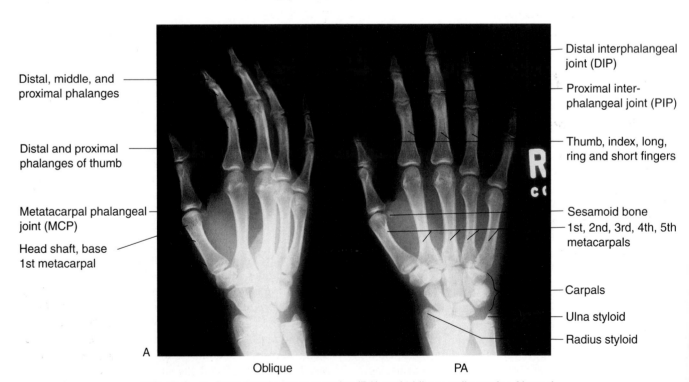

Distal, middle, and proximal phalanges

Distal and proximal phalanges of thumb

Metatacarpal phalangeal joint (MCP)

Head shaft, base 1st metacarpal

A

Oblique

Distal interphalangeal joint (DIP)

Proximal interphalangeal joint (PIP)

Thumb, index, long, ring and short fingers

Sesamoid bone

1st, 2nd, 3rd, 4th, 5th metacarpals

Carpals

Ulna styloid

Radius styloid

PA

FIG. 11-1. A: Right-hand posteroanterior (PA) and oblique radiographs. Normal.

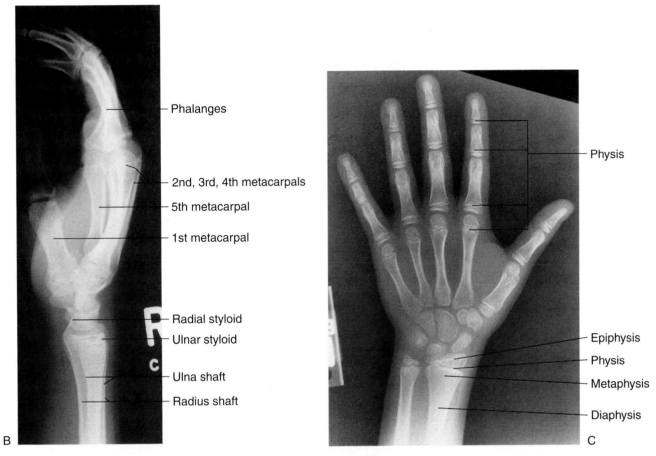

FIG. 11-1. *Continued.* **B:** Right-hand lateral radiograph. Normal. **C:** Left-hand PA radiograph. Normal physis, epiphysis, metaphysis, and diaphysis. The physis is a lucent area on a radiograph.

stand and treat fractures in these areas, a thorough knowledge of wrist and forearm anatomy is very important. The appearance, location, and names of each carpal bone must be learned, as well as their relationship to the distal radius and ulna. These relationships are well visualized on standard PA, lateral, and oblique radiographic views of the wrist (Fig. 11-2).

We generally obtain anteroposterior (AP) and lateral views of the forearm in children and adults (Fig. 11-3). Routine elbow radiographs consist of AP and lateral views (Fig. 11-4), but oblique views of the elbow may be requested on occasion (Fig. 11-5A) Radiographs of the humerus usually consist of AP (see Fig. 11-5A) and lateral views. Generally, an AP radiograph is obtained to evaluate the shoulder (Fig. 11-5B), and this is supplemented by either an axillary or lateral view of the shoulder depending on local practice. Musculoskeletal anatomy and disease can be nicely demonstrated by computed tomography (CT) and magnetic resonance imaging (MRI) (Table 11-2). CT imaging is especially good for bone detail, whereas MRI is good for soft tissue and bone marrow imaging.

MRI is especially helpful in displaying the shoulder rotator cuff anatomy (Fig. 11-6).

Lower Extremity

Now we approach lower extremity radiologic imaging by beginning with the foot and moving toward the hip. The standard views of the foot are AP, lateral, and oblique (Fig. 11-7). Naming of the toes is far easier than

text continues on page 241

TABLE 11-2. *Musculoskeletal CT and MRI indications*

Computed tomography
Bone detail
Fracture fragment evaluation
Bone tumor workup
Magnetic resonance imaging
Bone marrow imaging (white)
Soft tissue evaluation: ligaments, tendons, cartilages, and vessels (black)
Bone tumor workup

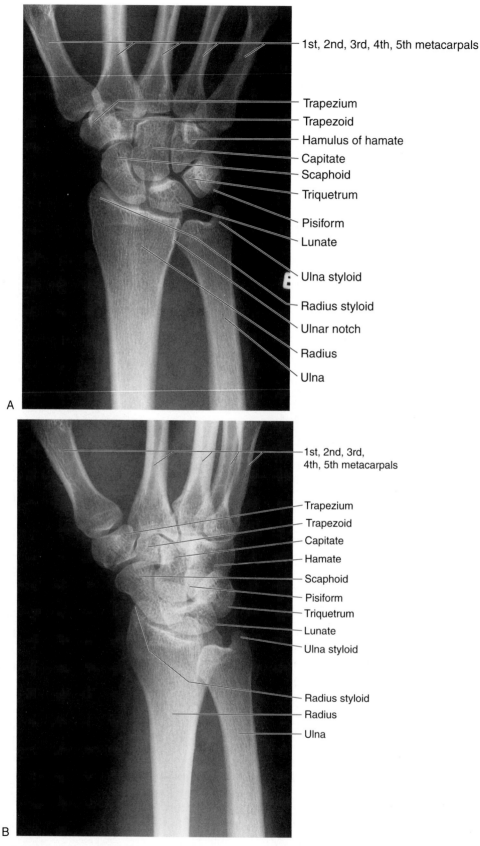

FIG. 11-2. Right wrist PA **(A)**, oblique **(B)**, and lateral **(C)** radiographs. Normal. Notice that the tip of the radial styloid is at least 1 cm distal to the tip of the ulnar styloid and the radius articulates distally with the scaphoid and lunate carpals and laterally with the ulna (ulnar notch). The distal radial articular surface slopes toward the ulna and anteriorly. The distal ulna articulates with the radius laterally and wrist cartilage distally. The ulna does not articulate directly with a carpal.

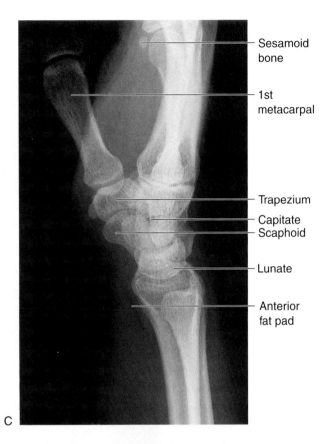

Sesamoid bone

1st metacarpal

Trapezium
Capitate
Scaphoid

Lunate

Anterior fat pad

FIG. 11-2. *Continued.* C

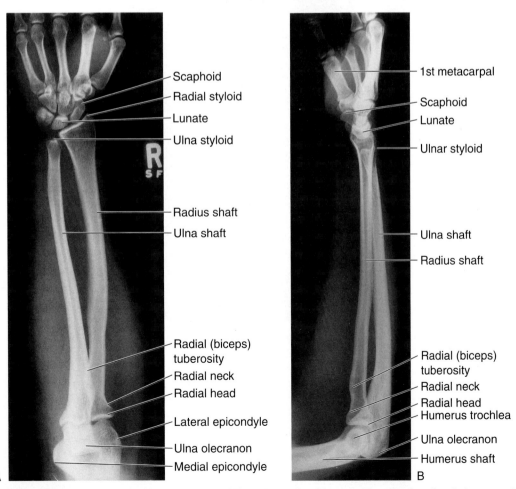

Scaphoid
Radial styloid
Lunate
Ulna styloid

Radius shaft
Ulna shaft

Radial (biceps) tuberosity
Radial neck
Radial head
Lateral epicondyle
Ulna olecranon
Medial epicondyle

1st metacarpal

Scaphoid
Lunate

Ulnar styloid

Ulna shaft

Radius shaft

Radial (biceps) tuberosity
Radial neck
Radial head
Humerus trochlea
Ulna olecranon
Humerus shaft

A   B

FIG. 11-3. Right forearm AP **(A)** and lateral **(B)** radiographs. Normal. The distal radius is large and the proximal radius is small while the distal ulna is small and the proximal ulna is large. The radius is far more important than the ulna in the wrist joint while the ulna is more important in the elbow joint than the radius.

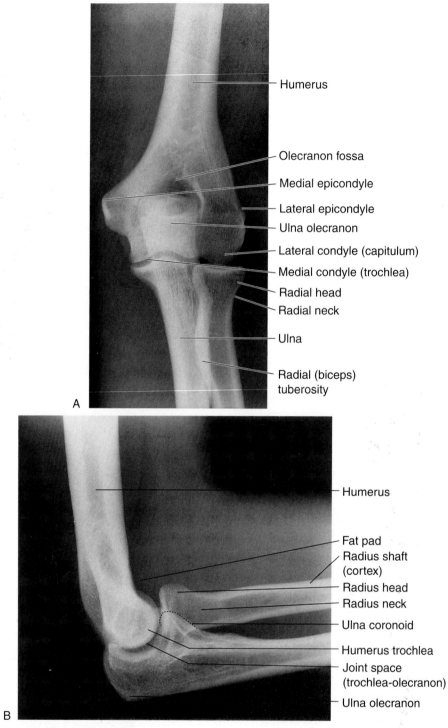

FIG. 11-4. Left elbow AP **(A)** and lateral **(B)** radiographs. Normal. The dotted line on (B) indicates the ulna coronoid process.

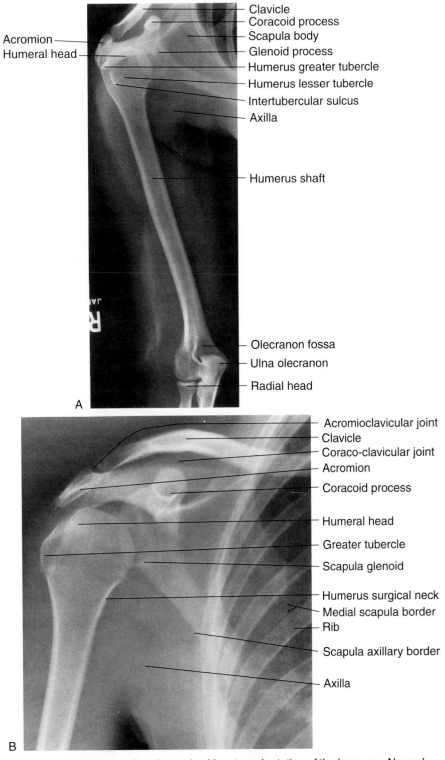

Clavicle
Coracoid process
Scapula body
Glenoid process
Humerus greater tubercle
Humerus lesser tubercle
Intertubercular sulcus
Axilla

Acromion
Humeral head

Humerus shaft

Olecranon fossa
Ulna olecranon
Radial head

A

Acromioclavicular joint
Clavicle
Coraco-clavicular joint
Acromion
Coracoid process

Humeral head

Greater tubercle

Scapula glenoid

Humerus surgical neck
Medial scapula border
Rib

Scapula axillary border

Axilla

B

FIG. 11-5. A: Right humerus and shoulder AP radiograph with external rotation of the humerus. Normal. The right elbow is in an oblique position. **B:** Right shoulder AP radiograph with external rotation of the humerus. Normal.

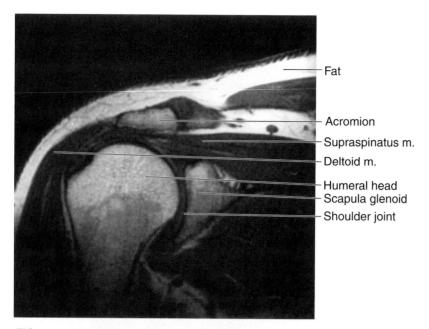

Fat

Acromion

Supraspinatus m.

Deltoid m.

Humeral head
Scapula glenoid
Shoulder joint

FIG. 11-6. Right shoulder coronal T1 MR image. Normal.

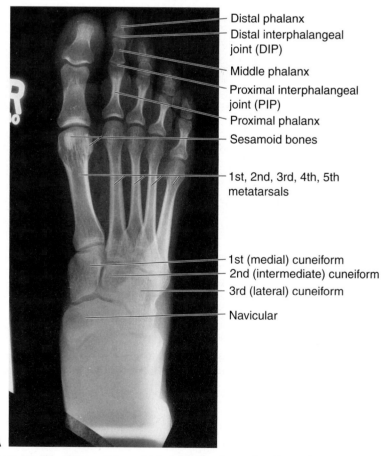

Distal phalanx
Distal interphalangeal joint (DIP)

Middle phalanx
Proximal interphalangeal joint (PIP)
Proximal phalanx
Sesamoid bones

1st, 2nd, 3rd, 4th, 5th metatarsals

1st (medial) cuneiform
2nd (intermediate) cuneiform
3rd (lateral) cuneiform

Navicular

A

FIG. 11-7. Right foot AP **(A)**, oblique **(B)**, and lateral **(C)** radiographs. Normal.

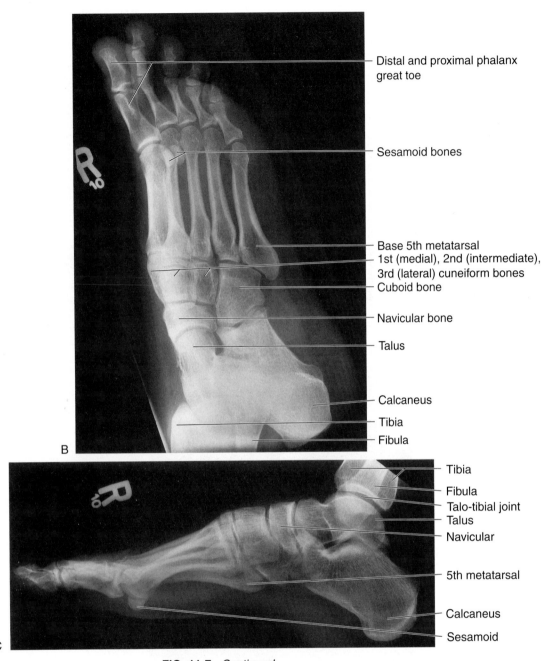

Distal and proximal phalanx great toe

Sesamoid bones

Base 5th metatarsal
1st (medial), 2nd (intermediate), 3rd (lateral) cuneiform bones
Cuboid bone

Navicular bone

Talus

Calcaneus
Tibia
Fibula

B

Tibia
Fibula
Talo-tibial joint
Talus
Navicular

5th metatarsal

Calcaneus
Sesamoid

C

FIG. 11-7. *Continued.*

that of the fingers. The big toe or great toe may be referred to as the 1st toe, and the remaining toes are numbered sequentially ending with the little or 5th toe. Similarly, the metatarsals are numbered sequentially with the great toe articulating with the 1st metatarsal and the 2nd toe articulating with the 2nd metatarsal, and so forth. The ankle is usually imaged by AP, lateral, and oblique radiographs (Fig. 11-8). However, MRI is used to image the ankle to detect soft tissue injury (Fig. 11-9). Radiographs of the tibia and fibula usually consist of AP and lateral views (Fig. 11-10). Routine knee radio-

graphs consist of AP and lateral views and they may be supplemented by AP standing radiographs (Fig. 11-11A, B, C) and/or oblique views. Sagittal and coronal MR images of the knee (Fig. 11-12) are commonly requested to evaluate nonosseous soft tissue injuries of the knee, including the medial and lateral menisci, articular cartilages, ligaments, tendons, and muscles. *Remember that ligaments, tendons, cartilages, and vessels have a low-intensity signal or appear black on MR images.*

text continues on page 246

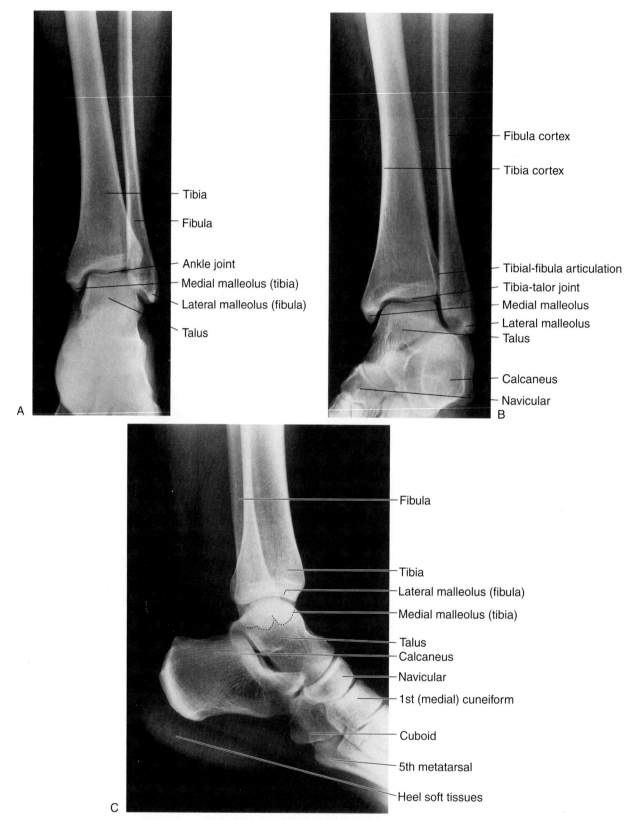

FIG. 11-8. Left ankle AP **(A)**, oblique **(B)**, and lateral **(C)** radiographs. Normal. Note how the oblique view (B) allows improved visualization of the distal tibia-fibula articulation.

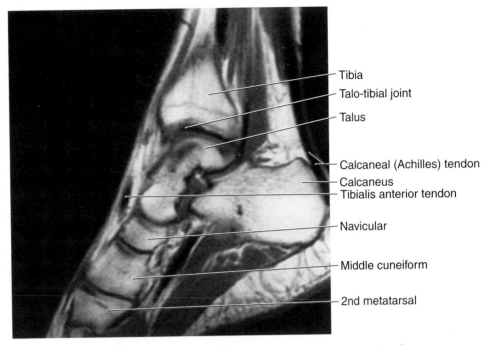

Tibia
Talo-tibial joint
Talus

Calcaneal (Achilles) tendon
Calcaneus
Tibialis anterior tendon

Navicular

Middle cuneiform

2nd metatarsal

FIG. 11-9. Right ankle sagittal T1 MR image. Normal. Note that the calcaneal (Achilles) tendon has a homogeneous low-intensity (black) signal.

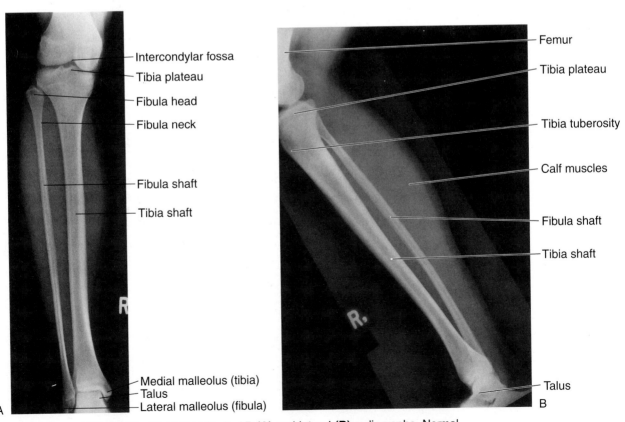

Intercondylar fossa
Tibia plateau
Fibula head
Fibula neck

Fibula shaft

Tibia shaft

Medial malleolus (tibia)
Talus
Lateral malleolus (fibula)

Femur

Tibia plateau

Tibia tuberosity

Calf muscles

Fibula shaft

Tibia shaft

Talus

FIG. 11-10. Right tibia-fibula AP **(A)** and lateral **(B)** radiographs. Normal.

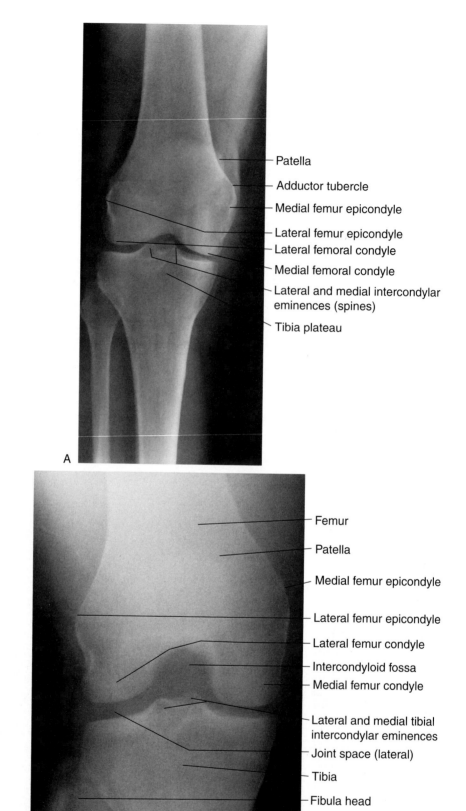

— Patella

— Adductor tubercle

— Medial femur epicondyle

— Lateral femur epicondyle
— Lateral femoral condyle

— Medial femoral condyle

— Lateral and medial intercondylar eminences (spines)

— Tibia plateau

A

— Femur

— Patella

— Medial femur epicondyle

— Lateral femur epicondyle

— Lateral femur condyle

— Intercondyloid fossa
— Medial femur condyle

— Lateral and medial tibial intercondylar eminences

— Joint space (lateral)

— Tibia

— Fibula head

— Fibula neck

B

FIG. 11-11. Right knee AP **(A)**, AP standing **(B)**, and lateral **(C)** radiographs. Normal.

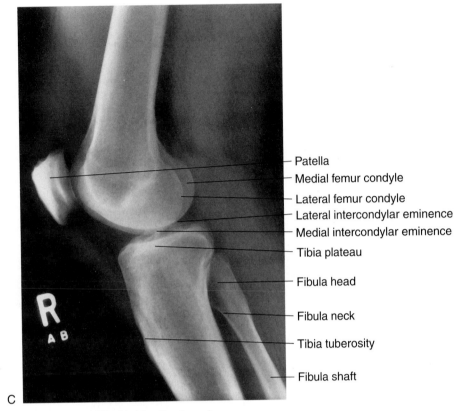

Patella
Medial femur condyle
Lateral femur condyle
Lateral intercondylar eminence
Medial intercondylar eminence
Tibia plateau
Fibula head
Fibula neck
Tibia tuberosity
Fibula shaft

C

FIG. 11-11. *Continued.*

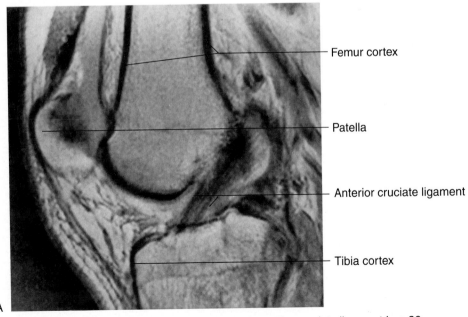

Femur cortex

Patella

Anterior cruciate ligament

Tibia cortex

A

FIG. 11-12. A: Right knee proton-dense sagittal MR image. Normal anterior cruciate ligament in a 36-year-old man.

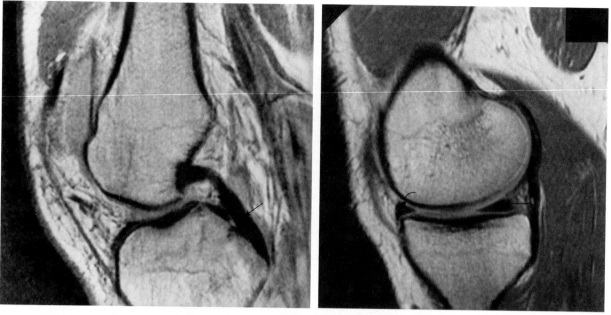

B

C

FIG. 11-12. *Continued.* **B:** Right knee proton-dense sagittal MR image in the same patient. Normal posterior cruciate ligament. The posterior cruciate ligament *(arrow)* is more homogeneous and has a lower intensity signal (blacker) than the anterior cruciate ligament. **C:** Right knee proton dense medial-sagittal MR image in a 32-year-old man. Normal posterior horn *(straight arrow)* and anterior horn *(curved arrow)* of the medial meniscus.

The femur and the hip joint are radiographed in the AP and lateral views (Fig. 11-13).

VARIATIONS OF NORMAL

There are several osseous variations of normal that can cause confusion for the novice (Table 11-3). One such variation of normal is the *sesamoid bone,* which is merely a normal extra bone within a tendon. Sesamoids occur at numerous sites and are commonly found in the plantar aspect of the foot near the head of the 1st metatarsal (see Fig. 11-7), and in the palmar aspect of the hand near the head of the 1st metacarpal (see Fig. 11-1A) (Fig. 11-14A–C). When you think about it, the patella is actually a sesamoid bone or a bone within a tendon. *Ossicles* are another variant of normal. They are small supernumerary or extra bones found in a variety of places in juxtaposition to the skeletal system and usually named after the neighboring bone (Fig. 11-14D, 11-19, and 12-14). The bipartite patella (Fig. 11-14E, F) is another example of an accessory bone that should not be

text continues on page 250

TABLE 11-3. *Normal osseous variations*

Sesamoid bones (located within a tendon like the patella)
Ossicles (extra small bones)
Supernumerary epiphyses

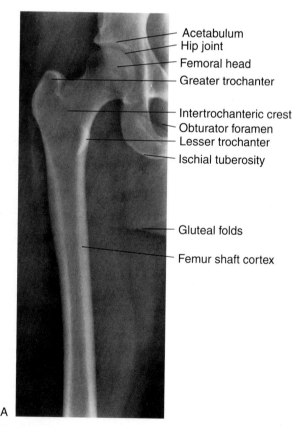

— Acetabulum
— Hip joint
— Femoral head
— Greater trochanter

— Intertrochanteric crest
— Obturator foramen
— Lesser trochanter
— Ischial tuberosity

— Gluteal folds

— Femur shaft cortex

A

FIG. 11-13. **A:** Right hip and proximal femur AP radiograph. Normal.

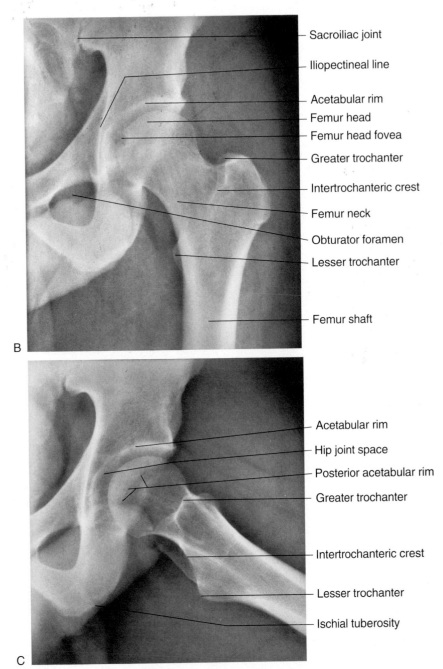

Sacroiliac joint
Iliopectineal line
Acetabular rim
Femur head
Femur head fovea
Greater trochanter
Intertrochanteric crest
Femur neck
Obturator foramen
Lesser trochanter
Femur shaft

B

Acetabular rim
Hip joint space
Posterior acetabular rim
Greater trochanter
Intertrochanteric crest
Lesser trochanter
Ischial tuberosity

C

FIG. 11-13. *Continued.* **B, C:** Left hip AP (B) and lateral (C) radiographs. Normal.

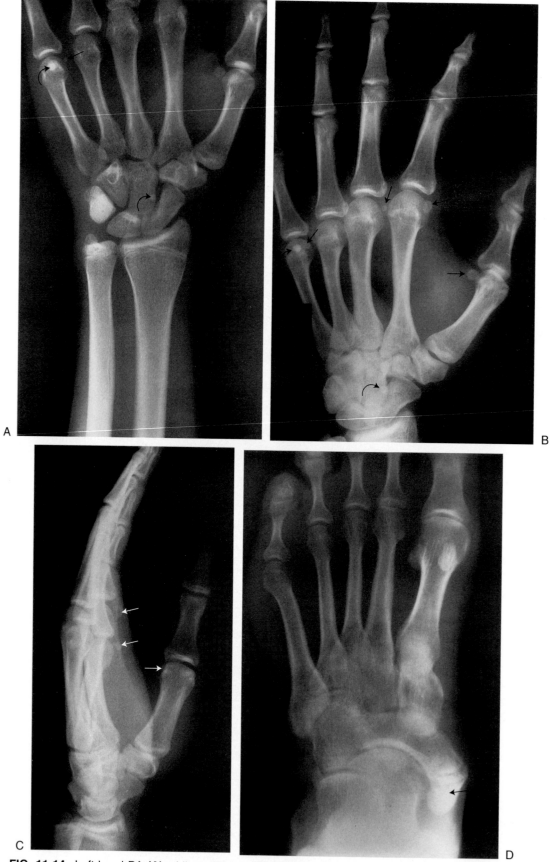

FIG. 11-14. Left-hand PA **(A)**, oblique **(B)**, and lateral **(C)** radiographs. Multiple sesamoids *(arrows)*. Bone islands *(curved arrows)* are present in the head of the 5th metacarpal and the capitate, and they have no clinical significance. **D:** Left foot AP radiograph. Os tibiale externum *(straight arrow)* and os peroneum *(curved arrow)*.

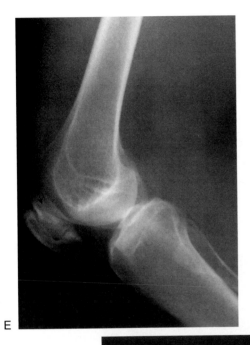

E

FIG. 11-14. *Continued.* **E, F:** Right knee lateral radiograph (E) and tangential radiograph of both knees (F). Bilateral bipartite patella. Note that the patella has two sections and the accessory bone *(straight arrows)* usually lies superior and lateral to the main body of the patella. **G:** Right wrist PA radiograph. Normal distal right radial epiphysis spur. This 21-year-old woman fell and had a painful wrist. This spur *(arrow)* is a variant of normal and must not be confused with a fracture. **H:** Right ankle AP radiograph. Accessory epiphysis near the tip of the distal tibia epiphysis in the region of the medial malleolus *(arrow).* This is a variant of normal.

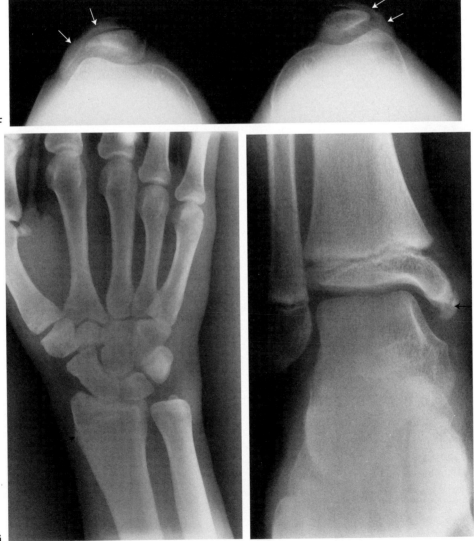

F

G

H

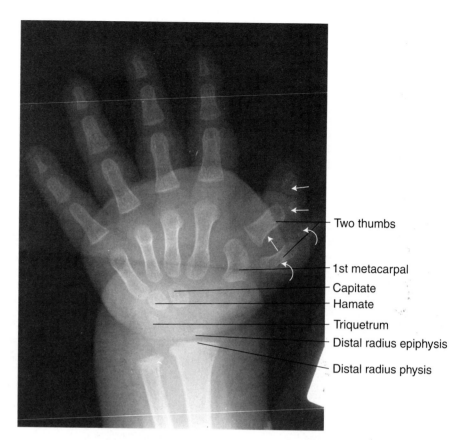

Two thumbs

1st metacarpal
Capitate
Hamate
Triquetrum
Distal radius epiphysis
Distal radius physis

FIG. 11-15. Left-hand PA radiograph (child). Polydactylism. There are two thumbs and one first metacarpal. One thumb has three phalanges *(straight arrows)*, and the other thumb has two phalanges *(curved arrows)*.

mistaken for a fracture. The condition results when one of the patella ossification centers fails to fuse with the main patellar body. The result is that the patella has two or more sections, and it occurs bilaterally approximately 75% of the time.

Epiphyses can vary in their number and appearance and still be normal (Fig. 11-14G, H).

ANOMALIES

Osseous congenital anomalies are not uncommon in our patients, and a few of the many variations are illustrated in Figs. 11-15 to 11-19 and listed in Table 11-4.

Osteogenesis imperfecta is a congenital, non-sex-linked, hereditary abnormality with the primary defect residing in the bone matrix (1). These patients have abnormal bones (Fig. 11-20) that are fragile, fracture easily, and are often deformed.

Achondroplasia is a hereditary, autosomal-dominant anomaly manifested by shortened long bones that results in dwarfism (Fig. 11-21). The hip joint is the most common site of congenital dislocation (1). Congenital dislocation of the hip (CDH) or congenital hip dysplasia

(CHD), shown in Fig. 11-22A, is usually diagnosed in infancy. CDH is an abnormal development of the hip joint resulting in an abnormal acetabulum and femoral head. There is displacement of the femoral head referable to the acetabular cartilage. The femoral head usually displaces superiorly but can displace posteriorly.

TABLE 11-4. *Some bone anomalies*

Upper extremity:
 Supernumerary digits or polydactylism
 Missing bones (fingers, radius)
 Large digits or macrodactyly
 Supracondylar process
Lower extremity:
 Polydactylism
 Talocalcaneal coalition
 Congenital hip dysplasia
 Slipped capital femoral epiphysis
 Legg-Calvé-Perthes disease (avascular necrosis)
 Talipes equinovarus (club foot)
Generalized:
 Osteogenesis imperfecta
 Achondroplasia

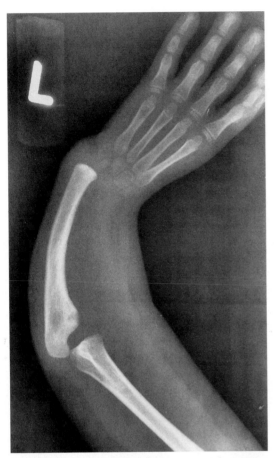

FIG. 11-16. Left forearm PA radiograph. Absence of the radius, 1st metacarpal, and thumb. This 6-year-old had left-hand and arm deformity at birth.

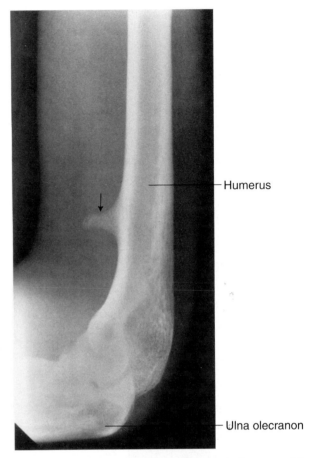

FIG. 11-17. Right humerus lateral radiograph. Supracondylar process or spur *(arrow)*. It is usually located in the antero-medial aspect of the distal humerus.

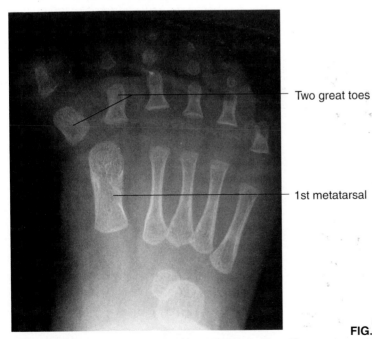

FIG. 11-18. Right foot AP radiograph. Polydactylism. There are two great toes but only one 1st metatarsal.

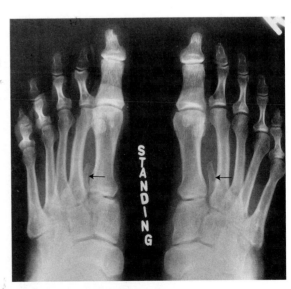

FIG. 11-19. Right and left feet standing AP radiograph. Os metatarsum. Accessory metatarsals *(arrows)* are present bi-laterally.

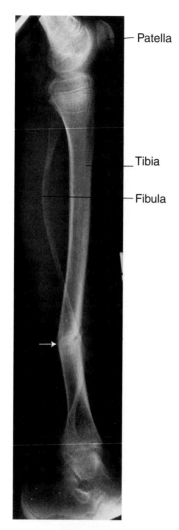

Patella

Tibia

Fibula

FIG. 11-20. Left tibia and fibula lateral radiograph. Osteogenesis imperfecta. There is a healing posteriorly angulated left tibia fracture *(arrow)*. Note the thin serpentine appearance of the fibula and generalized osteoporosis.

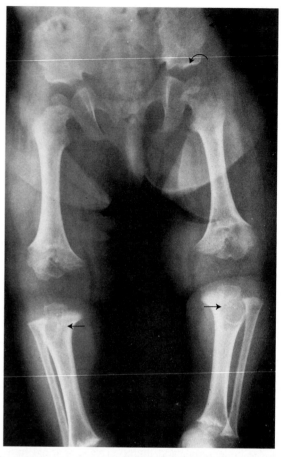

FIG. 11-21. Pelvis and lower extremities AP radiograph. Achondroplasia. The proximal long bones are shorter and wider than normal especially the proximal tibias *(straight arrows)*. The iliac bones are rounded *(double arrows)*, and the acetabula are flat *(curved arrow)*.

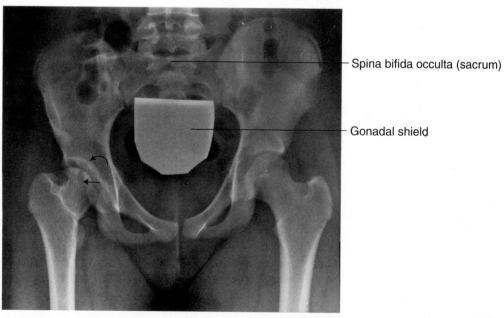

Spina bifida occulta (sacrum)

Gonadal shield

A

FIG. 11-22. A: Pelvis AP radiograph. Congenital dislocation of the right hip (CDH) or congenital hip dysplasia (CHD) in a 14-year old. The right hip is abnormal with a flattened femoral head *(single arrow)* and a poorly formed acetabulum *(curved arrow)*. Compare the right hip to the normal left hip.

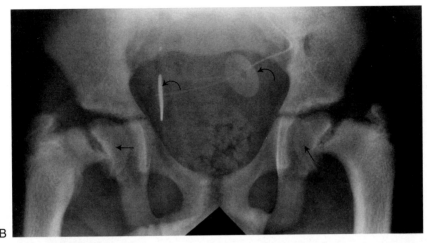

FIG. 11-22. *Continued.* **B:** Pelvis AP radiograph. Bilateral slipped capital femoral epiphyses (SCFE) in a 15-year-old with chronic renal failure and on dialysis. The capital femoral epiphyses or proximal femoral epiphyses *(straight arrows)* are displaced from their normal anatomic position, and they are usually displaced inferiorly and posteromedially (1). There are monitoring electrodes projecting over the pelvis *(curved arrows)*.

Two hip problems that can cause confusion are slipped capital femoral epiphysis and Legg-Calvé-Perthes disease (Table 11-5). Slipped capital femoral epiphysis (SCFE) (Fig. 11-22B) is a hip problem that occurs during adolescence and is often associated with hip pain. The etiology is not understood, but there may be a history of trauma. Apparently, the physis becomes weakened during the rapid growth around puberty. The radiographic findings show the femoral head slipping or displacing posteriorly, medially, and inferiorly relative to the femoral neck. The proximal epiphysis becomes widened. The early changes are similar to those of osteochondrosis or Legg-Calvé-Perthes disease and the late changes are similar to those of osteoarthritis.

Legg-Calvé-Perthes disease (Fig. 11-23A) is a form of avascular necrosis, and the etiology is unknown. It may be referred to as osteochondrosis and coxa plana. It typically occurs in a boy between 5 and 10 years of age who complains of hip pain and walks with a limp. It occurs less frequently in females. The pain may be referred to the ipsilateral knee or the knee on the same side. Radiographic findings vary, but may include increased density of the femoral capital epiphysis, femoral head flattening, rarefaction of the metaphysis, and me-

dial joint space narrowing. In general, avascular necrosis or aseptic necrosis can occur in any joint (Fig. 11-23B) and result from multiple other etiologies. Some of the other etiologies of avascular necrosis are listed in Table 11-6. The typical findings are sclerotic bone changes on one side of a joint that may go on to fragmentation and eventually to collapse or fracture.

TRAUMA

Fractures and Dislocations

Extremity fractures are very common, so now is the time to discuss fractures in general. *Because a fracture or other osseous abnormality may only be visible on one of the radiographs, always obtain at least two views of a bone or joint that are 90 degrees to each other.* Give yourself every opportunity to detect a fracture or other abnormality by obtaining as many views of an area as is practical. *Never accept just one radiographic view of a bone or joint.*

In general, fractures can be conveniently divided into two major clinical categories:

1. Simple or closed fracture means that there are bone fragments and the skin is intact.

TABLE 11-5. *Comparison of slipped capital femoral epiphysis (SCFE) and Legg-Calvé-Perthes disease (LCP)*

Feature	SCFE	LCP
Age	Adolescence	4–10 years
Gender	Boys more than girls (usually overweight)	Boys more than girls
Etiology	Unknown (usually during growth spurt)	Unknown
Symptoms	Hip and/or knee pain	Hip or knee pain and limping
Radiographic	Capital epiphysis slips posterior, medial, inferior to the femoral neck	Flat and sclerotic capital epiphysis

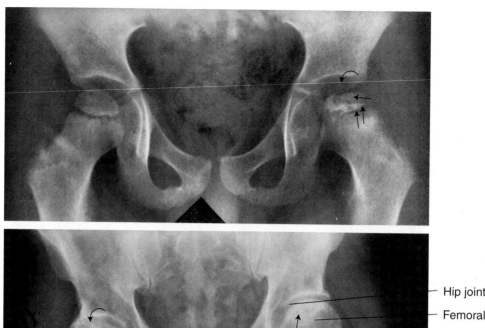

FIG. 11-23. A: Pelvis AP radiograph. Legg-Calvé-Perthes disease. The right femoral head is normal. Note the irregular contour, flattened articular surface, and increased density of the left femoral head *(straight arrow)*. The left hip joint space is widened *(curved arrow)*. The left proximal femoral epiphysis is widened *(double arrows)*, and the metaphysis is irregular. Note that the acetabulum is normal. **B:** Pelvis AP radiograph. Bilateral femoral head avascular necrosis of unknown etiology in a 42-year-old man. Both femoral heads *(straight arrows)* are sclerotic in appearance and the right femoral head is deformed due to mild collapse or fracture. The right hip joint is narrowed laterally *(curved arrow)*.

2. Compound or open fracture means the skin is not intact near the fracture. The skin has been penetrated by one or more of the bone fragments or by a penetrating foreign body.

Many terms applied to fractures are very descriptive and quite specific (Fig. 11-24A, B). Examples of straight-forward common terms for describing fractures include the following:

1. Spiral, transverse, oblique
2. Nondisplaced
3. Overriding
4. Distracted or pulled apart
5. Offset, usually described by the percentage of the fracture fragments abutting or touching each other

Some fracture terms (Fig. 11-24C) that are not quite so obvious include the following:

1. Torus fracture of the distal radius looks like the bump at the base of a Greek column and has nothing to do with a bull.
2. Comminuted or complex fracture indicates more than two bone fragments.

TABLE 11-6. *A partial list of avascular necrosis etiologies*

Steroids and antiinflammatory drugs	Alcohol
	Rheumatoid arthritis
Trauma including fractures and dislocations	Renal transplant
	Infection
Sickle cell anemia	Gout
Hemophilia	Diabetes

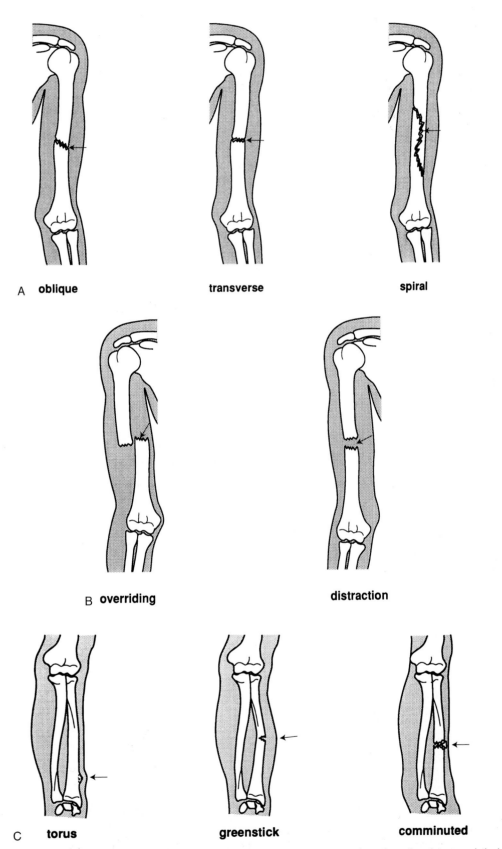

FIG. 11-24. A, B: Some common fractures *(arrows)* and the terms used to describe them and their alignment. **C:** Other common terms used to describe fractures *(arrows).*

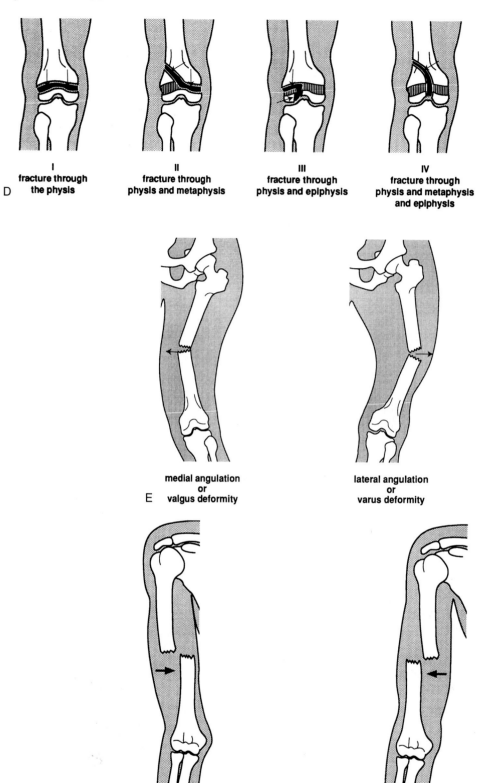

I
fracture through
the physis

II
fracture through
physis and metaphysis

III
fracture through
physis and epiphysis

IV
fracture through
physis and metaphysis
and epiphysis

V
fracture through
physis with
compression

D

medial angulation
or
valgus deformity

lateral angulation
or
varus deformity

E

medial
displacement

lateral
displacement

F

FIG. 11-24. *Continued.* **D:** The Salter-Harris classification of physis fractures. The solid black line indicates the fracture *(arrows)*, whereas the physis is indicated by the vertical black and white lines. **E:** Illustrations of the nomenclature used to describe fracture angulation. **F:** Nomenclature used to describe the direction of displacement of the distal fracture fragments.

3. Greenstick fractures describes a bone that fractures by bending like a green twig.
4. Pathologic fracture is one that passes through abnormal bone such as a metastasis, a primary bone tumor, or a bone cyst.
5. Stress fractures are secondary to unusual or excess stress, e.g., tibial fractures in runners who overdo it.
6. Insufficiency fractures describe a fracture in a bone with decreased strength, e.g., osteoporosis. Such a fracture may result from a normal stress such as merely walking across a room.
7. Avulsion fracture is usually a small chip fracture that can occur at the site of a tendon attachment. This fracture results when the tendon and muscle remain intact, while the bone gives way (avulses) at the site of the tendon attachment to the bone.

The Salter-Harris classification of fractures (Fig. 11-24D) is helpful to describe and understand fractures around a physis. *Remember that the physis represents the weakest point in a bone.*

Type 1: The fracture involves only the physis.
Type 2: The fracture involves the physis and metaphysis.
Type 3: The fracture involves the physis and epiphysis.
Type 4: The fracture involves the physis, metaphysis, and epiphysis.
Type 5: The fracture involves only the physis, and there is compression of the physis.

When describing the position of displaced fracture fragments, we use another set of terms. The apex of the angle created by the fracture fragments is the key to the nomenclature. If the apex of the fracture fragments points lateral, the fracture is laterally angulated. If the apex of the fracture fragments points medial, then it is medially angulated (Fig. 11-24E). The same applies to volar, dorsal, radial, ulnar, varus, valgus, or any other direction of angulation that you choose to use. Another useful rule for describing fracture alignment describes the direction in which the distal fracture fragment is displaced (Fig. 11-24F).

Fracture Healing

The rate at which a fracture heals depends on the fracture site, type of fracture, patient age, adequacy of immobilization, nutrition, and presence or absence of infection. When a fracture occurs, there usually is an associated hemorrhage into the fracture site with subsequent hematoma formation around and between the fracture fragments. The fibrin in a hematoma serves as a framework for fibroblasts, osteoblasts, and a general inflammatory reaction. Bone matrix or osteoid appears in the repair process after a few days, and this is called "soft callus" or "provisional callus." The soft callus is

not visible on a radiograph. As calcium salts precipitate in the soft callus and new bone grows, this is called callus. As the callus gradually becomes more dense it becomes visible on a radiograph. Eventually the callus becomes solid, and bone union is established between the fracture fragments.

In a few days following a fracture, some absorption or removal of bone occurs as a part of the repair process near the ends of the fracture fragments. Due to this bone absorption the fracture line becomes more visible on subsequent radiographs . This explains why some subtle fractures may not be visible on radiographs obtained immediately following injury but become visible approximately 7–10 days post injury.

Self-explanatory terms used to describe problems in the fracture healing process include the following:

1. Nonunion or nonhealing
2. Delayed union
3. Malunion

Upper Extremity

Fractures of the hands result from a wide variety of activities (Table 11-7). Some fractures and injuries are so obvious that the average citizen could spot them on a radiograph (Fig. 11-25). Subtle fractures can involve any bone and are common in the phalanges of the hand (Figs. 11-26 and 11-27). Joint dislocations occur in almost all joints, and the hand phalangeal joints are common dislocation sites especially in sports (Fig. 11-28). Metacarpal fractures are also common, and fractures of the 5th metacarpal often result from striking a hard object as in fisticuffs. These fractures are appropriately called Saturday night fractures (Fig. 11-29). The most commonly fractured carpal is the scaphoid (Fig. 11-30). The carpal scaphoid is often referred to as the navicular by clinicians, but anatomists correctly call it the carpal scaphoid. To add to the confusion, there is a tarsal navicular. Carpal scaphoid fractures result from the injury lines of force being transmitted along the long axis of the thumb, and the majority of these fractures are located in the scaphoid waist. Because of its variable blood supply, scaphoid fractures may develop complications such as posttraumatic arthritis, nonunion, and avascular necrosis. These complications are more apt to occur when there is delayed diagnosis and delayed or inadequate treatment. If a scaphoid fracture is suspected

TABLE 11-7. *Common causes of upper extremity fractures*

Work injuries	Sports
Home falls	Motor vehicle accidents
Recreational activities	Fisticuffs

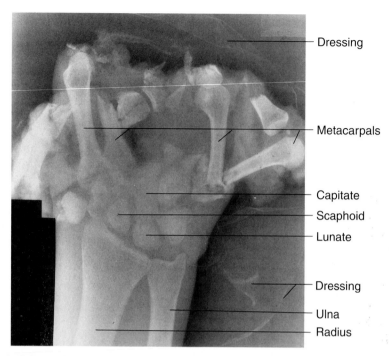

FIG. 11-25. Left-hand AP radiograph. Obvious severe hand injuries secondary to a corn-picking accident. The phalanges are essentially missing, and there are fractures of the metacarpals and carpals.

Dressing

Metacarpals

Capitate
Scaphoid
Lunate

Dressing

Ulna
Radius

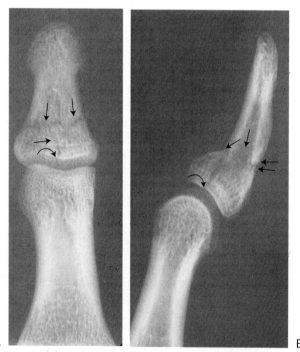

A   B

FIG. 11-26. Left thumb PA (A) and lateral (B) radiographs. Comminuted fracture (straight arrows) that extends to the articular surface of the interphalangeal joint (curved arrow). There is mild palmar angulation at the fracture site (double arrows).

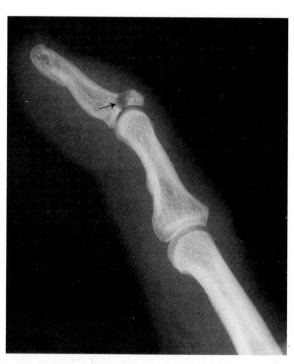

FIG. 11-27. Right index finger lateral radiograph. Mallet finger. The distal phalanx demonstrates a slightly flexed attitude due to fracture (arrow) at site of the insertion of the extensor digitorum mechanism. The loss of the extensor mechanism continuity with the distal phalanx allows the distal phalanx to assume a flexed position or a mallet finger.

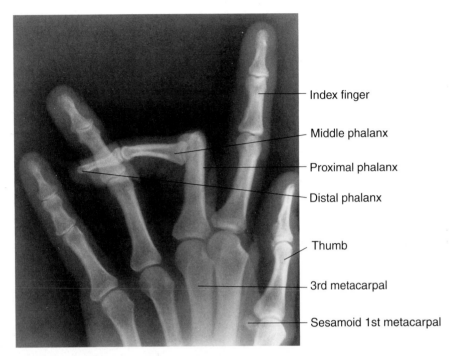

FIG. 11-28. Left-hand PA radiograph. Dislocation at the PIP joint of the left long finger. The middle and distal phalanges are completely dislocated relative to the proximal phalanx. There are no fractures.

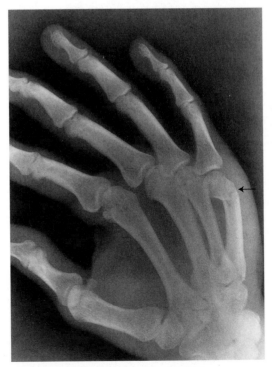

FIG. 11-29. Right hand PA oblique radiograph. Boxer or Saturday night fracture. The dorsal angulated fracture *(arrow)* is through the neck of the right 5th metacarpal.

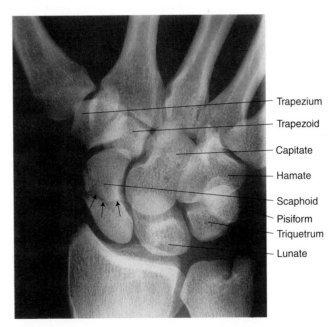

FIG. 11-30. Right wrist PA radiograph. Mildly distracted and comminuted fracture *(arrows)* of the scaphoid carpal.

but the initial radiographs are negative, additional radiography or CT is indicated.

Using arms and outstretched hands to cushion falls often results in fractures of the distal radius and ulna. One such common fracture is called the Colles fracture (Fig. 11-31). It is imperative to reduce these fractured bones as close to their normal anatomic alignment as possible, or "set them," as grandmother would say. Anything less than anatomic realignment may result in a painful and/or poorly functioning wrist. Therefore, it is important to know that the radial styloid tip is 1–1.5 cm distal to the ulnar styloid tip, and the distal radial articular surface slopes 15–25 degrees toward the ulna and 10–25 degrees volar or anteriorly (1). These important relationships are summarized in Table 11-8.

TABLE 11-8. *Important distal radius–anatomic relationships*

Radius styloid tip lies 1–1.5 cm distal to the ulnar styloid tip
Distal radius articular surface slopes 15–25 degrees toward ulna
Distal radius articular surface slopes 10–25 degrees anteriorly

A subtle fracture in the distal forearm is the torus fracture (Fig. 11-32). Torus does not refer to a bull but rather the convex molding/projection (torus) located at the base of a classical column (2). The torus fracture on a radiograph usually appears as a minimal bump on

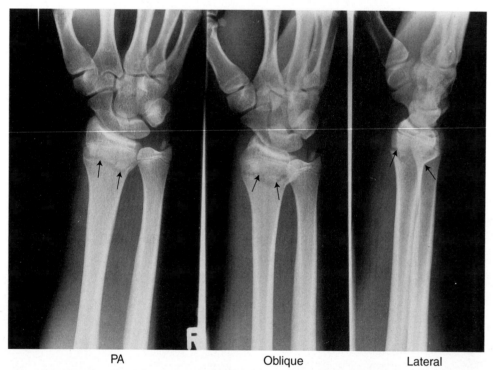

PA Oblique Lateral

FIG. 11-31. Right wrist PA, oblique, and lateral radiographs. Colles fracture. There are fractures of the distal radius *(straight arrows)* and the ulna styloid *(curved arrows)* with dorsal tilting of the distal radius fracture fragment and anterior angulation at the radial fracture site. The ulna styloid is mildly displaced radially. Note that the radial length is well maintained and the distal radius articular surface slopes toward the ulna on the PA view. However, the distal radius articular surface now slopes posteriorly on the lateral view, and this is unacceptable.

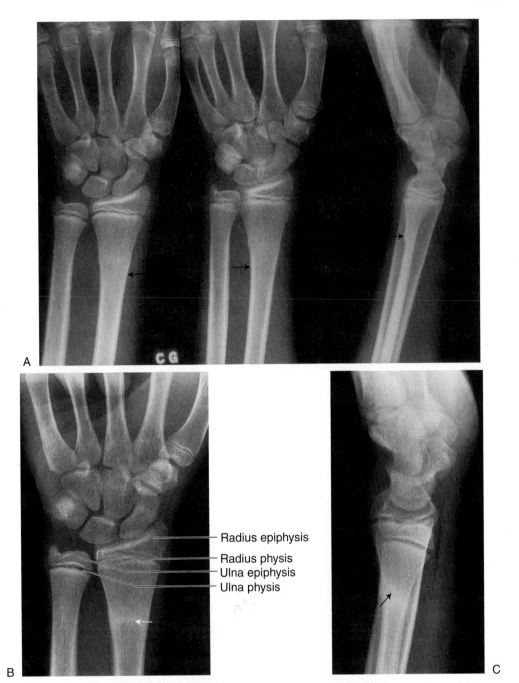

Radius epiphysis
Radius physis
Ulna epiphysis
Ulna physis

FIG. 11-32. A:. Left wrist PA, oblique, and lateral radiographs. Torus fracture *(arrows)* or a nondisplaced fracture of the distal left radius. **B, C:** Left wrist PA (B) and lateral (C) radiographs. Healing left radius torus fracture 6 weeks following the radiograph shown in A. The dense white zone *(arrows)* is the typical appearance of a healing fracture.

the bone without a visible fracture line. It represents a buckling of the bone cortex. However, most fractures of the radius and ulna that are encountered in practice are much more obvious (Fig. 11-33).

Elbow fractures (Figs. 11-34 to 11-36) and dislocations (Fig. 11-37A–D) can occur when children and adults fall directly on their elbow or on an extended arm or hand. Dislocations of the elbow are named for the direction the radius and ulna dislocate relative to the humerus. When the radius and ulna dislocate anterior to the humerus, it is an anterior dislocation.

The radiographic anatomy of the elbow is complicated. This is especially true in children due to the presence or absence of multiple ossification centers. *When in doubt about an elbow fracture or dislocation, always obtain the noninvolved elbow for comparative purposes.* This principle of comparative views applies to all areas of difficult anatomy. It is important to remember that fractures and dislocations of the elbow can be a threat to the brachial artery because of its proximity to the distal humerus (Fig. 11-37E).

A very common injury to the shoulder occurs when a senior citizen trips on the rug or stairs. If they land on their extended hand and do not fracture their wrist, they may sustain a fracture in the area of the humerus surgical neck (Fig. 11-38). Generally, this is very easily treated with a sling or a light hanging cast. A similar fracture can occur through the physis of the proximal humerus in children (Fig. 11-39). Dislocation of the

shoulder is another common injury that can occur in all age groups. In anterior dislocation of the shoulder the humeral head becomes caudad or inferior to the glenoid cavity on an AP radiograph (Fig. 11-40), whereas in a posterior dislocation the humeral head is cephalad to the glenoid cavity. Anterior shoulder dislocation of the shoulder is more common than a posterior dislocation. In shoulder dislocations there may or may not be fractures of the humerus or scapula associated. Occasionally, a severe fracture or other disease process of the proximal humerus necessitates a shoulder prosthesis (Fig. 11-41). Fractures of the scapula are not common and usually result from direct blunt trauma as in motor vehicle accidents (MVAs) (Fig. 11-42). Fractures of the clavicle are very common, especially in children who fall (Fig. 11-43). The most common site for clavicle fractures is at the junction of the middle and distal thirds.

MRI is a powerful tool to evaluate shoulder rotator cuff integrity, and a complete interruption of the rotator cuff is shown in Fig. 11-44. Remember that MRI is excellent for demonstrating the bone marrow and soft tissue detail, whereas CT imaging is good for bone detail.

Sudeck's atrophy or reflex sympathetic dystrophy (Fig. 11-45) is a poorly understood phenomenon that can be the result of a fracture or almost any type of mild or severe injury. It is frequently associated with pain, swelling, and stiffness.

text continues on page 271

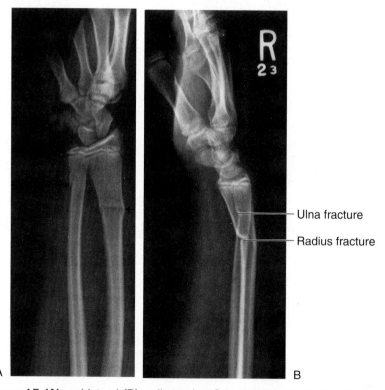

FIG. 11-33. Right forearm AP **(A)** and lateral **(B)** radiographs. Greenstick fractures *(straight arrows)* of the distal radius and ulna. The fractures simulate a broken green twig or branch wherein the twig bends or breaks but does not separate. On the lateral radiograph the fracture lines appear to involve only the anterior cortex of both bones. There is mild dorsal angulation.

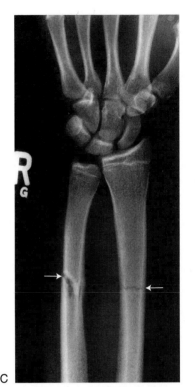

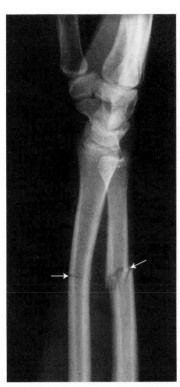

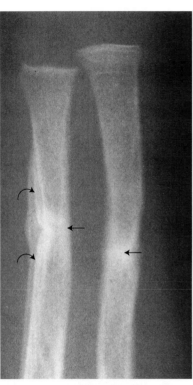

C   D   E

FIG. 11-33. *Continued.* **C, D:** Right forearm AP (C) and lateral (D) radiographs. Complete transverse fractures *(arrows)* of the distal shafts of the radius and ulna in a 15-year-old. There is mild volar or anterior angulation at the radius fracture site. The fracture fragments in the ulna are mildly offset. **E:** Right forearm AP radiograph. Healing fractures (straight arrows) of the radius and ulna. The fractures are in good alignment, and the curved arrows indicate periosteal reaction and new bone formation. The fracture lines are not visible, suggesting early bone union.

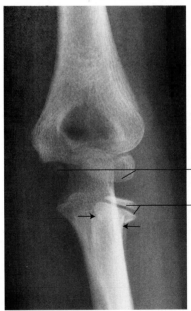

Trochlea and capitulum epiphyses

Radius epiphysis and physis

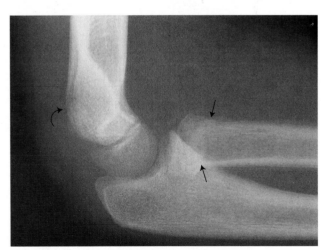

A   B

FIG. 11-34. Left elbow AP **(A)** and lateral **(B)** radiographs. Radial neck fracture. The straight arrows indicate the site of the fracture, and the radial head is tilted laterally on the AP view. The fracture is very difficult to see on the lateral view *(straight arrows)*. A positive fat pad sign is faintly visible posterior to the distal humerus *(curved arrow)* on the lateral view, and this always means that a fracture is present until proven otherwise. A visible fat pad anterior to the distal humerus is normal so long as it is not overly prominent.

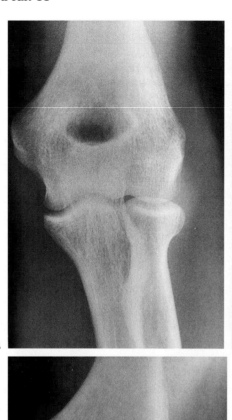

A

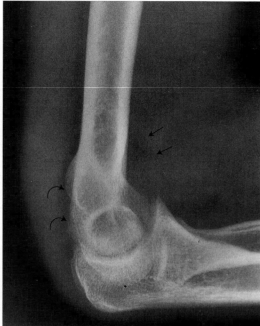

B

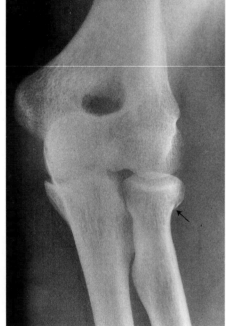

C

FIG. 11-35. Left elbow AP **(A)** and lateral **(B)**, and oblique **(C)** radiographs. Fracture of the radius neck. The patient fell from a bicycle and complained of a painful elbow. A fracture is not definitely visible on the AP and lateral radiographs; however, it should be strongly suspected because the anterior fat pad *(single arrows)* is more prominent than normal and a posterior fat pad *(curved arrow)* is present. The fracture *(straight arrow)* can be clearly visualized on the oblique radiograph. This demonstrates the importance of obtaining multiple views of a suspected fracture site and reiterates the significance of a positive posterior fat pad sign and a prominent anterior fat pad.

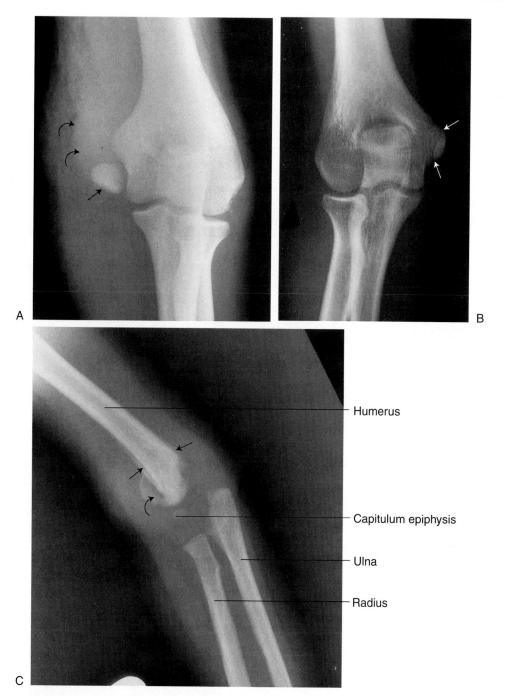

Humerus

Capitulum epiphysis

Ulna

Radius

FIG. 11-36. A: Left elbow AP radiograph. Avulsion fracture of the medial epicondyle epiphysis *(straight arrow)* in a 13-year-old. There is considerable soft tissue prominence *(curved arrows)* probably due to edema and hemorrhage secondary to the avulsion fracture. Remember that the pronators and flexors of the forearm attach to the medial epicondyle, and the extensors and supinators to the lateral epicondyle. Remember also that the pronators and flexors of the forearm attach to the medial epicondyle, and the extensors and supinators to the lateral epicondyle. **B:** Right elbow AP radiograph for comparison. Normal. The medial epicondyle epiphysis *(straight arrows)* is normal. **C:** Right elbow oblique radiograph. Bucket handle fracture of the distal humerus *(curved arrow)* in a 14-month-old child. Bucket-handle-type fractures can be found in child abuse situations. The straight arrows indicate periosteal reaction that occurs as a part of the healing process.

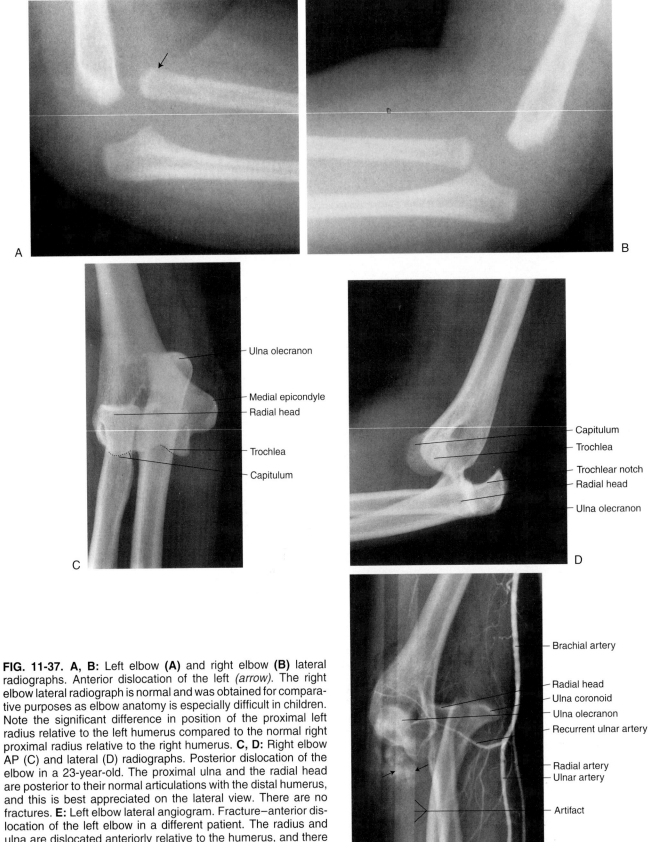

Ulna olecranon

Medial epicondyle
Radial head

Trochlea

Capitulum

Capitulum
Trochlea

Trochlear notch
Radial head

Ulna olecranon

Brachial artery

Radial head
Ulna coronoid
Ulna olecranon
Recurrent ulnar artery

Radial artery
Ulnar artery

Artifact

FIG. 11-37. A, B: Left elbow **(A)** and right elbow **(B)** lateral radiographs. Anterior dislocation of the left *(arrow)*. The right elbow lateral radiograph is normal and was obtained for comparative purposes as elbow anatomy is especially difficult in children. Note the significant difference in position of the proximal left radius relative to the left humerus compared to the normal right proximal radius relative to the right humerus. **C, D:** Right elbow AP **(C)** and lateral **(D)** radiographs. Posterior dislocation of the elbow in a 23-year-old. The proximal ulna and the radial head are posterior to their normal articulations with the distal humerus, and this is best appreciated on the lateral view. There are no fractures. **E:** Left elbow lateral angiogram. Fracture–anterior dislocation of the left elbow in a different patient. The radius and ulna are dislocated anteriorly relative to the humerus, and there is a comminuted fracture of the ulna olecranon *(straight arrows)*. The brachial artery is displaced anteriorly by the dislocation and the associated soft tissue edema and hemorrhage.

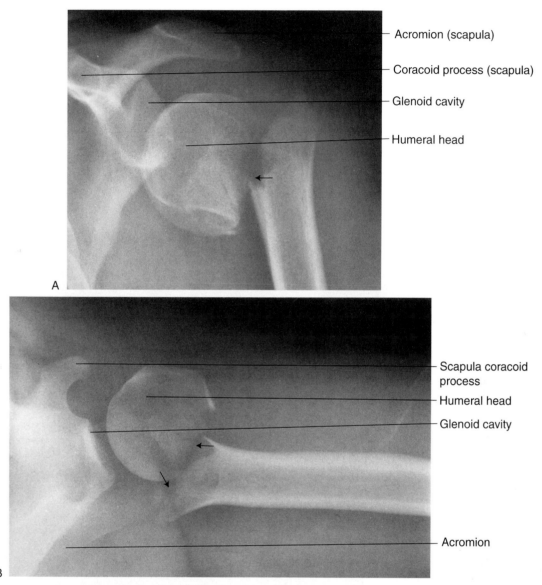

Acromion (scapula)

Coracoid process (scapula)

Glenoid cavity

Humeral head

A

Scapula coracoid process

Humeral head

Glenoid cavity

Acromion

B

FIG. 11-38. A: Left shoulder AP radiograph. Fracture *(straight arrow)* of the humerus surgical neck with offset of the fracture fragments in a 19-year-old. The humeral head is rotated and subluxed medially on the AP view resulting in an abnormal relationship between the humerus head and the scapula glenoid cavity. **B:** Left shoulder axillary radiograph of the same patient as A. The central x-ray beam travels through the axilla to nicely demonstrate the offset fracture fragments *(arrows)*. Note that the humeral head now is in a normal relationship with the scapula. The scapula coracoid process projects anterior and the scapula acromion projects posterior to the glenoid cavity on this view. Surgical internal fixation was required.

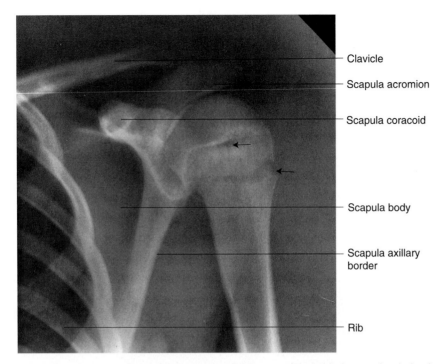

— Clavicle

— Scapula acromion

— Scapula coracoid

— Scapula body

— Scapula axillary border

— Rib

FIG. 11-39. Left shoulder AP radiograph. Salter 1 fracture *(straight arrows)* through the proximal physis of the left humerus in a 15-year-old. The patient fell on an outstretched arm. The major clue to the presence of a fracture is that the physis width is greater than normal.

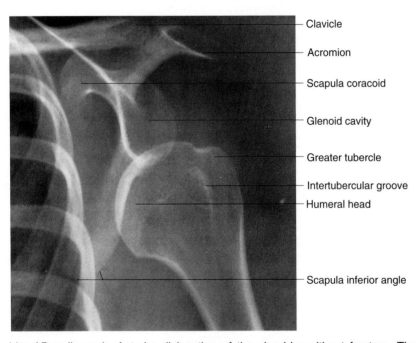

— Clavicle

— Acromion

— Scapula coracoid

— Glenoid cavity

— Greater tubercle

— Intertubercular groove

— Humeral head

— Scapula inferior angle

FIG. 11-40. Left shoulder AP radiograph. Anterior dislocation of the shoulder without fracture. The humeral head is inferior to the glenoid cavity, and this is the classic position of the humeral head in an anterior dislocation. The intertubercular (bicipital) groove is well visualized and within it rests the tendon of the long head of the biceps brachii.

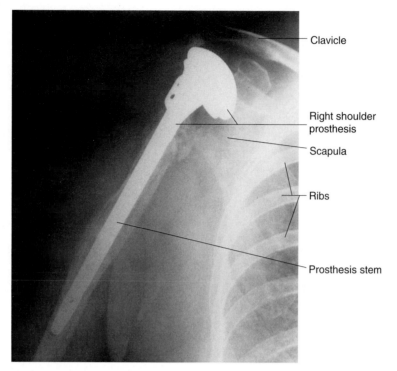

FIG. 11-41. Right shoulder AP radiograph. Right shoulder prosthesis. The prosthesis was necessitated by a severe old fracture deformity of the proximal humerus.

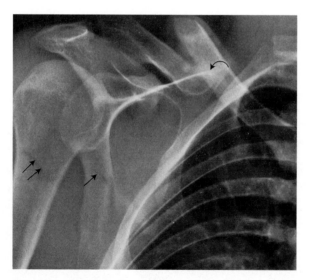

FIG. 11-42. Right shoulder AP radiograph. Acute fracture *(straight arrow)* of the scapula body and an old healed fracture *(curved arrow)* of the right midclavicle with deformity (malunion). The radiolucent line, or pseudofracture *(double arrows)*, in the proximal right humerus is secondary to overlying soft tissues.

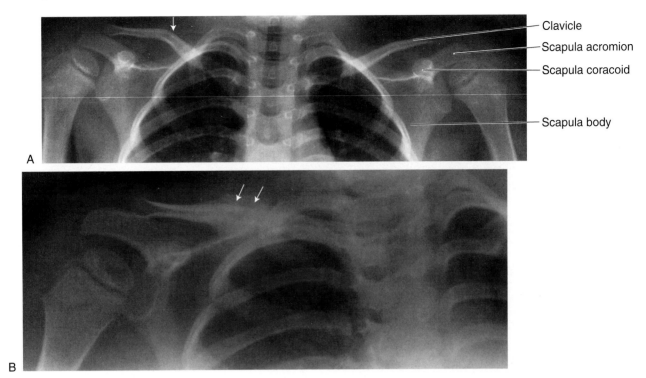

Clavicle
Scapula acromion
Scapula coracoid
Scapula body

A

B

FIG. 11-43. **A:** Right and left clavicles AP radiograph. Subtle greenstick fracture of the middle third of the right clavicle *(arrow)* in a 3-year-old child. There is minimal cephalad angulation at the fracture site. The fracture is more apparent when compared to the normal left clavicle. **B:** Right clavicle AP radiograph in the same patient 4 weeks later. Healing fracture. The white material surrounding the fracture site in the middle third of the right clavicle *(arrows)* is callus. The cephalad angulation has been corrected, and the clavicle alignment is normal.

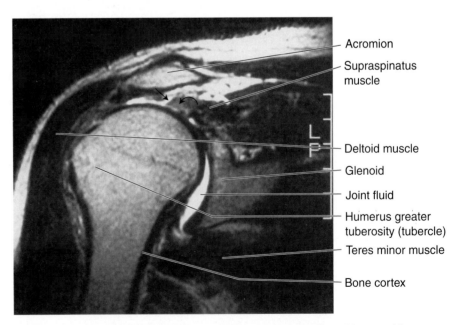

Acromion
Supraspinatus muscle

Deltoid muscle
Glenoid
Joint fluid
Humerus greater tuberosity (tubercle)
Teres minor muscle
Bone cortex

FIG. 11-44. Right shoulder T2 coronal MR image. Rotator cuff complete tear in a 60-year-old man. The area of high intensity or white signal *(straight arrow)* represents blood, edema, and joint fluid in the laceration of the supraspinatus tendon. The free margin of the torn supraspinatus tendon is indicated by the curved arrow. Note that the bone cortex is black on the MR image.

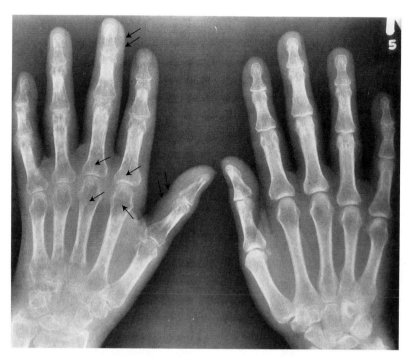

FIG. 11-45. Right- and left-hand PA radiographs. Sudeck's atrophy of the left-hand compared to the normal right hand. This patient's left upper extremity had been immobilized in a cast for 3 weeks. Sudeck's atrophy typically has patchy osteoporosis *(single arrows)* accompanied by soft tissue swelling *(double arrows)*, and the latter is minimal in this 58-year-old patient.

Lower Extremity

The etiologies of lower extremity injuries are similar to those in upper extremity injuries (see Table 11-7). Injuries to the feet are very common, as this is where our body meets mother earth (see Figs. 11-46 to 11-50 for a gallery of common foot injuries). Remember that a lateral radiolucent line near the base of the 5th metatarsal that runs parallel to the long axis of the metatarsal in a growing person represents a normal apophysis (see Fig. 11-47C), whereas *a transverse lucent line at the base of the 5th metatarsal always represents a fracture* (see Fig. 11-47D). An apophysis is a growth center (epiphysis) that does not contribute to bone length and usually is not located in a joint.

The ankle is frequently injured, and the injuries vary from minor sprains to severe trimalleolar fracture dislocations (Figs. 11-51 to 11-54). Fractures of the shafts of the tibia and fibula are common in sports, especially contact sports and skiing. A fracture that fails to heal is called a "nonunion fracture." Nonunion fractures have a variety of causes some of which are listed in Table 11-9. Nonunions are frequently found in the mid-

text continues on page 275

TABLE 11-9. *Causes of fracture nonunion*

Infection and osteomyelitis	Interposition of muscle or
Inadequate immobilization	other structure between
Poor blood supply	the fracture fragments
	Combinations of the above

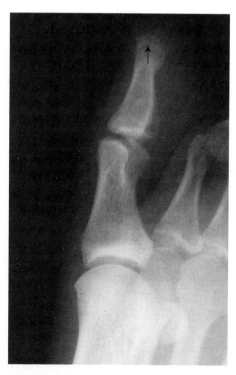

FIG. 11-46. Right great toe oblique radiograph. Nondisplaced fracture *(arrow)* of the distal phalanx tuft. As is commonly the case, this patient dropped a heavy object on the great or big toe.

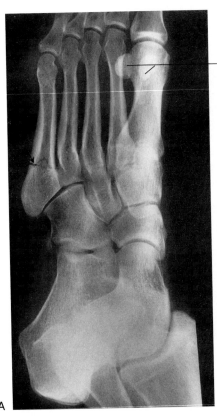

Medial and lateral
sesamoids

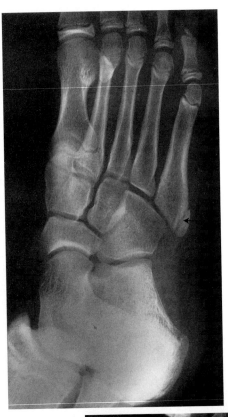

A

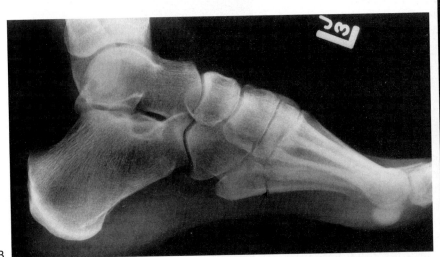

B

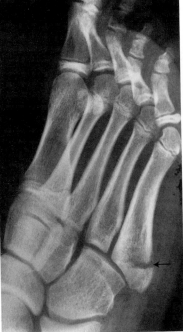

C

D

FIG. 11-47. Left foot oblique **(A)** and lateral **(B)** radiographs. Nondisplaced transverse fracture of the proximal left 5th metatarsal shaft *(arrows)*. **(C)** Right foot AP radiograph. Normal in a 14-year-old boy. The normal apophysis *(arrow)* at the base of the 5th metatarsal appears as a longitudinal radiolucent or black line and should not be confused with a fracture. **(D)** Right foot oblique radiograph. Transverse nondisplaced fracture *(straight arrow)* involving the 5th metatarsal base. This injury usually results from an inversion stress on the peroneus brevis that attaches to the base of the 5th metatarsal.

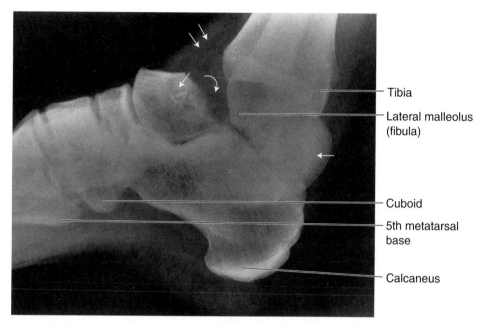

Tibia

Lateral malleolus
(fibula)

Cuboid

5th metatarsal
base

Calcaneus

FIG. 11-48. Right ankle lateral radiograph. Midtalus distracted fracture *(curved arrow)*. The fracture fragments *(straight arrows)* are markedly distracted, and the soft tissue edema and/or blood are indicated by the double arrows. The fracture resulted from a dorsiflexion injury

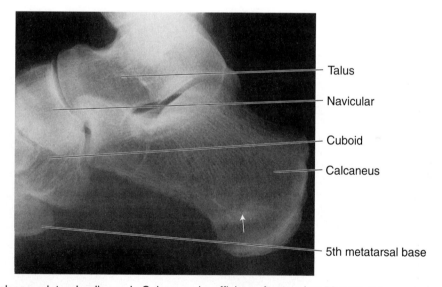

Talus

Navicular

Cuboid

Calcaneus

5th metatarsal base

FIG. 11-49. Right calcaneus lateral radiograph. Calcaneus insufficiency fracture in a 53-year-old woman. The white line *(arrow)* indicates a healing mildly impacted fracture that was not visible on radiographs 2 months prior to this study. The shape and height of the calcaneus are fairly well maintained. She had been on steroids for inflammatory bowel disease, and the steroids caused osteoporosis. As a consequence of the osteoporosis, the bone was not strong enough to prevent fracture.

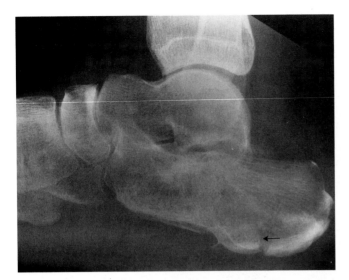

FIG. 11-50. Right calcaneus lateral radiograph. Calcaneus fracture *(arrow)* with impaction and collapse of the vertical height of the calcaneus in a 24-year-old. Compare the shape of the calcaneus in this patient to the calcaneus in Fig. 11-49.

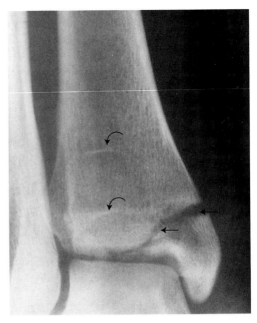

FIG. 11-51. Right ankle oblique radiograph. Mildly distracted fracture *(straight arrows)* through the base of the medial malleolus in an adult. The fracture extends onto the articular surface of the distal tibia. The white lines *(curved arrows)* are arrested growth lines and represent previous physis locations.

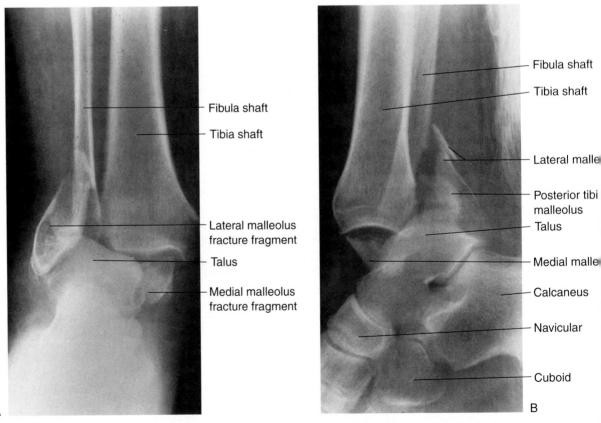

FIG. 11-52. Right ankle AP **(A)** and lateral **(B)** radiographs. Displaced trimalleolar fractures and talotibial dislocation. The medial and posterior tibial malleoli fracture fragments and the fibula lateral malleolus fracture fragments are all displaced. The talus is severely displaced laterally and posteriorly relative to the tibia. This is an eversion injury.

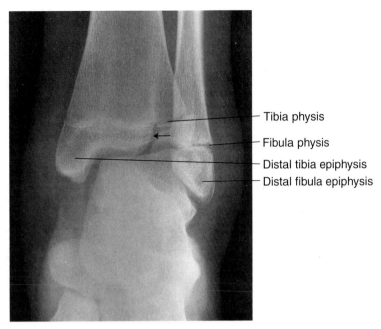

FIG. 11-53. Left ankle AP radiograph. Salter III fracture of the left distal tibia in a 12-year-old. The fracture line *(arrow)* extends from the physis through the distal tibial epiphysis to the articular surface.

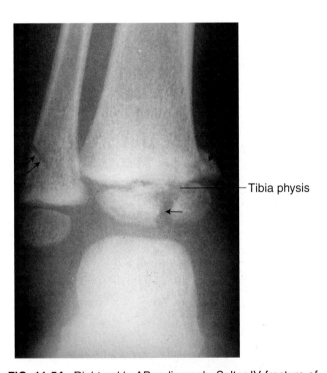

FIG. 11-54. Right ankle AP radiograph. Salter IV fracture of the distal tibia. The fracture line *(straight arrow)* extends from the distal tibial physis through the epiphysis to the tibial articular surface. The fracture also involves the medial tibia metaphysis *(curved arrow)*. There is an associated fracture of the distal fibula *(double arrows)*.

and distal tibia where the blood supply can be a problem (Fig. 11-55A, B). Severe fractures of the tibia may require internal fixation to facilitate immobilization and healing (Fig. 11-56). The tibia is also the site of stress fractures in all age groups, especially in runners (Fig. 11-57). A wide variety of fractures occur in and around the knee, and an example is demonstrated in Fig. 11-58. These figures demonstrate that not all fractures are visible on the initial radiographs around the time of injury. Whenever symptoms persist following an injury and the original radiographs were negative, you must consider follow-up imaging that might include radiographs, CT, radionuclide scans, or MRI.

Although 90% of child abuse deaths are secondary to head injuries, child abuse can involve all parts of the skeletal system. The metaphyseal fractures demonstrated in Fig. 11-59A are typical of the findings in some child abuse cases, and these metaphyseal fractures are probably due to a twisting mechanism. Subperiosteal hemorrhage on a radiograph is another twisting type of injury that should make you highly suspicious of child abuse (Fig. 11-59B). Bucket-handle fractures (see Fig. 11-36C) are also associated with child abuse. Skeletal injuries and fractures that should make the observer highly suspicious for child abuse are summarized in

text continues on page 278

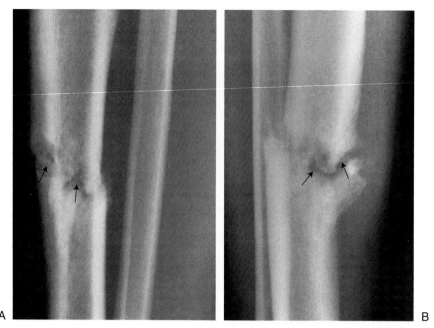

FIG. 11-55. Left tibia and fibula AP **(A)** and lateral **(B)** radiographs. Osteomyelitis and nonunion of a tibia fracture. The fracture line *(arrows)* is clearly visible 3 months following the injury, and this indicates a nonunion or nonhealing fracture. Infection at the fracture site caused the nonunion.

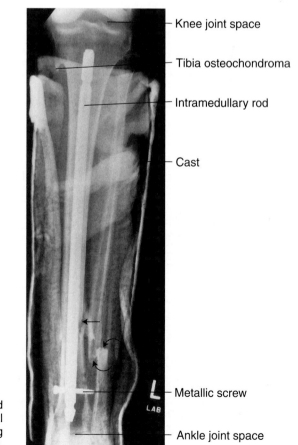

Knee joint space

Tibia osteochondroma

Intramedullary rod

Cast

Metallic screw

Ankle joint space

FIG. 11-56. Left tibia and fibula AP radiograph. Intramedullary rod internally fixating a transverse fracture in good alignment in the distal one-third of the left tibia *(straight arrow)*. There is an offset overriding transverse fracture in the distal one-third of the fibula *(curved arrows)*.

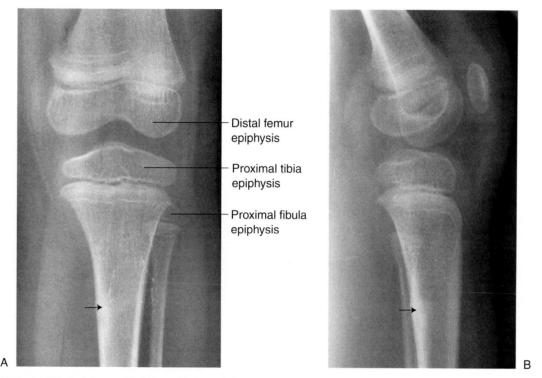

FIG. 11-57. Left knee AP **(A)** and lateral **(B)** radiographs. A healing stress fracture in this 5-year-old is indicated by the zone of increased density in the posteromedial proximal tibia *(arrows)*. The fracture resulted from excessive usage or stress.

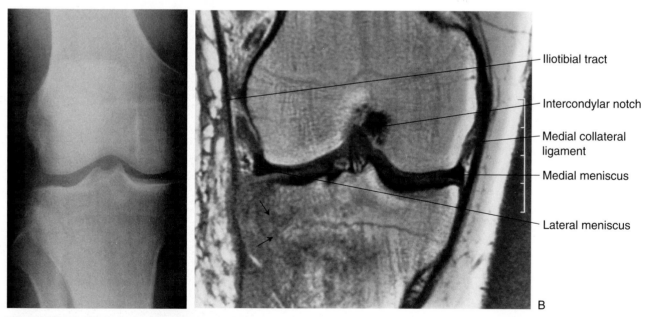

FIG. 11-58. A: Right knee AP radiograph. This AP radiograph and a lateral *(not shown)* radiograph were interpreted as normal. The radiographs were obtained because of right knee pain immediately following knee trauma in a 31-year-old man. **B:** Right knee coronal T1 MR image. Lateral tibial plateau fracture. This study was obtained 2 weeks following the initial radiograph in A because of persistent knee pain and a clinical suspicion of an anterior cruciate ligament injury. The arrows indicate an area of low-intensity signal (dark) caused by blood and edema replacing the bone marrow fat (white) in the tibial plateau fracture site. The anterior cruciate ligament was intact. The fracture eventually became apparent on subsequent radiographs.

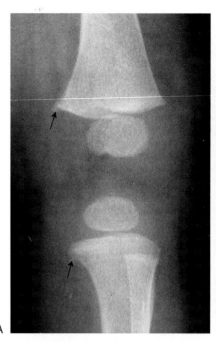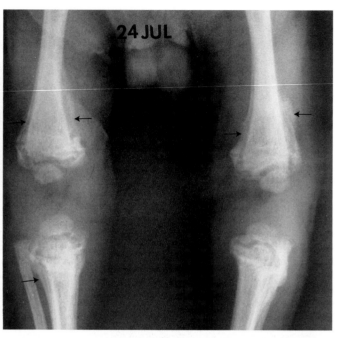

A

B

FIG. 11-59. A: Left knee AP radiograph. Metaphyseal corner fractures *(arrows)*. This battered child complained of knee pain and had an obvious limp. **B:** Right and left lower extremities radiograph. Subperiosteal hemorrhage. The straight arrows indicate the appearance of blood beneath the periosteum secondary to severe squeezing and twisting of the extremities. This appearance is highly suspicious for child abuse and should be investigated further.

Table 11-10, and the common child abuse fracture sites outside the skull are shown in Table 11-11.

Although the patella is a sesamoid bone, it is not uncommonly fractured in falls and MVAs (Fig. 11-60).

Osteochondritis dissecans (Fig. 11-61) is a common abnormality involving the knee in adolescents and young adults. It occurs most frequently along the lateral aspect of the medial femoral condyle, but it can be found elsewhere in the knee and in other joints including the hip, shoulder, ankle, and elbow. It is a localized ischemic or avascular necrosis that often occurs after injury and results in a button of necrotic bone that may or may

TABLE 11-10. *Osseous injuries suspicious for child abuse*

| Corner fractures |
| Periosteal hemorrhage |
| Bucket-handle fractures |

TABLE 11-11. *Common fracture sites in abused children*

| Lower extremity: femur (commonest), tibia |
| Elbow |
| Shoulder |
| Ribs |

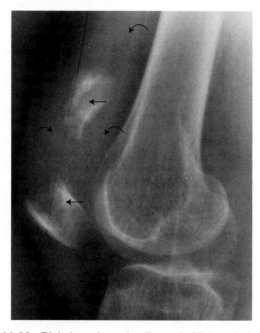

FIG. 11-60. Right knee lateral radiograph. Midpatella fracture secondary to a motor vehicle accident. There are two distracted fracture fragments *(straight arrows)* secondary to the fracture through the midpatella. The curved arrows indicate blood and increased synovial fluid in the supra-, pre-, and retropatellar spaces of the knee.

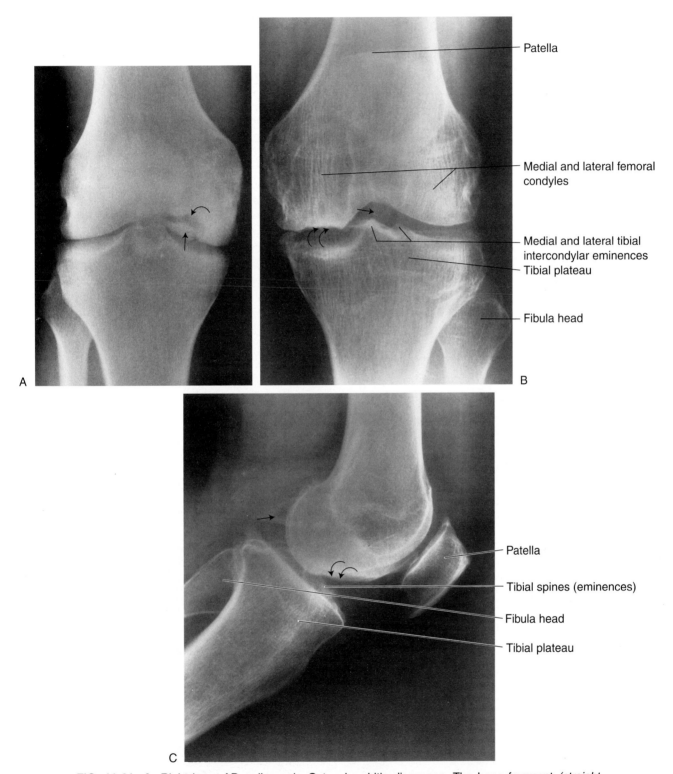

Patella

Medial and lateral femoral condyles

Medial and lateral tibial intercondylar eminences

Tibial plateau

Fibula head

Patella

Tibial spines (eminences)

Fibula head

Tibial plateau

FIG. 11-61. A: Right knee AP radiograph. Osteochondritis dissecans. The bone fragment *(straight arrow)* is not displaced from the donor site *(curved arrow)* on the lateral aspect of the medial femoral condyle. **B, C:** Left knee AP **(B)** and lateral **(C)** radiographs in a different patient. Osteochondritis dissecans. There is a displaced bone fragment or loose body *(straight arrows)* in the joint space. The radiolucent defect surrounded by the sclerotic zone *(curved arrows)* in the weight-bearing portion of the medial femoral condyle is the donor site of the loose body.

TABLE 11-12. *Some clinical presentations of bone ischemia (3)*

Osteochondrosis	Avascular necrosis
Osteochondritis dissecans	Aseptic necrosis
Legg-Calvé-Perthes disease	Bone infarcts

not detach from the donor site. When it becomes detached, it is a joint loose body. Avascular necrosis is bone ischemia. The clinical presentations of avascular necrosis (Table 11-12) vary with the bone site and size as well as bone age (3).

As a general rule, femoral shaft fractures are easy to detect both clinically and radiographically, as the patient experiences severe pain at the fracture site and is usually unable to bear weight (Fig. 11-62).

The hip is another area commonly injured in MVAs and falls, especially in the elderly (Fig. 11-63). Dislocations of the hip are not common and require violent trauma as in MVAs (Fig. 11-64). However, patients with a hip prosthesis may on occasion dislocate

the prosthetic head with a minimal amount of stress (Fig. 11-65).

Soft Tissue Injury

One of the commonest injuries of the lower extremity is the sprained ankle. A sprain is simply an injury to a ligament around the ankle (or any other joint), and it varies in severity from a strain or stretching of the ligament to a complete disruption. Sprains usually result from a turning or twisting of the ankle joint while walking or running. When the foot turns outward, it is an eversion or abduction injury. When the foot turns inward, it is an inversion or adduction injury. Sprains occur with and without associated fractures. A dramatic example of a severe sprain is demonstrated in Fig. 11-66. Because ankle sprains are usually treated by casting in the United States, MRI is not commonly used to image ankle sprains, and the imaging usually is limited to radiographs. However, MRI of the ankle is used for specific problems such as a peroneus or Achilles tendon tears. The Achilles tendon or calcaneal tendon is a com-

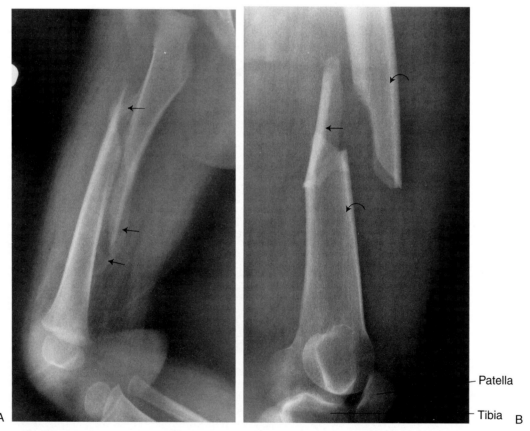

FIG. 11-62. A: Right femur lateral radiograph. Healing spiral fracture of the femur in a 14-month-old abused child. The arrows indicate callus at the fracture sites. **B:** Left femur lateral radiograph. Comminuted offset fracture middle third left femur in another patient. There is a large extra fracture fragment *(arrow)* between the major fracture fragments *(curved arrows).*

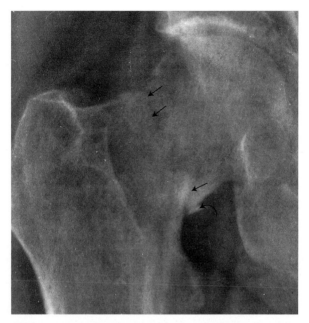

FIG. 11-63. Right hip AP radiograph. Femoral neck fracture. There is a mildly impacted fracture *(arrow)* through the mid-femoral neck. The curved arrow denotes a small fracture fragment. The patient complained of right hip pain and inability to bear weight on the right leg following a minor fall.

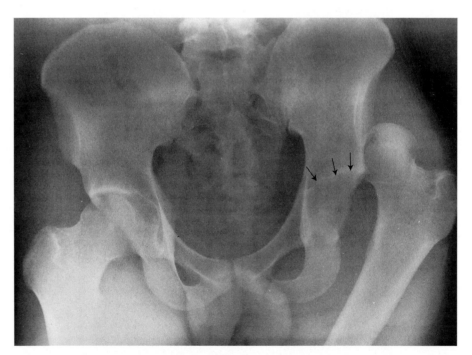

FIG. 11-64. Pelvis AP radiograph. Posterior dislocation of the left hip without fracture secondary to a motor vehicle accident. The left femoral head is displaced cephalad and lateral relative to the acetabulum *(straight arrows)*. The right hip is normal and makes an excellent comparison.

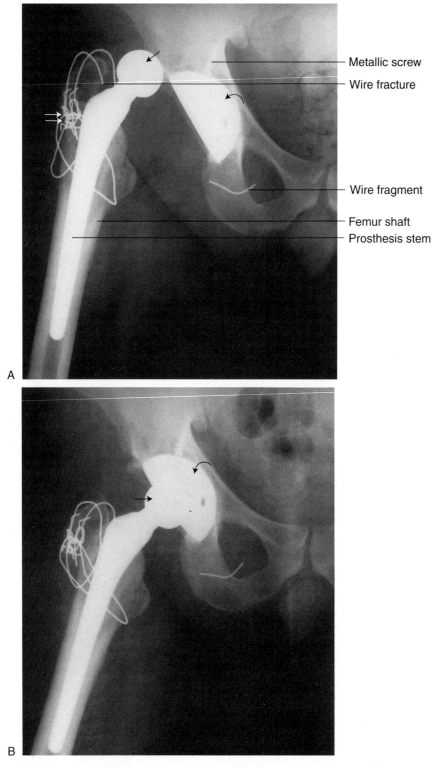

Metallic screw

Wire fracture

Wire fragment

Femur shaft
Prosthesis stem

A

B

FIG. 11-65. AP radiographs of the right hip. **A:** There is posterior dislocation of the right hip prosthesis head *(straight arrow)* in relation to the acetabular component *(curved arrow)*. The dislocation occurred while bending over to pick up a grandchild. Wires *(double arrows)* anchor the greater trochanter to the femur and at least one of the wires is fractured. A fragment of loose wire lies inferior to the prosthesis acetabular component. **B:** Following closed reduction (no surgery) under general anesthesia, the prosthetic head has been returned to its proper position relative to the acetabular prosthetic component.

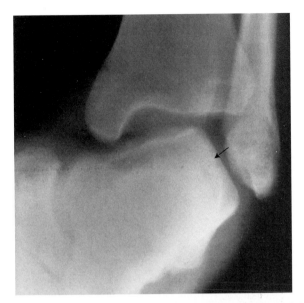

FIG. 11-66. Left ankle inversion stress AP radiograph. Ankle sprain. The talus is tilted laterally *(arrow)* secondary to disruption of the lateral collateral ligament in an inversion or adduction injury. There are no fractures.

mon injury site (Fig. 11-67). This injury can result from violent sport activities or simply stepping in a hole, and the diagnosis usually is made by the history of pain in the Achilles tendon. When there is a complete tear or disruption of the Achilles tendon, physical examination often shows pinpoint tenderness at the site of injury and inability to plantarflex the foot. An MRI is usually requested to confirm a clinical diagnosis or suspicion.

Following injury to muscles there may be subsequent calcification and/or ossification at the injury site called *myositis ossificans.*

MRI is a wonderful imaging tool to evaluate cartilages, tendons, and ligaments in and around the knee. Usually, the radiographs are negative in such injuries, but based on the physical findings and the patient's symptoms, an MR image is requested for a more definitive answer (Figs. 11-68 and 11-69).

Many foreign bodies in soft tissue and bone are radiopaque and readily identified on radiographs (Fig. 11-70A, B). Occasionally, a nonopaque foreign body in an extremity is suspected. If a foreign body is not visible on a radiograph, a CT or an MR study can be requested to assist in the detection and location of the foreign body (Fig. 11-70C).

text continues on page 286

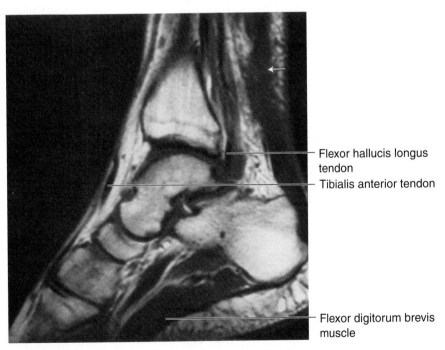

Flexor hallucis longus tendon
Tibialis anterior tendon
Flexor digitorum brevis muscle

FIG. 11-67. Right ankle midsagittal T1 MR image. Calcaneal (Achilles) tendon tear. The tear site is manifest by a high-intensity signal due to blood and edema within the tear *(arrow).*

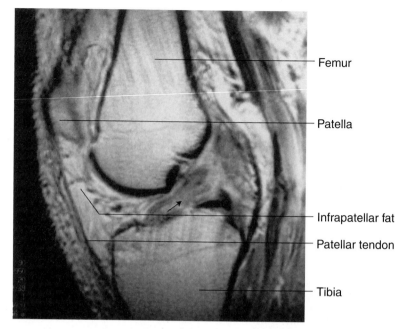

Femur

Patella

Infrapatellar fat

Patellar tendon

Tibia

FIG. 11-68. Right knee sagittal proton-dense MR image. Anterior cruciate ligament tear in a 41-year-old man. The arrow indicates the site of the anterior cruciate ligament tear manifest by a wavy high-intensity (white) signal.

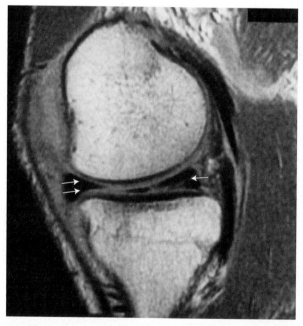

FIG. 11-69. Right knee medial sagittal proton-dense MR image. Tear of the posterior horn of the medial meniscus *(arrow)* in a 36-year-old man. The high-intensity signal (white) in the tear site probably represents edema, blood, or joint fluid within the tear. The double arrows indicate the normal anterior horn of the medial meniscus.

FIG. 11-70. Left foot AP **(A)** and lateral **(B)** radiographs taken through the boot. Metallic nail *(arrows)* piercing the boot and lodged in the calcaneus. The nail was driven into its present location by a power tool. **(C)** Left foot axial T2 MR image. Foreign body *(straight arrow)* in a different patient. The site of the foreign body entry wound *(curved arrow)* is marked by the white pill containing fat. The foreign body tract *(double arrows)* is white, probably because it is filled with edema, blood, or infection.

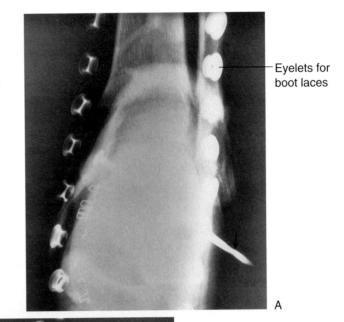

Eyelets for boot laces

A

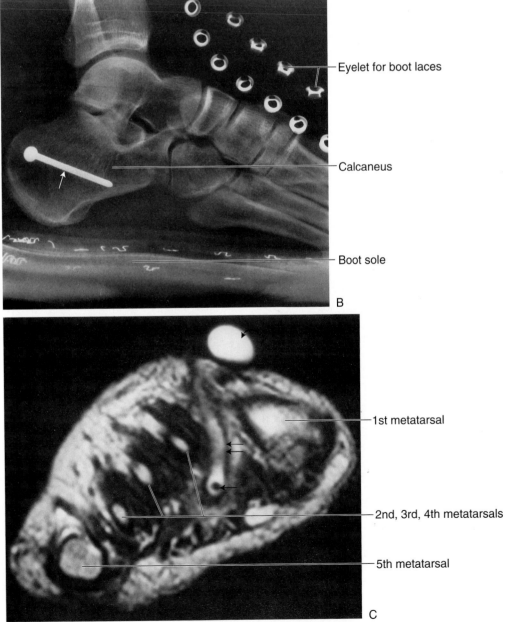

Eyelet for boot laces

Calcaneus

Boot sole

B

1st metatarsal

2nd, 3rd, 4th metatarsals

5th metatarsal

C

ARTHRITIDES

Osteoarthritis

Osteoarthritis (degenerative arthritis) is the most common form of arthritis. You can categorize osteoarthritis into two types. Secondary osteoarthritis, or degenerative joint disease (DJD), can occur at all ages, but tends to appear with increasing age as a result of wearing-out processes. It involves almost all of the joints of the extremities and spine (Figs. 11-71 to 11-73). Primary osteoarthritis is probably familial and involves the DIP joints of the hands, hips, and the first metacarpal-carpal joint.

The radiograph is the primary tool for evaluating osteoarthritis as well as all other arthritides. Some important facts and radiographic findings of osteoarthritis

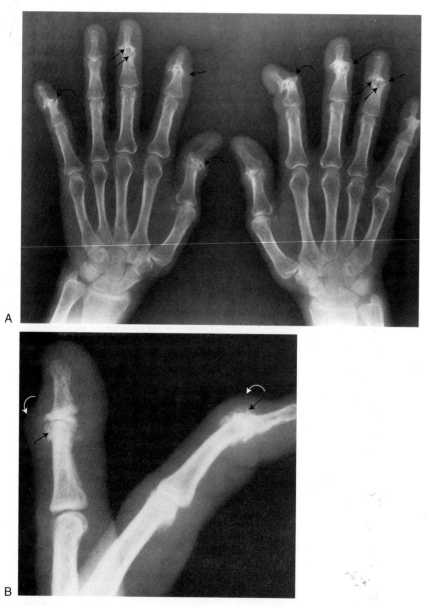

FIG. 11-71. A: Right- and left-hand PA radiograph. Osteoarthritis or erosive osteoarthritis. This 63-year-old woman worked as a typist for 20 years. Note the advanced osteoarthritic changes *(straight arrows)* involving the distal interphalangeal (DIP) joints of both hands. The DIP joints are markedly narrowed and osteophytes *(curved arrows)* are present. Erosions are also present *(double arrows)*. **B:** Left index and long finger lateral radiograph. Osteoarthritis DIP joints. For many years this 60-year-old woman operated an adding machine with her left hand. There is narrowing of the DIP joint spaces due to articular cartilage destruction. There are soft tissue prominences *(curved arrows)* overlying bone excrescences near the DIP joints. These bone excrescences or protuberances are called Heberden nodes *(straight arrows)*.

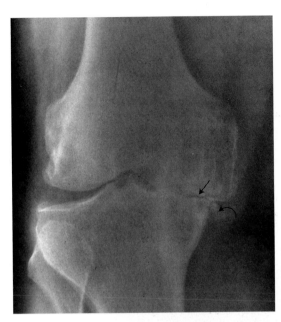

FIG. 11-72. Right knee AP radiograph. Osteoarthritis. The medial joint space or medial knee compartment is markedly narrowed, the articular surfaces are irregular *(straight arrow)*, osteophyte formation *(curved arrow)* is present, and there is varus deformity. Note that the medial joint space has all but disappeared compared to the lateral joint space.

TABLE 11-13. *Typical symptoms and radiographic findings in osteoarthritis and rheumatoid arthritis*

Osteoarthritis:
    Pain, deformity, and limitation of joint motion
    Involves all joints of the extremities and spine
    Typically involves the hand DIP joints and the 1st MCP joint
    Irregular joint narrowing
    Sclerotic bone changes
    Cysts or pseudocysts
    Osteophyte formation
    Usually absence of osteoporosis
    Genu valgus and varus deformities
    Cephalad and sometimes lateral migration of the femoral head
Rheumatoid arthritis:
    Pain, stiffness, limitation of motion, especially in the hands and feet
    Involves all joints of the extremities and spine and all synovial joints
    Typically involves the hand PIP joints
    Symmetric joint narrowing
    Periarticular osteoporosis (prominent feature)
    Periarticular soft tissue thickening and fusiform swelling
    Marginal and central osseous erosions
    MCP subluxation and ulnar deviation
    Medial migration of the femoral head and acetabular protrusio
    Pencil appearance of the distal clavicle

DIP, distal interphalangeal joint; PIP, proximal interphalangeal joint; MCP, metacarpal phalangeal.

are listed in Table 11-13 and include irregular joint narrowing due to articular cartilage destruction, osteosclerosis, and osteophyte formation. When advanced osteoarthritis involves the medial knee compartment, a genu varus deformity or bowed leg usually results. When advanced osteoarthritis involves the lateral knee compartment, a genu valgus deformity or knock-knee often results. When advanced osteoarthritis involves the hip, the femoral head migrates cephalad due to irregular cartilage destruction, whereas in rheumatoid arthritis the femoral head tends to drift medially resulting in acetabular protrusio.

Rheumatoid Arthritis

Rheumatoid is another type of arthritis that is frequently encountered in the everyday practice of medicine (Figs. 11-74 to 11-77). It is an inflammatory arthritis of unknown etiology that involves synovial joints and is characterized by symmetric joint narrowing secondary to articular cartilage destruction by pannus. Some important facts and radiographic findings are listed in Table 11-13. As in osteoarthritis, any or all of the joints in the extremities and spine can be involved. Often the initial symptoms of rheumatoid arthritis are stiffness, pain, limitation of movement, and swelling in the hands and/or feet. Usually, the first joints involved are the hand PIP and MP joints, and this tends to be symmetric. Potentially the earliest abnormality detectable on a ra-

diograph is periarticular soft tissue thickening. Additional radiographic findings include symmetrical joint narrowing, marginal and central erosions, and periarticular osteoporosis due to hyperemia. As the disease progresses, joint deformity may develop due to subluxation and ulnar deviation of the fingers at the MCP and PIP joints. This later finding is quite characteristic of rheumatoid arthritis. When joint cartilage destruction becomes far advanced, bony ankylosis of the joint may result. The differential diagnosis of rheumatoid arthritis is shown in Table 11-14. In gout, osteoporosis is usually absent, and articular and juxtaarticular erosions are more sharply defined. In osteomyelitis and infectious arthritis the osteoporosis is greatest near the infection site. In Sudeck's atrophy the osteoporosis is severe but the articular margins remain sharp. In osteoarthritis, osteoporosis is usually absent and osteophytes are often present.

text continues on page 290

TABLE 11-14. *The differential diagnosis of rheumatoid arthritis*

Gouty arthritis	Osteoarthritis
Infectious arthritis	Ankylosing spondylitis
Sudeck's atrophy	Scleroderma
Sarcoid	Systemic lupus erythematosus

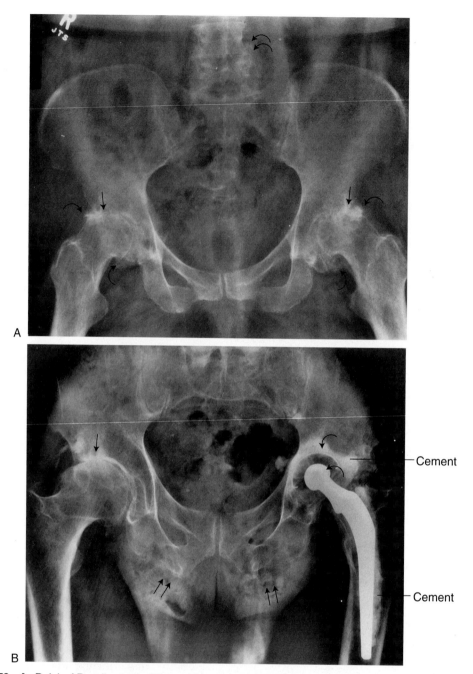

Cement

Cement

FIG. 11-73. A: Pelvis AP radiograph. Bilateral hip osteoarthritis in a 61-year-old. The hip joint spaces are irregularly narrowed, and the femoral heads are typically migrating in a cephalad direction *(straight arrows)*. The femoral heads are cystic and sclerotic in appearance. Osteophyte formation is present along the periphery of the joints *(curved arrows)*. Osteophyte formation is also present in the lower lumbar spine *(double curved arrows)*. **B:** Pelvis AP radiograph. Osteoarthritis of the right hip, left hip prosthesis, and bilateral inguinal hernias. There is irregular narrowing of the right hip joint and cephalad migration of the femoral head *(straight arrow)*. A left hip prosthesis is in place. The curved arrows indicate the prosthetic femoral head and acetabular components. Large bilateral inguinal hernias contain air-filled loops of bowel *(double arrows)*.

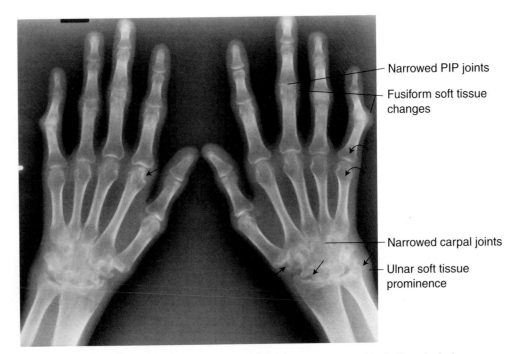

Narrowed PIP joints

Fusiform soft tissue changes

Narrowed carpal joints

Ulnar soft tissue prominence

FIG. 11-74. Right- and left-hand PA radiograph. Rheumatoid arthritis. The radiographic findings include periarticular osteoporosis *(curved arrows)*, swan neck deformities of the little fingers, narrowing of the PIP joints with associated fusiform soft tissue swelling, narrowing of the carpal and PIP joints, and soft tissue thickening or prominence around the distal ulna. Also, there are erosions involving the carpals, ulnar styloids, and metacarpal heads *(straight arrows)*. The fusiform soft tissue swelling surrounding the joints represents edema and effusion. The soft tissue prominence around the distal ulna is secondary to edema and thickening around the external carpi ulnaris.

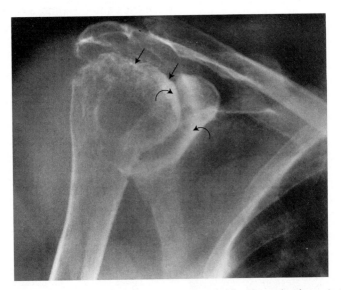

FIG. 11-75. Right shoulder AP radiograph. Rheumatoid arthritis. There is characteristic osteoporosis, a pointed distal clavicle, and mild cephalad drift of the humeral head. The cephalad drift of the humeral head suggests rotator cuff damage that is common in this disease. There are articular bone erosions *(straight arrows)* and sclerosis *(curved arrows)*.

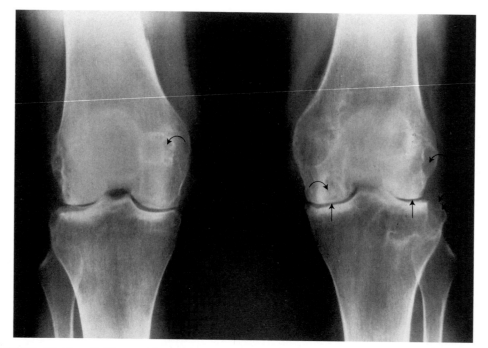

FIG. 11-76. Right and left knees AP radiograph. Rheumatoid arthritis in a 27-year-old. There is symmetric narrowing of the knee joints *(straight arrows)*, periarticular cysts *(curved arrows)*, erosions *(double arrows)*, and osteoporosis.

Ankylosing Spondylitis

Ankylosing spondylitis or Marie-Strumpell disease is another type of chronic inflammatory arthritis (Fig. 11-78). It is most common in young men and most frequently attacks the spine and sacroiliac (SI) joints. The

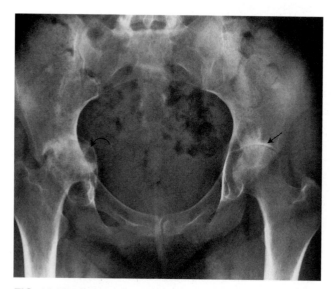

FIG. 11-77. Pelvis AP radiograph. Rheumatoid arthritis in a 27-year-old. There is generalized osteoporosis. The entire left hip joint space is symmetrically narrowed *(straight arrow)*. There is characteristic medial drift of the right femoral head and acetabular protrusio *(curved arrow)*. Note that the sacroiliac joints are not involved.

SI joints become narrowed or completely obliterated. Ankylosing spondylitis in the spine often results in squaring of the vertebral bodies and paravertebral ossifications, and these changes simulate a piece of bamboo or the bamboo spine. The bamboo spine is best appreciated on lateral spine radiographs. Ankylosing spondylitis may involve other joints, and these joints will have an appearance similar to rheumatoid arthritis. Psoriatic arthritis and Reiter's syndrome are inflammatory arthritides that may appear similar.

Gout Arthritis

Some arthritides that are associated with metabolic diseases and blood dyscrasias are listed in Table 11-15. Gout arthritis (Fig. 11-79) is secondary to hyperuricemia or elevated serum uric acid levels, and it is characterized by exacerbations and remissions. The patients classically present with podagra or pain and inflammatory changes near the medial aspect of the 1st metatarsal phalangeal joint (MTP). The disease usually is present for a number of years before it is detectable on a radiograph, and the

TABLE 11-15. *Arthritides associated with metabolic diseases and blood dyscrasias*

Gout
Calcium pyrophosphate dihydrate crystal deposition disease (CPPD)
Hemophilia

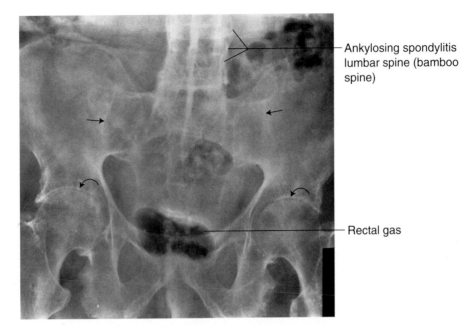

Ankylosing spondylitis lumbar spine (bamboo spine)

Rectal gas

FIG. 11-78. Pelvis AP radiograph. Ankylosing spondylitis. The sacroiliac joints *(straight arrows)* are obliterated, and there is concentric narrowing of the hip joints similar to the findings of rheumatoid arthritis *(curved arrows)*. Note the classic appearance of ankylosing spondylitis in the lower lumbar spine or the bamboo spine.

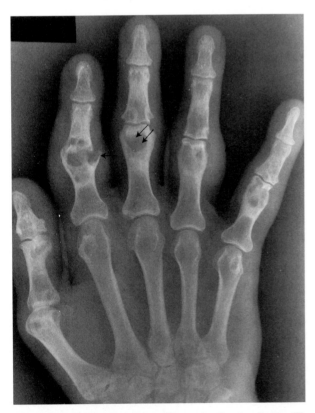

FIG. 11-79. Right-hand PA radiograph. Gout arthritis. The PIP joint spaces are at least partially preserved, and the lucent areas *(double arrows)* are typical of the sharply marginated periarticular erosions. Erosions that extend into the joint often have an overhanging edge *(single straight arrow)*. Note the classic appearance of a tophus *(curved arrow)*. A tophus is an asymmetric swelling about the joint that may or may not be calcified.

radiographic findings of gout are listed in Table 11-16. On the other hand, the joints in patients with hemophilia are gradually injured by repeated bleeding into the joints. Cystic changes develop in the bones neighboring the injured joints, and osteoporosis is a common feature (Fig. 11-80). In general, osteoporosis is a common feature in rheumatoid arthritis, blood dyscrasias, and osteomyelitis.

Chondrocalcinosis means calcification of joint cartilage, especially in the knee. It can be associated with a number of conditions that are listed in Table 11-17. CPPD, or pseudogout, is found in middle-aged or older people and is caused by the deposition of calcium pyrophosphate dihydrate crystals in the soft tissues of a joint, including menisci, ligaments, articular cartilage, and the joint capsule (Fig. 11-81).

TABLE 11-16. *Radiographic features of gout*

Sharply marginated and sometimes sclerotic bordered erosions with overhanging edges near a joint
Tophus formation or shoft tissue nodules
Usually osteoporosis is absent
Occasionally joint deformity

TABLE 11-17. *Causes of chondrocalcinosis*

CPPD (calcium pyrophosphate dihydrate crystal deposition)	Degenerative arthritis
Gout	Hyperparathyroidism

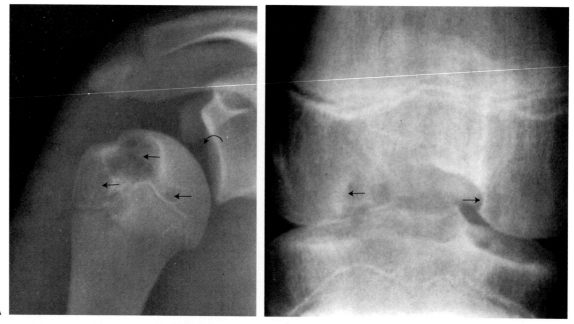

FIG. 11-80. A: Right shoulder AP radiograph. Hemophilia in a 15-year-old boy. There are cystic changes *(straight arrows)* in the humeral head secondary to repeated bleeds, and there is widening of the shoulde joint *(curved arrow)* due to hemarthrosis. **B:** Knee AP radiograph. Hemophilia in the same patient as in A. He has a widened intercondylar notch *(arrows)* secondary to repeated episodes of hemarthrosis. There is osteoporosis.

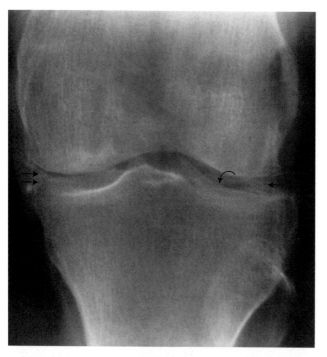

FIG. 11-81. Left knee AP radiograph. CPPD (calcium pyrophosphate dihydrate) crystal deposition disease or pseudogout. There are calcifications in the lateral meniscus *(single straight arrow)* and the medial meniscus *(double straight arrows)*. There is also calcification of the articular cartilage *(curved arrow)*.

Neuropathic Joints

Chronic trauma to a joint that has lost pain sensation can result in a neuropathic or Charcot's joint (Fig. 11-82). Some common causes are shown in Table 11-18. Diabetic neuropathic joints are most common in the lower extremity and syringomyelia neuropathic joints are usually found in the shoulders and upper extremities. The radiographic findings include joint space narrowing, fragmentation of sclerotic subchondral bone, articular bone cortex destruction, joint loose bodies, and bone mass formation at the articular margins (3). Some of the neuropathic joint findings are similar to those found in osteoarthritis.

Periarticular calcifications can result from acute and chronic trauma (Fig. 11-83). Although they do not involve joints, bone spurs could be considered a form of arthritis. Bone spurs cause pain and may be clinically difficult to differentiate from arthritis (Fig. 11-84). Also, bursitis may cause periarticular pain and can sometimes be demonstrated radiographically. Scleroderma is a connective tissue disorder that potentially involves the musculoskeletal system. Multiple soft tissue calcifications

TABLE 11-18. *Causes of neuropathic or Charcot's joints*

Diabetes mellitus	Spina bifida
Syringomyelia	Peripheral nerve injury
Congenital indifference to pain	

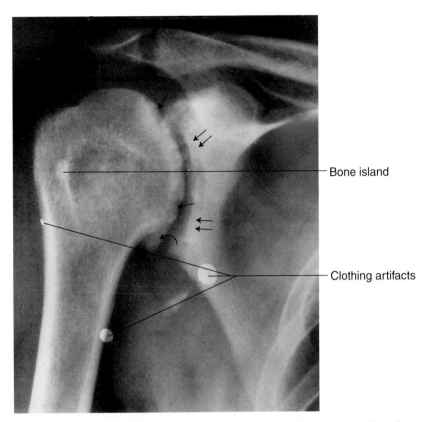

FIG. 11-82. Right shoulder AP radiograph. Neuropathic joint or Charcot's joint in a patient with syringomyelia. There is characteristic irregularity of the articular surfaces secondary to destruction of bone and joint cartilage *(single arrows)*. There are sclerotic changes or increased density *(double arrows)* of the bone surrounding the joint and an osteophyte *(curved arrow)*.

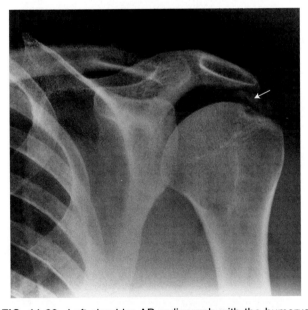

FIG. 11-83. Left shoulder AP radiograph with the humerus in external rotation. Calcific tendonitis. There is posttraumatic calcification *(arrow)* in the region of the supraspinatous mechanism.

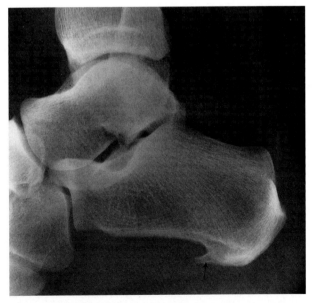

FIG. 11-84. Right calcaneus lateral radiograph. Degenerative calcaneal spur *(arrow)* in a 38-year-old. The spur is probably a traction osteophyte at the insertion of the plantar fascia.

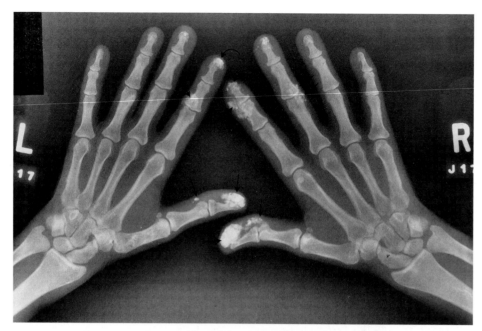

FIG. 11-85. Right and left hands PA radiograph. Scleroderma. Scleroderma is a connective tissue disease that may involve the musculoskeletal system. There are soft tissue calcifications *(straight arrows)*, and the soft tissues at the tip of the fingers are atrophic *(curved arrows)*. The joints are normal.

are commonly seen in these patients (Fig. 11-85). Other radiographic changes in scleroderma include atrophy of the finger tips and loss of bone at the tips of the distal phalanges. If joint changes are present, they may simulate rheumatoid arthritis.

TUMORS

Benign

There are a number of benign bone lesions and it is important to recognize them as such (Table 11-19). An osteochondroma or osteocartilaginous exostosis is the most common benign bone lesion and can occur in nearly all bones. They are bony projections from the external surface of a bone with a cartilage cap (Fig. 11-86) and are most commonly found in the metaphysis of long bones, especially around the knee and shoulder. These lesions can result in bone deformities and/or cause pressure on surrounding structures. The cartilaginous cap of osteochondromas undergoes malignant transformation to chondrosarcoma in less than 1% of the cases (1). Multiple osteochondromas or multiple osteocartilaginous exostoses or familial multiple exosto-

ses is a hereditary autosomal-dominant disorder (Fig. 11-87). Growth abnormalities and malignant transformation (5% to 15%) are more common in multiple osteochondromas than in a single osteochondroma (1).

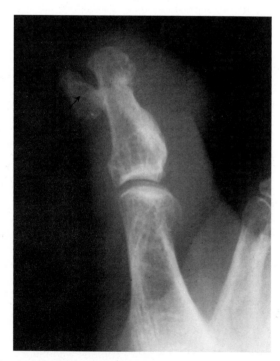

FIG. 11-86. Right great toe lateral radiograph. Subunguinal exostosis or osteochondroma *(arrow)* of the distal phalanx. The patient complained of something growing under the big toe nail.

TABLE 11-19. *Some benign bone lesions*

Osteochondroma	Fibrous dysplasia
Osteoma	Chondroblastoma
Osteoid osteoma	Osteoblastoma (Fig. 12-47)
Enchondroma	Hemangioma (Fig. 12-45)
Bone cyst	

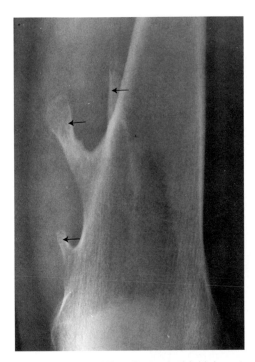

FIG. 11-87. Left femur AP radiograph. Multiple osteochondromas or familial multiple exostoses. The osteochondromas (arrows) point away from the knee joint simulating a coat rack.

Another benign bone lesion is the enchondroma (Fig. 11-88A). It is a slow-growing cartilaginous tumor usually found in the hand phalanges and in the distal metacarpals. Small calcifications may be present within the lesions, and they may be difficult to differentiate from bone infarcts. Bone infarcts (Fig. 11-88B) are most commonly present in long bones, and they may or may not be symptomatic. Bone infarcts usually have a well-defined and sclerotic border, whereas enchondromas do not (4). On occasion, infarcts may have a more permeative appearance mimicking a malignant primary bone tumor that necessitates a bone biopsy. The etiologies of bone infarcts include Caisson's disease, sickle cell anemia, systemic lupus erythematosus, and pancreatitis.

A simple benign bone cyst (Fig. 11-89) is commonly found in the proximal humerus and femur, but it can occur in almost all bones. Usually this lesion occurs in patients before the age of 25, and a common complication is a pathologic fracture.

Fibrous dysplasia is a benign fibrous-osseous lesion that arises centrally in the bone, and it can affect one bone (monostotic) or multiple bones (polyostotic). The exact etiology is unknown and these lesions may or may not be symptomatic. The radiographic features include: expansive bone lesions, bone cortex thinning, radiolucent lesions of variable density, and pathologic fractures. The differential diagnosis includes Paget's disease, hyperparathyroidism, and simple bone cyst.

TABLE 11-20. *Using the radionuclide bone scan to differentiate bone lesions*

Positive bone scans:	Negative bone scans:
Osteoid osteoma	Multiple myeloma
Primary bone tumors	Bone island
Metastases	
Paget's disease	

Osteoid osteoma (Fig. 11-90) is a benign bone lesion of unknown etiology and the typical symptom is night pain relieved by aspirin. It can occur in almost every bone, but is most often found in the femoral neck and the tibia. Approximately 75% to 80% of these lesions are intracortical and have multiple radiographic appearances, but the classical appearance is sclerosis surrounding a radiolucent center or nidus. In some instances, there may be calcifications within this lucent zone mimicking a sequestra of osteomyelitis. The differential diagnosis would also include stress fracture, bone island, multiple myeloma, and metastatic disease. Radionuclide bone scans are helpful to exclude multiple myeloma and bone island lesions as neither of these entities demonstrate increased uptake on radionuclide scans, whereas osteoid osteomas, primary bone tumors, and metastases usually show increased uptake on radionuclide bone scans (Table 11-20).

A chondroblastoma (Fig. 11-91) is an uncommon benign bone lesion found in the epiphysis usually before skeletal maturity. These radiolucent lesions generally have sclerotic borders and sometimes contain scattered calcifications. The differential diagnosis should include giant cell tumor, infection, osteoid osteoma, and metastatic disease.

Malignant

Metastatic lesions (Fig. 11-92A–C) are the most common malignant bone tumors and represent spread from a wide variety of primary neoplasms. Bone metastases may be single, multiple, osteolytic (radiolucent or black), or osteoblastic (white). The majority of metastases are osteolytic radiolucent, but osteoblastic metastases frequently result from cancers of the prostate and breast (Table 11-21). A bone island (Fig. 11-92D) should not be confused with an osteoblastic metastatic

text continues on page 299

TABLE 11-21. *Radiographic appearance of bone metastases*

Osteoblastic or sclerotic:	Mixed (lytic and blastic):
Prostate	Breast
Breast	Cervix
Carcinoid	Bladder
Neuroblastoma	**Osteolytic:**
	Nearly all neoplasms

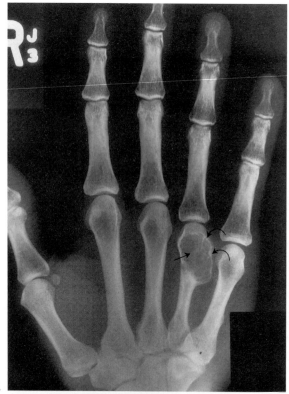

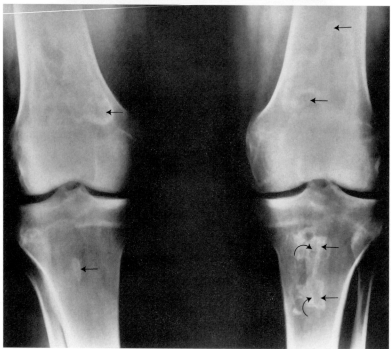

FIG. 11-88. **A:** Right-hand PA radiograph. Enchondroma of the distal 4th metacarpal *(straight arrow)*. This slow-growing tumor typically causes thinning and scalloping *(curved arrows)* of the inner bone cortex. **B:** Right and left knees AP radiograph. Multiple bone infarcts. The multiple infarcts are manifest by thin zones of sclerosis surrounding lucencies *(straight arrows)* and marrow calcifications *(curved arrows)*. The etiology in this patient is unknown.

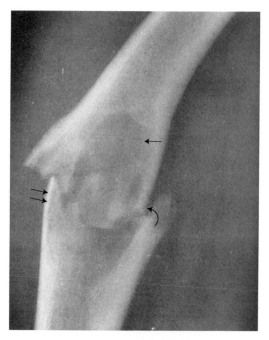

FIG. 11-89. Right femur AP radiograph. Benign cyst *(straight arrow)* with pathologic fracture *(curved arrow)* in a 10-year-old child. There is lateral angulation and mild offset of the fracture fragments. Note the thinning of the bone cortex *(double straight arrows)* caused by the expanding benign cyst.

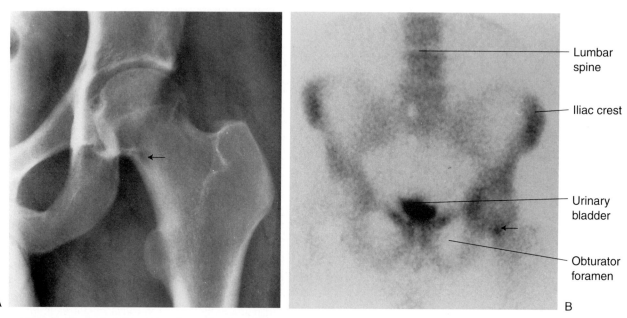

FIG. 11-90. A: Left hip AP radiograph. Osteoid osteoma in a 20-year-old. The patient experienced left hip night pain that was typically relieved by aspirin. The lucent zone *(arrow)* in the inferior aspect of the left femur subcapital region is the osteoid osteoma. **B:** Anterior pelvis radionuclide scan on the same patient. The single area of increased radionuclide uptake *(arrow)* in the left femoral neck corresponds to the radiolucent abnormality visualized in A. The bone scan is otherwise normal.

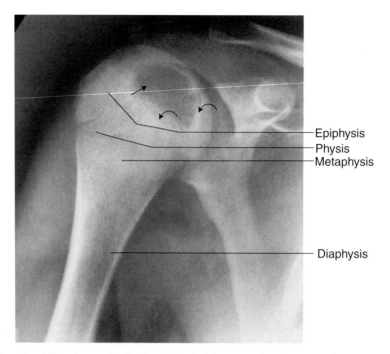

FIG. 11-91. Right shoulder AP radiograph. Benign chondroblastoma *(straight arrow)* of the proximal humerus epiphysis in a 14-year-old. The typical sclerotic border is present *(curved arrows).*

Epiphysis
Physis
Metaphysis

Diaphysis

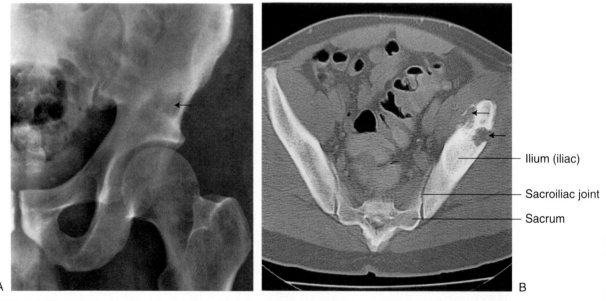

Ilium (iliac)

Sacroiliac joint

Sacrum

A

B

FIG. 11-92. A: Left hip AP radiograph. Metastatic carcinoma of the lung. The radiolucent area in the left iliac bone *(arrow)* represents a suspected osteolytic metastasis. **B:** Pelvis axial CT image in the same patient. Two osteolytic metastases *(arrows)* in the left iliac bone. The CT image confirmed the presence of two bone lesions, when only one was suspected on the radiograph.

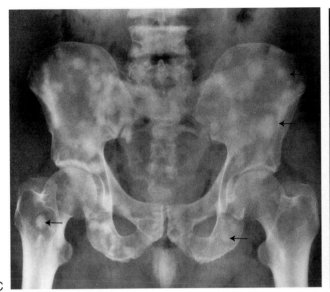
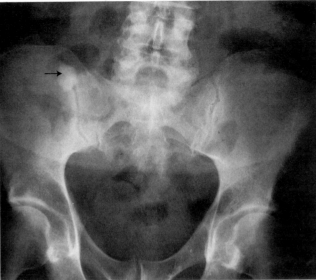

C

D

FIG. 11-92. *Continued.* **C:** Pelvis AP radiograph. Osteoblastic metastases from carcinoma of the prostate. The arrows indicate multiple bilateral osteoblastic (white) metastatic lesions *(arrows)*. **D:** Pelvis AP radiograph. Bone island *(straight arrow)*. Bone islands are usually ovoid or oblong with a spiculated contour. They are benign and generally asymptomatic.

lesion. These lesions are benign, asymptomatic, and distributed widely in the skeletal system.

Multiple myeloma originates in the bone marrow and is the most common primary malignant bone tumor (Table 11-22). The patient usually complains of pain in the involved area. Although any bone can be involved, the most commonly affected sites include the skull, spine, ribs, and pelvis. Unlike Ewing's sarcoma, this disease occurs in the over-40 age group. The typical radiographic appearance (Fig. 11-93) consists of multiple osteolytic areas with a punched-out appearance. At times it is difficult to differentiate multiple myeloma from osteolytic metastatic disease. *Remember that metastatic disease generally causes increased uptake on a radionuclide scan, whereas multiple myeloma usually does not.*

Giant cell tumors occur in young adults following skeletal maturity (Fig. 11-94). These lesions are eccentrically located in the end of long bones such as the tibia, femur, radius, and humerus. They usually have sharp nonsclerotic borders without periosteal reaction, and occasionally they abut the articular surface. Based on

TABLE 11-22. *Some malignant bone lesions*

Primary:	Secondary:
Multiple myeloma	Metastases
Giant cell tumor	
Osteosarcoma	
Ewing's sarcoma	
Chondrosarcoma (Fig. 12-52)	

their radiographic appearance, it is difficult to determine if they are benign or malignant. Approximately 15% are malignant, and they are considered malignant when metastases occur or the tumor recurs following surgery (4). Radiographically these lesions may be impossible to differentiate from metastases and other primary malignant bone tumors.

Osteosarcoma is a primary malignant bone tumor that commonly occurs during the second decade of life. It can occur in many locations but is usually found near the end of a long bone. It has a wide variety of radiographic appearances (Fig. 11-95). In some primary bone tumors a Codman's triangle (Fig. 11-95) may be identified, and the triangle represents periosteal new bone formation reacting to the growing tumor. Osteosarcomas may have a Codman's triangle as well as a sunburst or ray appearance that is secondary to bone formation in the tumor (Fig. 11-95). On occasion, it can be difficult to differentiate osteosarcomas from metastatic disease and other primary bone tumors, especially Ewing's sarcoma.

Ewing's sarcoma usually occurs in children and young adults (Fig. 11-96.) The classic appearance is a permeative or moth-eaten pattern, but it may have a variety of other associated bone changes such as sclerosis. Occasionally, Ewing's sarcoma has a layered periosteal reaction secondary to the tumor's presence that looks like onion skin. Other lesions in children with periosteal reaction would include osteomyelitis, fracture, eosinophilic granuloma, neuroblastoma, and osteosarcoma. The soft tissue extension of Ewing's sarcoma usually will not contain bone or cartilage calcification, whereas

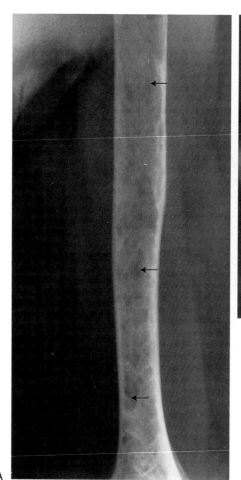

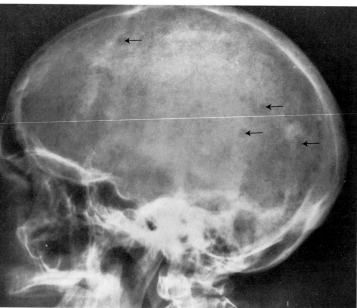

FIG. 11-93. Left humerus AP radiograph **(A)** and lateral skull radiograph **(B)**. Multiple myeloma. The lucent or black areas indicated by the arrows represent the classic appearance of multiple myeloma in bone.

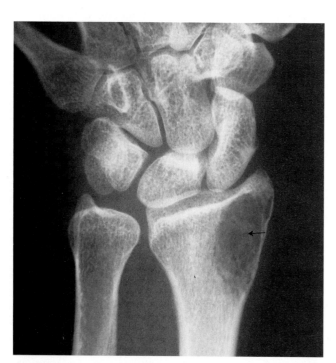

FIG. 11-94. Left wrist PA radiograph. Giant cell tumor *(arrow)* of the distal radius. This is the classic appearance and common location of this tumor.

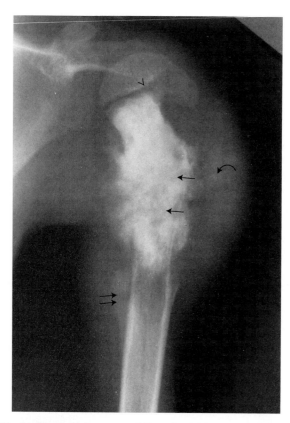

FIG. 11-95. Left humerus AP radiograph in a 6-year-old. Large osteosarcoma of the humerus metaphysis and diaphysis. The tumor *(single straight arrows)* has not crossed the physis. Codman's triangle *(double straight arrows)* represents periosteal new bone formation reacting to the tumor growth, and the sunburst or ray appearance *(curved arrow)* represents tumor bone.

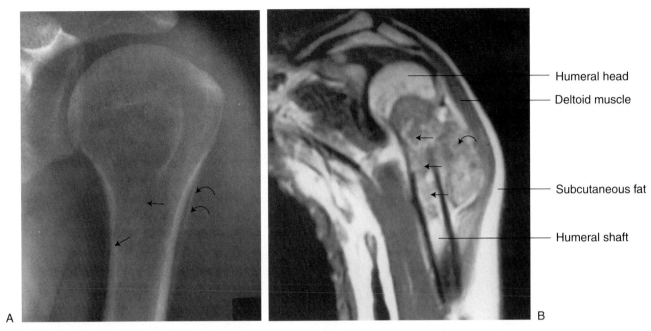

FIG. 11-96. A: Left humerus AP radiograph. Ewing's sarcoma. This 27-year-old presented with left arm and shoulder pain, and the radiographic appearance is typical: with a permeative or moth-eaten appearance *(straight arrows)*, ill-defined borders, and periosteal reaction *(curved arrows)*. **B:** Left humerus coronal T1 MR image on the same patient. Ewing's sarcoma. The tumor replaces nearly all the proximal humerus bone marrow *(straight arrows)*. Note how much of the tumor extends into the soft tissue surrounding the proximal humerus *(curved arrow)*. This latter finding cannot be fully appreciated on the radiograph.

the soft tissue extensions of osteosarcomas tend to produce bone (3).

METABOLIC DISEASES

Some metabolic diseases have the potential to significantly effect bones and a few examples are listed in Table 11-23.

Paget's Disease

Paget's disease is a common, chronic, and progressive metabolic bone disease of unknown etiology that occurs in adults over the age of 40. This disease can involve all bones but curiously often spares the fibula (Fig. 11-97). The radiographic features of Paget's disease are listed in Table 11-24. On radiographs the bone cortices are thick and sclerotic in appearance, and the trabecular pattern is thickened and prominent. Rarefaction and bone destruction may occur. Occurring secondary to

bone softening are bone deformities such as bowing of long bones and acetabular protrusio. The two most significant complications are pathologic fractures and sarcomatous degeneration. The differential diagnosis should include osteoblastic metastatic disease, fibrous dysplasia, lymphoma, and osteosclerosis.

Hypothyroidism

The radiographic findings in hypothyroidism of infants and children involves the physis, epiphysis, and metaphysis (Fig. 11-98). The epiphyses appear late and often are fragmented. This can result in delayed skeletal maturation, improper growth, and, occasionally, dwarfism (1). The epiphyseal changes are sometimes confused with other disease processes involving the epiphyses, including epiphyseal dysplasias and rickets.

Osteopenia is the increased radiolucency of bone on a radiograph, and it is a common radiographic finding that may be present in all age groups. It is often difficult
text continues on page 304

TABLE 11-23. *Some metabolic diseases that may affect bones*

Paget's disease	Acromegaly
Hypothyroidism	Rickets
Scurvy	Diabetes mellitus

TABLE 11-24. *Radiographic features of Paget's disease*

Thick and sclerotic bone cortices	Long bone bowing
Thick and prominent trabecular pattern	Acetabular protrusio
	Pathologic fractures

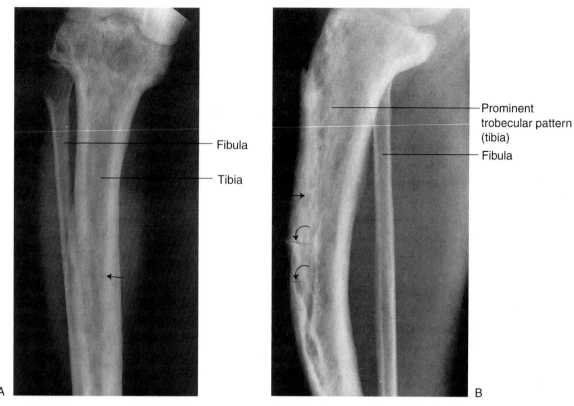

FIG. 11-97. Right tibia and fibula AP **(A)** and lateral **(B)** radiographs. Paget's disease. The tibia cortices are sclerotic in appearance *(straight arrows)* due to widening and thickening of the cortices and a prominent trabecular pattern. The tibia is bowed anterolaterally. The fibula is spared. The typical transverse pathologic fractures are best visualized on the lateral radiograph *(curved arrows)*, and they are the most common complication of this disease. There is osteoporosis.

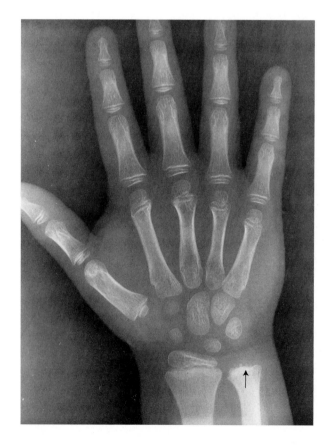

FIG. 11-98. Right-hand PA radiograph. Hypothyroidism in an 11-year-old. The distal ulna metaphysis is irregular, fragmented, poorly formed *(arrow)*, and has increased density. The epiphysis is absent.

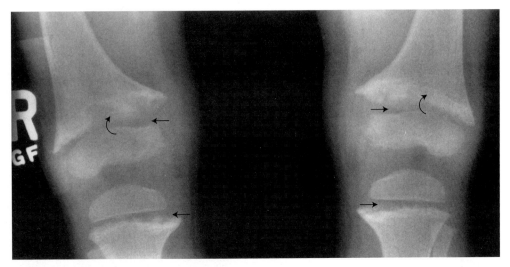

FIG. 11-99. Right and left knees AP radiographs. Rickets. The physes are widened *(straight arrows)*, and the metaphases are cupped *(curved arrows)*.

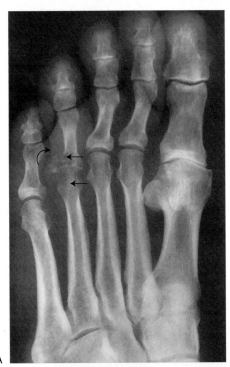

FIG. 11-100. A: Left foot AP radiograph. Osteomyelitis in a patient with diabetes mellitus. There are destructive changes *(straight arrows)* involving the base of the proximal phalanx of the 4th toe as well as the 4th metatarsal head. Also, there are destructive changes in the 4th metatarsal-phalangeal joint manifest by narrowing of the joint space. The infection has characteristically caused destructive joint changes as well as bone destruction on both sides of the joint. Loose bone fragments have resulted from the osteomyelitis *(curved arrows).* **B:** Left foot axial T1 MR image in the same patient. When compared to the other metatarsal heads the 4th metatarsal head is not visible because the infection *(arrow)* has destroyed and replaced the bone marrow.

A

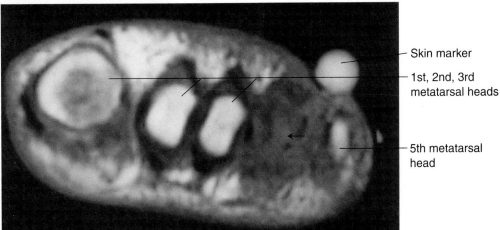

Skin marker

1st, 2nd, 3rd metatarsal heads

5th metatarsal head

B

TABLE 11-25. *Some etiologies of osteoporosis*

Immobilization	Hyperparathyroidism
Sudek's atrophy	Diabetes mellitus
Estrogen-deficient or post-	Anemias
menopausal	Paget's disease
Steroid therapy	Malnutrition
Cushing's disease	Osteogenesis imperfecta

to pinpoint the exact etiology of osteopenia on a radiograph alone. Osteopenia may be secondary to osteoporosis or osteomalacia.

Osteoporosis and Osteomalacia

Osteoporosis (see Figs. 11-20, 11-45, 11-74 to 11-77, 11-80B) is secondary to a reduced amount of bone matrix (osteoid) with normal mineralization, whereas osteomalacia is a normal bone matrix (osteoid) with a reduced amount of mineralization. Osteoporosis has become a major public health problem with countless related fractures per year and probably costing billions of dollars per year. There is a long list of osteoporosis etiologies, and a partial list of etiologies is shown in Table 11-25.

Rickets

Rickets is a good example of osteomalacia and osteopenia in children. It is found in the growing portions of infant bones and is caused by poor calcification of the osteoid matrix that may result from vitamin D deficiency, renal disease, and intestinal malabsorption diseases. The radiographic findings include widened and irregular physes, cupping of the metaphyses, bowing of the legs, and osteopenia (Fig. 11-99). This disease occurs in adults with similar etiologies but is called osteomalacia.

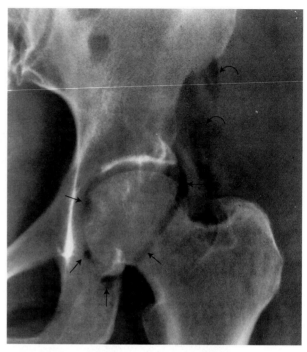

FIG. 11-101. Left hip AP radiograph. Gas-producing infection of the left hip. The black areas *(straight arrows)* represent gas produced by the infectious organisms involving the left hip joint. The curved arrows represent gas in the soft tissues outside the hip joint.

INFECTION

Osteomyelitis (Fig. 11-100) can occur in all age groups, and the classic clinical presentation is bone or joint pain and fever. There are multiple etiologies including trauma and hematogenous spread of infection. The radiographic appearance of osteomyelitis can be similar to a bone tumor with bone and joint destruction, periosteal reaction, and a soft tissue component. Unlike tumors, infections may have gas in the soft tissues secondary to gas forming organisms (Fig. 11-101). MRI is a very useful tool for the demonstration of bone and soft tissue involvement by infection.

Key Points

- It is important to recognize sesamoid bones and ossicles as normal variants. Sesamoids are bones within a tendon. Ossicles are extra or supernumerary bones next to the skeleton and usually named after the neighboring bone.
- MRI is useful for injuries to the shoulder rotator cuff, knee ligaments, and menisci, ankle ligaments, and Achilles tendon. CT imaging is good for bone detail, fracture diagnosis, and locating fracture fragments.
- The Salter-Harris classification describes fractures around the physis, which is considered the weakest point in a growing bone.
- Because fractures and other abnormalities may not be visualized on all radiographic views, always insist on at least two views of an injured or diseased area that are 90 degrees to each other.
- Fractures may not be visible on the first radiographs but may become visible after time (7 days) due to bone absorption at the ends of the fracture fragments.
- The complicated anatomy of the elbow and other anatomic sites often necessitates a comparable view of the opposite bone or joint. This is especially true in children.
- A transverse lucent line at the base of the 5th metatarsal always represents a fracture, whereas the normal apophysis in this area is lateral and parallel to the long axis of the metatarsal.
- Osteoarthritis is the most common form of arthritis and often results from wearing out.
- The radiographic features of osteoarthritis include irregular joint narrowing, sclerosis, absence of osteoporosis, and osteophyte formation.
- The radiographic features of rheumatoid arthritis include periarticular thickening, symmetric joint narrowing, marginal erosions, periarticular osteoporosis, and joint deformity.
- Metastatic cancer is the most common malignant bone tumor. The majority of metastatic lesions are osteolytic or radiolucent. Osteoblastic metastatic lesions most commonly are secondary to prostate and breast neoplasms.
- Multiple myeloma is the most common primary malignant bone tumor, and it originates in the bone marrow.
- Ewing's sarcoma usually occurs in children and young adults. They may have a permeative type of lesion and an onion-skin-like periosteal reaction.
- Osteomyelitis and septic joints typically present with localized pain and fever. The radiographic features include bone and joint destruction, periosteal reaction, and, occasionally, a soft tissue component.

REFERENCES

1. Greenspan A. *Orthopedic Radiology*, 2nd ed. Philadelphia: JB Lippincott, 1992.
2. *The American Heritage Dictionary*, 2nd College ed. Boston: Houghton Mifflin, 1976, p. 1280.
3. Edeiken J. *Roentgen Diagnosis of Diseases of Bone*, 4th ed. Baltimore: Williams and Wilkins, 1990.
4. Helms C. *Fundamentals of Skeletal Radiology*. Philadelphia: WB Saunders, 1989.

FURTHER READINGS

1. El-Khoury GY, Bergman RA, Montgomery WJ. *Sectional Anatomy by MRI*, 2nd ed. New York: Churchill Livingstone, 1995.
2. Griffiths HJ. *Basic Bone Radiology*, 2nd ed. Norwalk, CT: Appleton and Lange, 1987.

CHAPTER 12

Spine and Pelvis

William E. Erkonen

Backache is a problem for the majority of our patients at some time in their lives. Most people recover from their back pain with little or no medical care. Occupational-related back injuries are common and other common etiologies of back pain are listed in Table 12-1. When patients do seek medical care for back pain, radiologic imaging often becomes an important diagnostic tool. Following a thorough history and physical examination, routine anteroposterior (AP) and lateral radiographs often are the first radiologic consultation to be requested to evaluate the symptomatic region of the spine. These images may be supplemented with oblique and coned-down views to better visualize an area, and occasionally lateral flexion and extension views are requested to document spine motion and stability.

Computed tomography (CT) and magnetic resonance imaging (MRI) are extremely useful noninvasive diagnostic tools in visualizing the spine, and their use is

TABLE 12-1. *Back pain etiologies*

Congenital:
  Spina bifida
  Meningocele and myelomeningocele
  Scoliosis
Acquired:
  Trauma—fracture, muscle and ligament injury, spondylolysis, and spondylolisthesis
  Neoplasm—benign and malignant primary bone tumors, metastatic
  Arthritis—degenerative, rheumatoid, ankylosing spondylitis
  Metabolic—osteoporosis, osteomalacia, Paget's disease, sickle cell anemia
  Infection—staphylococcus, tuberculosis
Extraspinal:
  Psychosomatic or functional
  Gastrointestinal disease—pancreatic cancer
  Cardiovascular system—referred myocardial pain, aortic aneurysm
  Genitourinary system—renal and ureteral pain

TABLE 12-2. *Indications for the use of imaging modalities in the spine and pelvis*

Radiographs:
  Routine
    Cervical spine—**AP** and lateral
    Dorsal spine—AP and lateral
    Lumbar spine—AP and lateral
    Pelvis—AP
  Optional when indicated
    Cervical spine—AP open mouth view and/or swimmer's view in trauma, flexion, and extension views for mobility and stability, oblique views for the neural foramina
    Lumbar spine—flexion and extension views for stability and mobility, oblique views for spondylolysis
CT
  Fractures and disc disease
Conventional tomography
  Fractures
MRI
  Soft tissues and bone marrow
  Spinal cord and disc disease
  Fractures with suspected cord injury
Myelogram
  Disc disease, spinal stenosis, cord and extradural tumors

TABLE 12-3. *Checklist for spinal radiograph observations*

  Lateral radiograph
    Alignment (3 lines in cervical spine)
    Must visualize 7 cervical vertebrae
    Vertebral body heights
    Disc space heights
    Osseous density
  AP radiograph
    Alignment
    Vertebral body heights
    Disc space heights
    Bone density
    Pedicles

increasing while utilization of the invasive myelogram is decreasing. CT delineates anatomy and pathology more clearly than does myelography. One significant shortcoming of myelography is its inability to demonstrate lateral disc herniations and lateral stenosis. CT is superior for bone detail and is useful for diagnosing subtle fractures not visible on plain radiographs. CT is helpful for localizing the exact position of vertebral fracture fragments, especially when the fracture fragments are displaced into the spinal canal. CT is also useful in screening for disc disease and degenerative disease. Magnetic resonance imaging (MRI) is especially good for imaging soft tissues, the bone marrow, and allows a wonderful view of the spinal cord and the intervertebral discs. MRI is also used when a spine fracture is present and an associated cord injury is suspected. However, MRI costs approximately twice as much as CT imaging (Table 12-2).

NORMAL IMAGES

Cervical Spine

As previously emphasized in other anatomic regions, a systematic approach for evaluating the spine is needed. You will eventually develop your own system, but the following one will work until you do (Table 12-3). Start with the lateral radiograph (Fig. 12-1A) as it is the most important cervical spine radiograph. Glance at the entire image to see if something obvious jumps out at you. On the lateral radiograph the normal cervical curve should be mildly convex anteriorly. When the patient has significant pain, straightening of the spine may occur secondary to muscle spasm. Make note of the normal lines that should be intact on this view (Fig. 12-1B). Now simply count the cervical vertebrae. Things you must see include: all seven cervical vertebrae, the C7 and T1 intervertebral disc space, and ideally the T1 vertebral body. This is especially important in trauma situations as a fracture could be lurking in nonvisualized areas of the spine, and the result could be catastrophic. For example, if the C7 vertebra is not included on the lateral cervical spine radiograph, a fracture of C7 might go unrecognized. An unrecognized and displaced fracture has the potential to cause a serious cord injury. *Always* gauge the vertical heights of the vertebral bodies and the intervertebral disc spaces. The vertical heights of each vertebral body and intervertebral disc space should be approximately equal to those immediately above and below. Note the osseous densities in general. Some common causes for decreased (osteopenia) and increased bone density are shown in Table 12-4. Metastatic bone disease from prostate, breast, and other malignancies can result in an increased bone density or osteoblastic appearance.

Next look at the AP radiograph (Fig. 12-2A) and again check the alignment of the cervical spine. The spine should be straight on this view. Again note the heights of the vertebral bodies and intervertebral disc spaces. An extremely important observation to make is the presence or absence of the vertebral pedicles. Pedicles look like the headlights of the vertebrae. They are often involved by metastatic disease because of their abundant blood supply. *If one or more pedicles are absent, metastatic involvement or some other destructive process must be strongly suspected.* When disease or injury is suspected at the C1 and C2 levels, an AP radiograph of the upper cervical spine is obtained by directing the central x-ray beam through the open mouth. This is called the *open mouth view* (Fig. 12-2B), and its primary function is to visualize the dens or odontoid process of the C2 vertebra. Additionally, this view allows visualization of the C1 and C2 alignments and joints. Occasion-

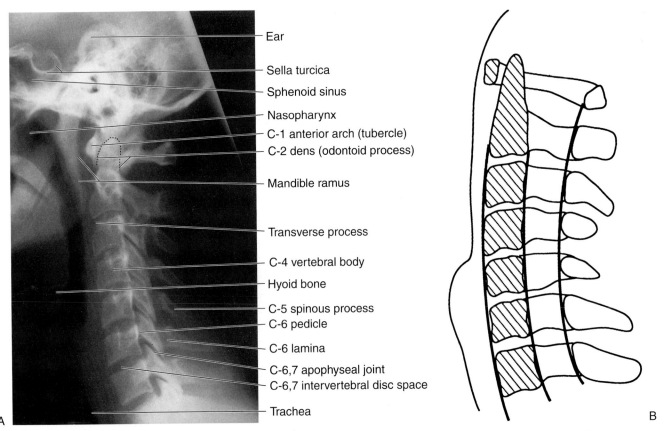

Ear
Sella turcica
Sphenoid sinus
Nasopharynx
C-1 anterior arch (tubercle)
C-2 dens (odontoid process)
Mandible ramus
Transverse process
C-4 vertebral body
Hyoid bone
C-5 spinous process
C-6 pedicle
C-6 lamina
C-6,7 apophyseal joint
C-6,7 intervertebral disc space
Trachea

A

B

FIG. 12-1. A: Cervical spine lateral radiograph. Normal. **B:** Cervical spine lateral illustration. Normal lines found on the normal lateral radiograph.

TABLE 12-4. *Some common causes for increased and decreased bone density*

Decreased
Neoplasm:
    Primary bone tumor, especially multiple myeloma
    Osteolytic metastases
Rheumatoid arthritis, ankylosing spondylitis
Osteomyelitis
Osteoporosis
Osteomalacia
Increased
Neoplasm:
    Osteoblastic metastases (prostate and breast)
    Lymphoma
    Primary bone tumors (<5% of multiple myeloma)
Callus formation—fractures
Bone infarcts
Bone island
Fibrous dysplasia
Paget's disease
Osteopetrosis

FIG. 12-2. A: Cervical spine AP radiograph. Normal. **B:** Cervical spine AP open mouth radiograph of the upper cervical spine. Normal.

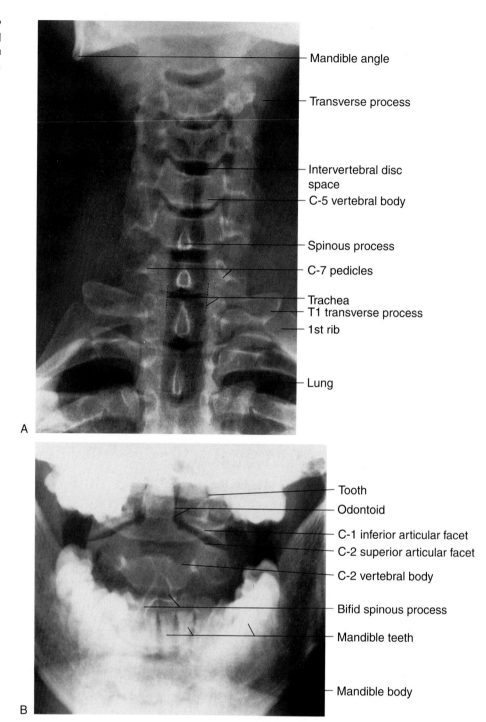

Mandible angle

Transverse process

Intervertebral disc space
C-5 vertebral body

Spinous process

C-7 pedicles

Trachea
T1 transverse process
1st rib

Lung

A

Tooth
Odontoid
C-1 inferior articular facet
C-2 superior articular facet
C-2 vertebral body

Bifid spinous process

Mandible teeth

Mandible body

B

ally, nonroutine oblique views (Fig. 12-3) are obtained, and the same observations are made as on the other views. However, the most important thing to observe is the patency of the intervertebral foramina through which the spinal nerves pass. Any disease process that narrows the foramina could potentially cause pressure on the nerve exiting through the neural foramen, resulting in radiculopathy or pain along the distribution of the involved nerve. Some processes that can impinge on the intervertebral foramina include herniated intervertebral disc disease, arthritides, and primary and sec-

ondary neoplasms. Occasionally, flexion and extension views are necessary to evaluate flexibility and stability of the spine. The majority of motion occurs in the upper cervical spine. When situations arise wherein the lower cervical vertebrae cannot be visualized on the lateral view, then a swimmer's view is indicated (Fig. 12-4). CT is often used to diagnose occult cervical spine fractures, determine the extent of fractures, and to localize fracture fragments. As already mentioned, MRI is especially useful to evaluate the spinal cord and the intervertebral discs (Fig. 12-5).

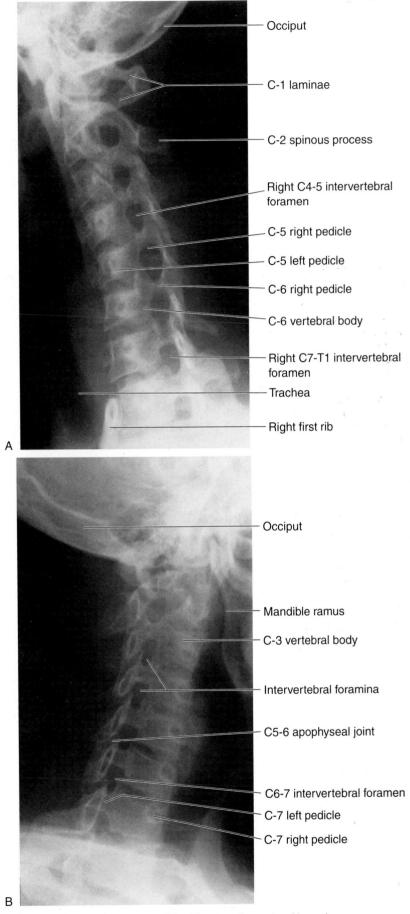

Occiput

C-1 laminae

C-2 spinous process

Right C4-5 intervertebral foramen

C-5 right pedicle

C-5 left pedicle

C-6 right pedicle

C-6 vertebral body

Right C7-T1 intervertebral foramen

Trachea

Right first rib

A

Occiput

Mandible ramus

C-3 vertebral body

Intervertebral foramina

C5-6 apophyseal joint

C6-7 intervertebral foramen

C-7 left pedicle

C-7 right pedicle

B

FIG. 12-3. Cervical spine right **(A)** and left **(B)** oblique radiographs. Normal.

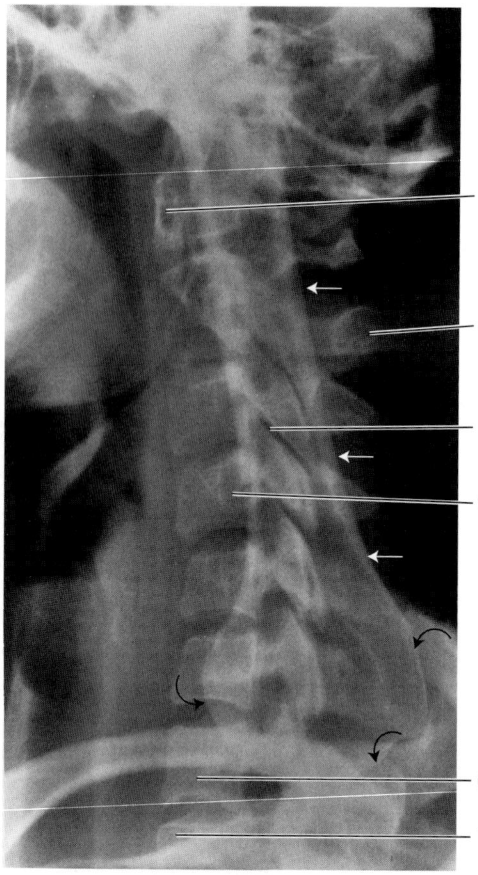

C-1 anterior arch

C-2 spinous process

Apophyseal joint

C-4 vertebral body

C-7 vertebral body

T-1 vertebral body

FIG. 12-4. Cervical spine lateral swimmer's view. Normal. The patient is almost always radiographed supine with one arm, usually the left, abducted upward alongside the head whereas the other arm is lowered. This position makes patients appear as if they are swimming the backstroke. The central x-ray beam is directed to the C7-T1 level from the patient's side on which the arm is lowered, usually the right. The straight arrows indicate the raised arm humerus projecting over the spine. The curved arrows outline the humeral head. Note how well the C7 vertebra is visualized as well as a portion of the T1 vertebra and the apophyseal joints. In this view it is considered good technique when you can see all of the C7 vertebra and at least the upper one-third of the T1 vertebral body.

Thoracic (Dorsal) Spine

Routine radiographic study of the dorsal spine consists of AP and lateral radiographs (Fig. 12-6). When viewing the dorsal spine, it is easiest to begin with the lateral view and follow the same method of evaluation as used for the lateral cervical spine radiograph. The normal dorsal curve should be mildly convex posterior. Again, assess the vertical heights of the dorsal vertebral bodies and intervertebral disc spaces. As always, check the overall densities of the bones.

Next, evaluate the AP dorsal spine radiograph wherein the spinal alignment should be straight. Assess the vertical height of each dorsal vertebral body and each dorsal intervertebral disc space. As in the AP cervical spine, the pedicles look like headlights on the vertebral bodies, and every attempt should be made to visualize all of them. On AP radiographs the spinous processes project over the midvertebral bodies at all levels in the spine.

MRI and CT (Fig. 12-7) imaging are useful in the dorsal spine for the same indications as in the cervical spine.

Lumbar Spine

Pain in the lumbar spine region is a major cause of disability, lost work time, and health dollar expenditure.

The etiology of back pain is complicated, varied, and poorly understood. Following a careful history and physical examination of the lower back, the next step in the evaluation process usually includes radiographs. Routine lumbar radiographs generally consist of AP and lateral views (Fig. 12-8). As previously noted, look first at the lateral view using the same system as described for the lateral cervical and dorsal spine radiographs. In general, note the lumbar spine alignment, which is normally convex anterior. When muscle spasm or disease processes are present this normal curvature may be lost and the spine appears straight. In addition, observe the overall osseous densities. Next, carefully evaluate the vertical heights of the lumbar vertebral bodies and the invertebral disc spaces; they should be approximately equal to those immediately above and below. As a general rule, the L4–5 intervertebral disc space height is greater than the other lumbar disc spaces. If the L4–5 disc space is the same height as those above or below, you should suspect L4–5 disc disease.

Always observe the pars interarticularis region of each vertebra for a possible defect, as an interruption of bone continuity in the pars interarticularis is abnormal and called *spondylolysis*. Similar observations are made on the AP radiograph regarding alignment, density, vertical heights of the lumbar vertebral bodies and the lumbar intervertebral disc spaces. Again, be

text continues on page 316

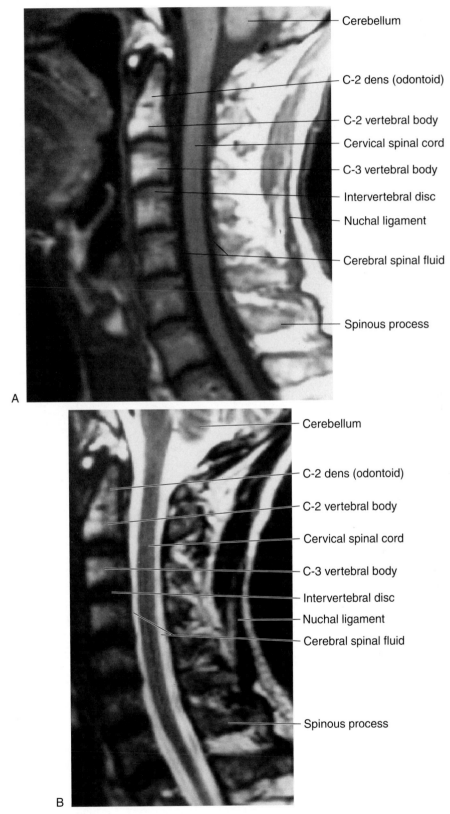

— Cerebellum

— C-2 dens (odontoid)

— C-2 vertebral body
— Cervical spinal cord
— C-3 vertebral body
— Intervertebral disc
— Nuchal ligament
— Cerebral spinal fluid

— Spinous process

A

— Cerebellum

— C-2 dens (odontoid)
— C-2 vertebral body
— Cervical spinal cord
— C-3 vertebral body
— Intervertebral disc
— Nuchal ligament
— Cerebral spinal fluid

— Spinous process

B

FIG. 12-5. A: Cervical spine sagittal T1 MR image. Normal. The cerebral spinal fluid is black on a T1 image and white on a T2 image. The bone marrow fat appears whiter (high-intensity signal) on a T1 image than on the T2 image. **B:** Cervical spine sagittal T2 MR image. Normal.

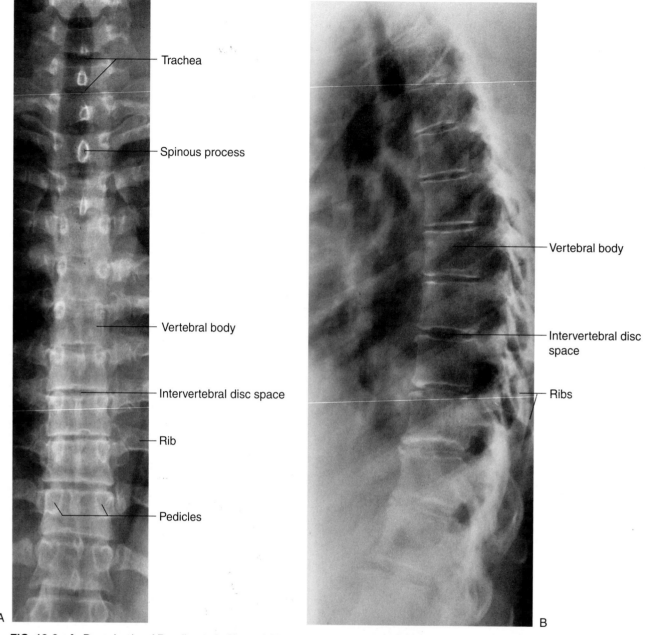

Trachea

Spinous process

Vertebral body

Intervertebral disc space

Rib

Pedicles

Vertebral body

Intervertebral disc space

Ribs

A

B

FIG. 12-6. A: Dorsal spine AP radiograph. Normal. The pedicles on each vertebra have an appearance similar to automobile headlights. **B:** Dorsal spine lateral radiograph. Normal.

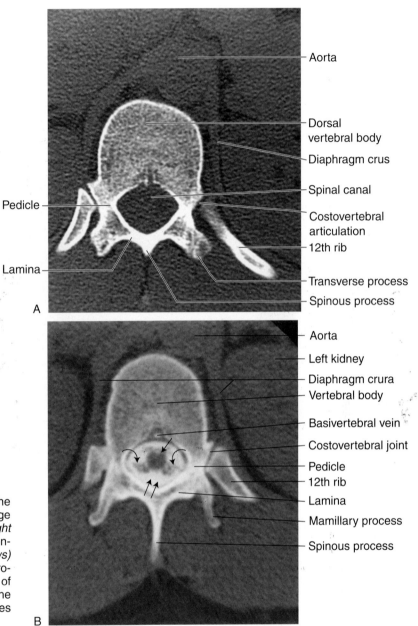

Aorta

Dorsal
vertebral body

Diaphragm crus

Spinal canal

Costovertebral
articulation

12th rib

Transverse process

Spinous process

Pedicle

Lamina

A

Aorta

Left kidney

Diaphragm crura

Vertebral body

Basivertebral vein

Costovertebral joint

Pedicle

12th rib

Lamina

Mamillary process

Spinous process

B

FIG. 12-7. **A:** Dorsal spine axial CT image at the T12 level. Normal. **B:** Dorsal spine axial CT image at the T12 level. Normal. The spinal cord *(straight arrow)*, nerve roots *(curved arrows)*, and the contrast-filled subarachnoid space *(double arrows)* are well visualized. The contrast media was introduced into the subarachnoid space as part of a myelogram, and the CT imaging followed the myelogram. Note how well the osseous structures of the spine are demonstrated.

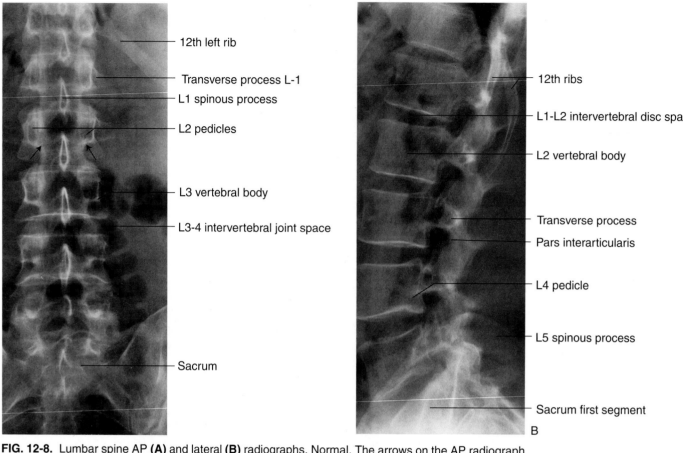

FIG. 12-8. Lumbar spine AP **(A)** and lateral **(B)** radiographs. Normal. The arrows on the AP radiograph indicate the pars interarticularis region.

certain that all of the pedicles are present. Occasionally, lateral flexion and extension radiographs are requested to assess mobility and stability of the lumbar spine. The majority of motion is in the upper lumbar spine. Note also that, oblique radiographs (Fig. 12-9) are sometimes necessary to better assess the pars interarticularis when spondylolysis is suspected. Once again, the observation checklist for spine radiographs is outlined in Table 12-3.

MRI of the lumbar spine is requested to evaluate the vertebrae, intervertebral disc spaces, and the spinal cord (Fig. 12-10).

As elsewhere in the spine, CT imaging may be requested to determine the presence and extent of fractures and the presence of intervertebral disc disease (Fig. 12-11).

In the past the myelogram was the gold standard for the diagnosis of disease in and around the neural canal. The myelogram is an invasive procedure that is accompanied by discomfort and requires some hospitalization time. It is accomplished by injecting contrast material into the subarachnoid space via a lumbar or cervical puncture and typical images are shown in Fig. 12-12. Fortunately, the new water-soluble myelographic con-

trast agents do not require removal, as they are absorbed in the same manner as cerebral spinal fluid. Understandably, CT and MR examinations are far more acceptable to the patient than the invasive spinal puncture associated with myelography.

Pelvis

An AP pelvis radiograph is the standard view (Fig. 12-13). A lateral view is not obtained but on occasion up- and down-tilt AP views are indicated when occult fractures are suspected, but not visualized on the standard AP radiograph. As elsewhere, you must know the anatomy and have a system for looking at the pelvis radiograph. First look at the sacrum and coccyx followed by the iliac bones bilaterally. Compare the sacroiliac joints as they may be narrowed, or even absent in diseases like ankylosing spondylitis. Then check out the ischial bones bilaterally as well as the pubis rami and the symphysis pubis. *Remember that the hamstring muscles arise from the ischial tuberosity,* and this explains why someone with a hamstring injury runs off the athletic field clutching his or her buttock. As you know, all of *text continues on page 321*

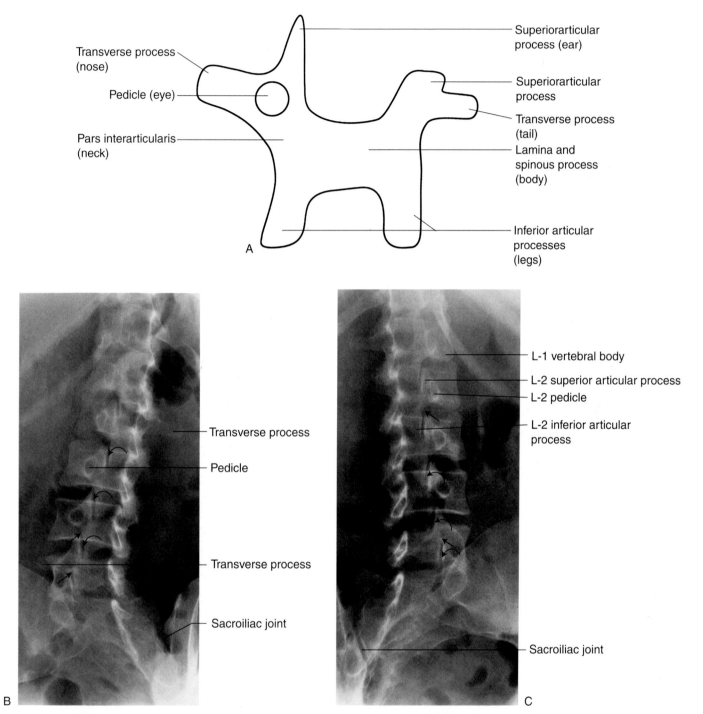

FIG. 12-9. A: Visible "scotty dog" and the anatomy that it represents on oblique lumbar spine radiographs. The neck of the scotty dog represents the pars interarticularis. When the scotty-dog neck is absent, the condition is called spondylolysis. **B, C:** Lumbar spine right (B) and left (C) oblique radiographs. Normal. Note on these oblique views how well you visualize the normal pars interarticularis or the neck of the scotty dog *(straight arrows)* and the normal apophyseal joints between the superior and inferior articular processes *(curved arrows)*.

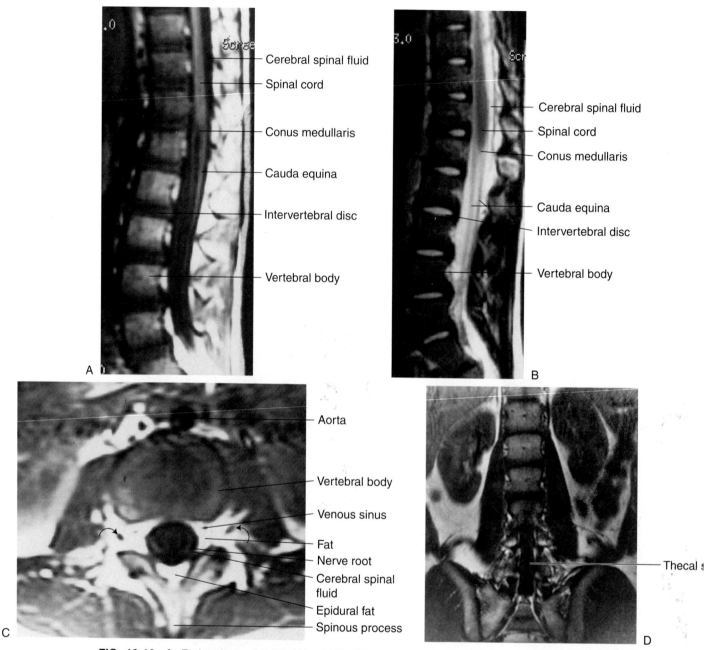

FIG. 12-10. A, B: Lumbar spine T1 (A) and T2 (B) sagittal MR images. Normal. Notice again that the cerebral spinal fluid is black on a T1 image and white on a T2 image. Also, the bone marrow fat is whiter (high-intensity signal) on the T1 image. The intervertebral disc is whiter on the T2 image. **C:** Lumbar spine T1 axial image. Normal. Note that the nerve roots *(curved arrows)* are well visualized. **D:** Lumbar spine T1 coronal MR image. Normal. The coronal plane passes through the upper lumbar vertebral bodies and the lower lumbar neural sac.

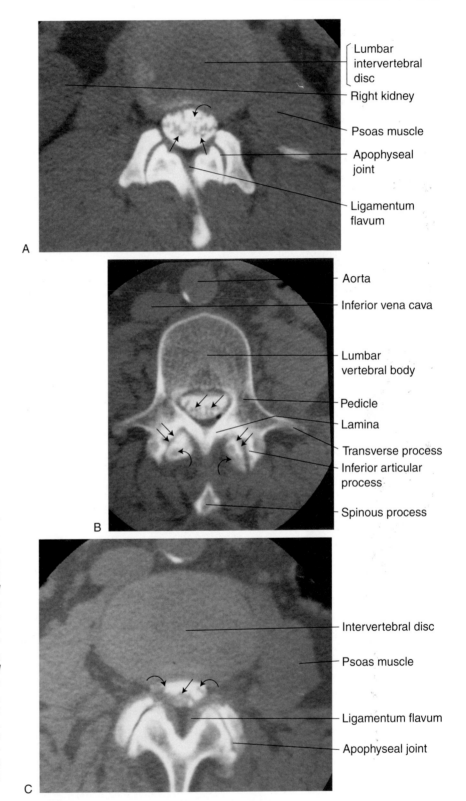

Lumbar intervertebral disc

Right kidney

Psoas muscle

Apophyseal joint

Ligamentum flavum

A

Aorta

Inferior vena cava

Lumbar vertebral body

Pedicle

Lamina

Transverse process

Inferior articular process

Spinous process

B

Intervertebral disc

Psoas muscle

Ligamentum flavum

Apophyseal joint

C

FIG. 12-11. A: Lumbar spine axial CT image through the L1-2 intervertebral disc level. Normal. The straight arrows indicate the cauda equina surrounded by contrast media in the subarachnoid space cerebral spinal fluid (curved arrow). B: Lumbar spine axial CT image through a lumbar vertebra. Normal. The straight arrows indicate multiple nerve roots. Notice how the inferior articular processes of the vertebra articulate with the superior articular processes (curved arrows) from the vertebra below to form the apopyseal joints (double arrows). C: Lumbar spine axial CT image through a lumbar intervertebral disc. Normal. The straight arrow indicates nerve roots in the posterior aspect of the subarachnoid space whereas the curved arrows indicate nerve roots about to exit through the neural foramina.

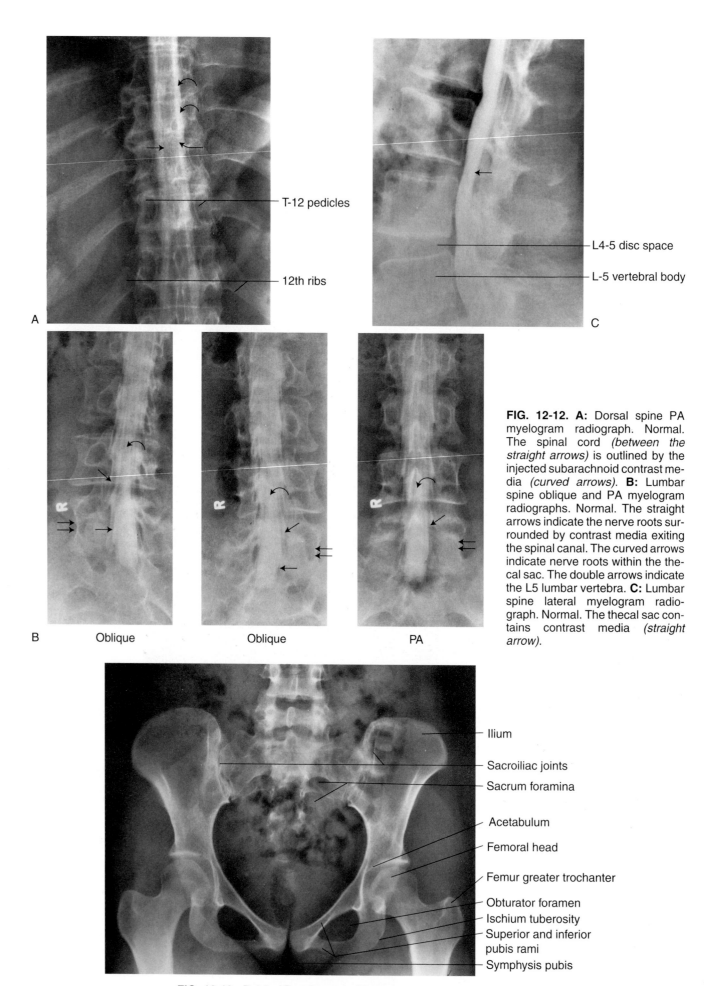

FIG. 12-12. A: Dorsal spine PA myelogram radiograph. Normal. The spinal cord *(between the straight arrows)* is outlined by the injected subarachnoid contrast media *(curved arrows)*. **B:** Lumbar spine oblique and PA myelogram radiographs. Normal. The straight arrows indicate the nerve roots surrounded by contrast media exiting the spinal canal. The curved arrows indicate nerve roots within the thecal sac. The double arrows indicate the L5 lumbar vertebra. **C:** Lumbar spine lateral myelogram radiograph. Normal. The thecal sac contains contrast media *(straight arrow)*.

T-12 pedicles

12th ribs

L4-5 disc space

L-5 vertebral body

A

B   Oblique   Oblique   PA

C

Ilium

Sacroiliac joints

Sacrum foramina

Acetabulum

Femoral head

Femur greater trochanter

Obturator foramen

Ischium tuberosity

Superior and inferior pubis rami

Symphysis pubis

FIG. 12-13. Pelvis AP radiograph. Normal.

the pelvic bones must be evaluated for fractures, density, anomalies, and metastatic lesions.

ANOMALIES

Anomalies of the spine and pelvis (Table 12-5) vary in severity from mild to severe. *As a general rule, most mild spinal anomalies are asymptomatic.* Small extra bones or supernumerary bones called **accessory ossicles** are usually asymptomatic, and they may be located near many different bones including the spine. Examples of accessory ossicles are shown in Fig. 12-14A, B and 11-14D. Accessory ossicles are simply normal variants and should not be confused with a fracture.

Occasionally, extra ribs arise from the cervical spine, and they are called *cervical ribs* (Fig. 12-14C). Cervical ribs are generally asymptomatic, but have the potential to cause symptoms secondary to extrinsic pressure on the brachial plexus and the vessels of the upper extremities. A common anomaly is partial sacralization of L5,

TABLE 12-5. *A partial list of spine and pelvis anomalies*

Mild:
Accessory ossicles
Cervical ribs
Transitional vertebrae
Spina bifida
Hemivertebra
Osteitis condensans ilii
Severe:
Meningocele and myelomeningocele
Absence of the sacrum
Symphysis diastasis
Scoliosis
Osteopetrosis

wherein fusion exists between a portion of the L5 vertebra and the sacrum (Fig. 12-15A). Usually one of the L5 transverse processes is fused with the sacrum, but there are many variations. When the L5 vertebra begins to have the appearance of the sacrum or the sacrum begins to look like a lumbar vertebra, this general situa-

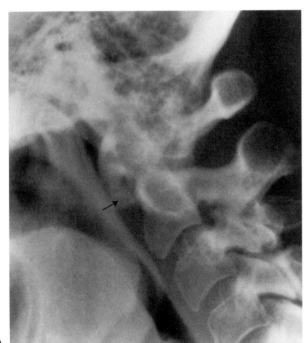

A

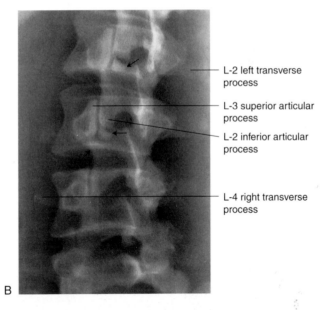

— L-2 left transverse process

— L-3 superior articular process

— L-2 inferior articular process

— L-4 right transverse process

B

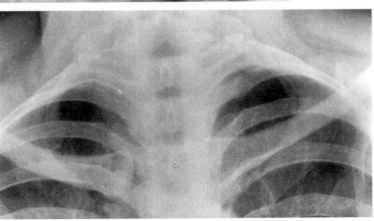

C

FIG. 12-14. A: Cervical spine lateral radiograph. This accessory ossicle is located inferior to the anterior arch of the atlas or C1. This supernumerary bone or os *(straight arrow)* is a normal variant. **B:** Lumbar spine right oblique radiograph. Lumbar spine accessory ossicles *(straight arrows)*. This 22-year-old gymnast experienced a sudden onset of back pain. The accessory ossicles are variants of normal and had nothing to do with the patient's back pain. They are usually found around the L2 and L3 levels. **C:** Lower cervical and upper dorsal spine AP radiograph. Bilateral cervical ribs. The small bilateral ribs (arrows) arise from the C7 vertebra; hence the name cervical ribs.

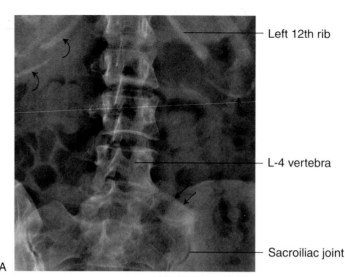

— Left 12th rib

— L-4 vertebra

— Sacroiliac joint

A

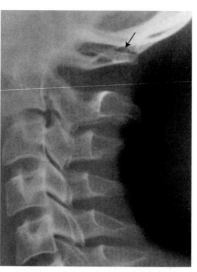

B

FIG. 12-15. A: Lumbar spine AP radiograph. Partial sacralization of L5. L5 articulates with the left sacrum in an anomalous fashion *(straight arrows)*. This is commonly referred to as a transitional vertebra. Transitional vertebrae describe a situation wherein L5 begins to look like a part of the sacrum or the sacrum begins look like a part of the lumbar spine. The curved arrows indicate calcifications within the costocartilaginous structures. **B:** Cervical spine lateral radiograph. Partial occipitalization of C1. The spinous process of C1 articulates with the occiput *(arrow)*. Normally the spinous process of C1 does not articulate with the occiput.

tion is called a *transitional vertebra.* This may become symptomatic especially after excessive back strain. A less common anomaly is an abnormal articulation between the C1 spinous process and the occiput (Fig. 12-15B). A more severe anomaly of the cervical spine is total absence of the posterior vertebral arch.

An important anomaly is spina bifida (Fig. 12-16), which occurs in approximately 5% of the population. Spina bifida is a midline defect of the vertebral arch (usually posterior), and it is generally asymptomatic. When spina bifida has an associated soft tissue mass

associated, it is called a meningocele. Meningoceles contain cerebral spinal fluid and the sac envelope consists of the meninges. When the sac contains spinal cord and/or nerve roots, it is called a myelomeningocele ("myelo-" refers to the cord). A meningocele (Fig. 12-17) is a herniation of neural tissue through a bone defect. The size of these herniations is variable, and the herniation direction most commonly is posterior, but can be anterior or lateral. The symptoms vary from nonexistent to extensive and disabling. Visceral innervation of the bladder and/or rectum may be affected, as

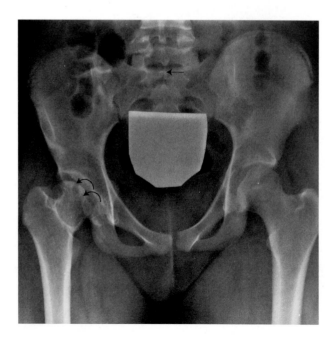

FIG. 12-16. Pelvis AP radiograph. Spina bifida occulta and congenital dislocation of the hip (congenital hip dysplasia). Spina bifida occulta is indicated by the straight arrow and represents incomplete fusion of the posterior sacral segments. Incidentally noted is right hip congenital dislocation *(curved arrows)*. Note the presence of a gonadal shield.

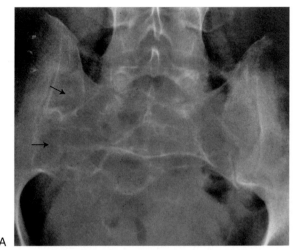 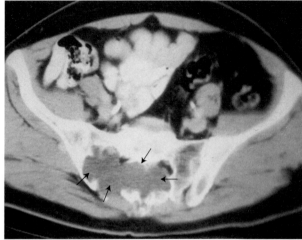

A   B

FIG. 12-17. A: Pelvis AP radiograph. Sacral meningocele. This 54-year-old patient consulted a physician because of urinary retention. The lucent areas in the sacrum *(straight arrows)* indicate the bone defect secondary to the meningocele mass. **B:** Pelvis axial CT image. The full extent of the meningocele mass within the sacrum is indicated by the straight arrows.

well as sensory and motor nerves. Another unfortunate anomaly in this category is complete absence of the sacrum, and it is often associated with a variety of other anomalies. Another severe anomaly is exstrophy of the urinary bladder, which is associated with abnormal widening of the symphysis pubis. This widening of the symphysis pubis or diastasis can occasionally be associated with some bone dysplasias, epispadias, hypospadias, and the prune belly syndrome (loss or absence of abdominal wall muscles).

One of the most clinically important anomalies of the spine is scoliosis. Some of the many etiologies of scoliosis include idiopathic, neuromuscular diseases, trauma, infections, tumors, radiation therapy, acromegaly, and underlying congenital problems such as hemivertebrae.

A significant vertebral anomaly that can result in scoliosis is the *hemivertebra* (Fig. 12-18). A hemivertebra is a vertebra with a missing part secondary to absence of a lateral ossification center. Usually a hemivertebra has only one rib that is located on the normally developed side (Fig. 12-19). The majority of the cases are idiopathic (Fig. 12-20), whereas approximately 10% are congenital with associated vertebral and rib abnormalities as shown in Fig. 12-19.

Osteitis condensans ilii (Fig. 12-21) is a well-marginated area of increased bone density found predominately in women of childbearing years. It is located in the iliac bone just lateral to the sacroiliac joint, but the sacrum and sacroiliac joints are not involved. This abnormality may or may not be symptomatic. The differential diagnosis should include osteoblastic metastatic disease, ankylosing spondylitis, and other inflammatory arthritides such as rheumatoid arthritis. It usually can be differentiated from metastatic disease that commonly involves multiple widespread sites. The sacroiliac joints

are usually narrowed or absent in ankylosing spondylitis and often appear irregular in the other inflammatory arthritides such as rheumatoid arthritis.

Another inherited bone disease is osteopetrosis or marble bone. It is a congenital anomaly involving bone development and maturation. Fortunately, this is very rare and is included here as a dramatic manifestation of disease. The clinical features include optic atrophy, anemia, and overall marble-like increased density of

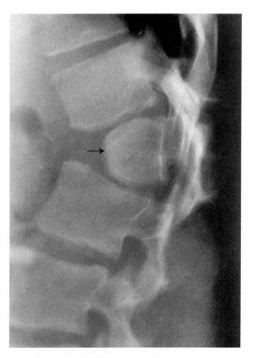

FIG. 12-18. Lumbar spine lateral radiograph. L1 posterior hemivertebra *(arrow)*. They are usually asymptomatic.

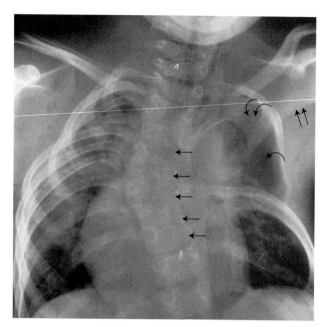

FIG. 12-19. Thoracic spine AP radiograph. Congenital scoliosis. The dorsal spine is convex to the right *(straight arrows)*, and the thorax is markedly asymmetric. Underlying the scoliosis are multiple hemivertebrae or incompletely formed dorsal vertebrae *(straight arrows)*. There are multiple absent left ribs *(curved arrows)* and several left upper ribs are fused *(double curved arrows)*. The left scapula is abnormally elevated *(double straight arrows)*.

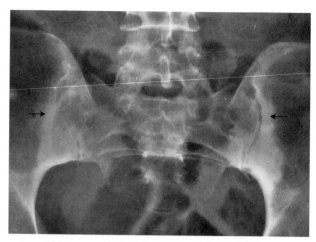

FIG. 12-21. Pelvis AP radiograph. Osteitis condensans ilia. The sharply marginated bilateral increased densities (sclerosis) involve the iliac sides of the sacroiliac joints and spares the sacrum. This is a benign condition that is usually found in women in their childbearing years and seldom found in older women. This can be an incidental finding on a radiograph or the patient may present with acute or chronic back pain.

the bones (1). The bone appears marble-like as the increased density obliterates the normal trabecular pattern, and it is difficult to differentiate between the bone cortex and medulla. When the spine is involved, there is a characteristic sandwich vertebrae appearance on a lateral radiograph caused by increased density or sclerosis in the vertebral endplates (Fig. 12-22).

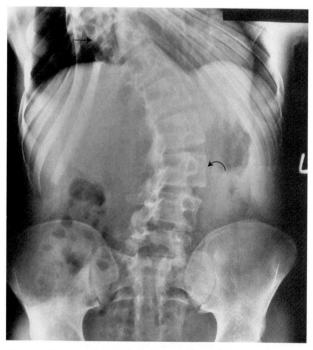

FIG. 12-20. Thoracolumbar spine AP radiograph. Idiopathic scoliosis of the thoracic and lumbar spine. The lumbar spine is convex to the left *(curved arrow)*, and the lumbar vertebrae are markedly rotated. This rotation component causes the lumbar vertebra to appear oblique on the radiograph. The lower thoracic spine is convex to the right *(straight arrow)* resulting in asymmetry of the ribs and thorax.

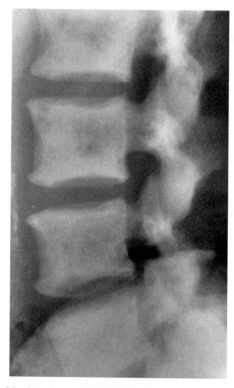

FIG. 12-22. Lumbar spine lateral radiograph. Osteopetrosis. The overall density of the bones is uniformly increased.

TRAUMA (FRACTURES, DISLOCATIONS, AND SOFT TISSUE)

Fractures

Fractures of the spine and pelvis are common and result from a wide variety of traumas including motor vehicle accidents, sports, and falls. Fractures of the spine are obviously important as the spinal cord and cauda equina are vulnerable to injury because of their close proximity to the vertebrae. Roughly 50% of cervical spine fractures have neurologic complications.

Cervical Spine Injuries

A variety of injuries occur when the cervical spine undergoes acute hyperflexion and hyperextension (Table 12-6). The tear-drop fracture (Fig. 12-23) is one type of injury that results from acute cervical spine hyperflexion. The tear-drop-shaped fracture fragment is an avulsion from the anterior inferior aspect of the vertebral body. This fracture is usually accompanied by disruption of the anterior longitudinal ligament and the interspinal ligaments between the spinous processes, thus making the spine very unstable. Other ligaments

TABLE 12-6. *Cervical spine flexion injuries*

Ligament disruption
Facet locking
Tear-drop fracture
Odontoid process fractures (also in extension injuries)
Anterior wedge fracture

that may be involved are the supraspinal ligament and the ligamenta flava. The involved vertebral body may be displaced posterior, and this situation is a good indication for CT imaging to determine the extent of the fracture line or lines and to determine the precise location of the fracture fragments, especially their relationship to the cervical spinal cord.

Facet locking (Fig. 12-24) is another hyperflexion injury. Locking will occur when the inferior articular process of the upper vertebra moves forward or anteriorly over the superior articular process of the lower vertebra, and this results in an anterior dislocation of the upper vertebra. Once again, the spine is unstable as there usually is posterior and sometimes anterior ligamentous disruption, and cervical spinal cord injury is common. The lateral radiograph is usually sufficient to make the

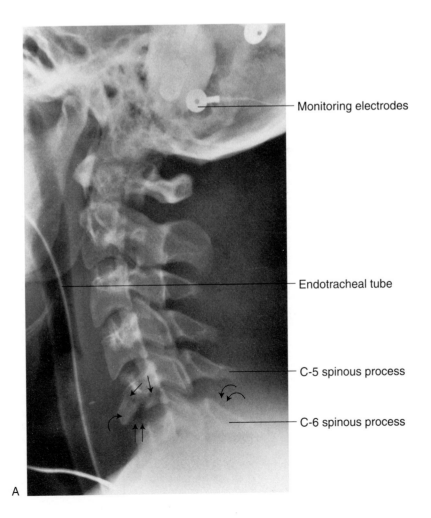

FIG. 12-23. A: Lateral cervical spine radiograph. C5 flexion tear-drop fracture. This 21-year-old man was involved in a motor vehicle accident. There is mild compression anteriorly of the C5 vertebral body secondary to the comminuted fracture *(straight arrows)*, and there is mild separation of the fracture fragments. The major fracture fragment has a tear-drop shape *(curved arrow)* due to avulsion at the site of the anterior longitudinal ligament. The hyperflexion injury has resulted in a mild separation or fanning of the space between the C5 and C6 spinous processes secondary to ligamentous disruption *(double curved arrows)*. The disrupted ligaments are the interspinal and supraspinal ligaments and possibly the ligamentum flavum. Also, the hyperflexion injury created minimal widening of the C5-C6 disc space *(double straight arrows)* and mild angulation of the spine at this level with minimal retrolisthesis of C5 on C6. This type of cervical fracture usually is associated with severe cord injury as the vertebral body is often displaced posteriorly into the spinal canal.

Monitoring electrodes

Endotracheal tube

C-5 spinous process

C-6 spinous process

FIG. 12-23. *Continued.* **B:** Cervical spine axial CT image of the C5 vertebra. The comminuted fracture lines in the vertebral body are separated or distracted *(straight arrows)*, and the anterior fracture fragments are displaced anteriorly approximately 3 mm *(curved arrow)*. **C:** Lateral cervical spine radiograph. Posterior wire stabilization of the cervical spine between the spinous processes of C5 and C6 vertebrae *(curved arrow)*. The major fracture fragment *(straight arrow)* is in fairly good alignment with mild offset of the fragments *(double straight arrows)*. The spine is now in good alignment.

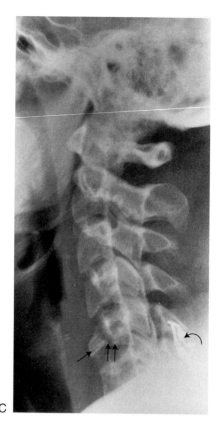

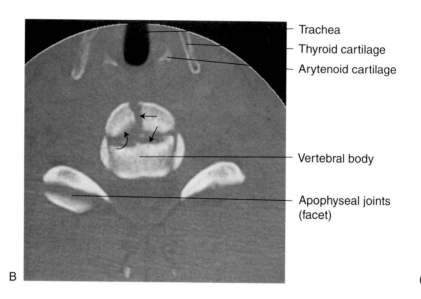

— Trachea
— Thyroid cartilage
— Arytenoid cartilage

— Vertebral body

— Apophyseal joints (facet)

B

C

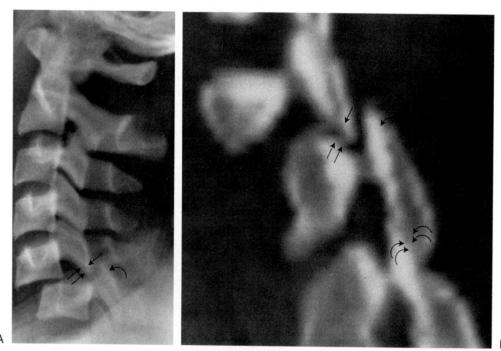

A

B

FIG. 12-24. A: Cervical spine lateral radiograph. Bilateral facet locking at the C5–6 level. The inferior articular process of C5 *(straight arrow)* is anterior to the superior articular process of C6 *(curved arrow)*. The double straight arrows indicate the expected normal position for the superior articular process of the C6 vertebra. There is obvious posterior dislocation of the C6 vertebral body referable to the C5 vertebral body. No fractures are apparent. **B:** Cervical spine sagittal reconstructed CT image on a different patient. Bilateral facet lock. The inferior articular processes of the upper vertebra *(straight arrow)* is in an abnormal relationship with the superior articular process of the lower vertebra *(curved arrow)*. The double straight arrows indicate the expected normal location of the displaced superior articular process. A normal apophyseal articulation is visible at the level below *(double curved arrows)*.

diagnosis (see Fig. 12-24A), but occasionally a reconstructed sagittal CT image (see Fig. 12-24B) is necessary to confirm the diagnosis.

Occasionally hyperflexion injury results in ligamentous injury without fracture (Fig. 12-25). As with other hyperflexion injuries, this has the potential for spinal instability and cord injury.

Dens or odontoid process fractures are unstable and they may result from hyperflexion or hyperextension injuries. The best methods for the diagnosis of odontoid process fracture are AP open mouth and lateral cervical radiographs, plain film tomography, and CT imaging. The odontoid fracture in Fig. 12-26 is probably a hyperextension injury as the odontoid is displaced posteriorly.

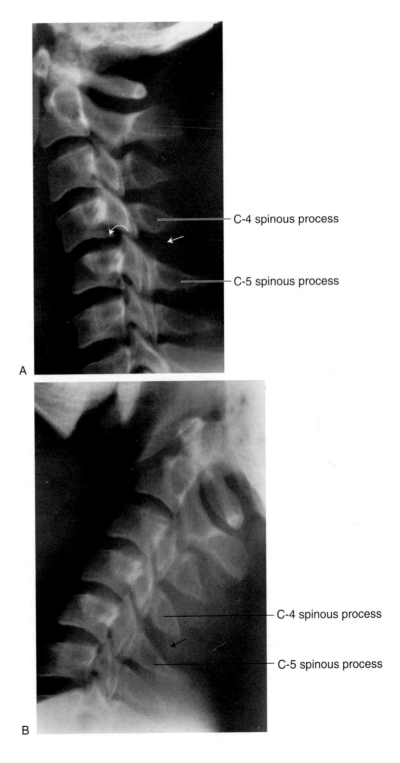

FIG. 12-25. A: Cervical spine cross-table lateral radiograph with the patient supine. Posterior ligament disruption at C4–5. There is an increase in the height of the interspinous space between the C4–5 spinous processes *(straight arrow)* secondary to disruption of the C4–5 interspinal ligament, supraspinal ligament, and possibly the ligamenta flava. Compare the height of the C4–5 interspinous space to those above and below. The mild anterior spondylolisthesis of C4 referable to C5 *(curved arrow)* has resulted in mild dorsal angulation and reverse of the normal cervical curvature at the C4 level. **B:** Cervical spine extension lateral radiograph in the same patient. When the cervical spine is in full extension, the C4–5 interspinous space *(straight arrow)* is now normal in height and the anterolisthesis of C4 on C5 has been reduced.

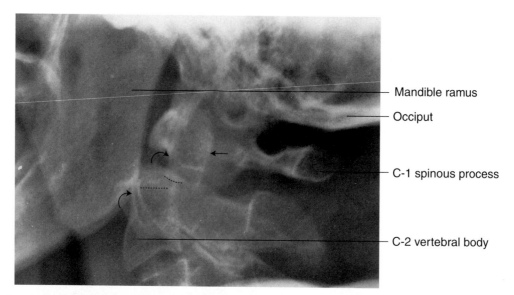

FIG. 12-26. Cervical spine lateral radiograph. Displaced fracture through the caudad or inferior aspect of the dens or odontoid process of C2. The actual fracture edges are indicated by the dotted lines and the dens *(arrow)* is displaced posteriorly approximately 8 mm. The curved arrows indicate the amount of displacement of the dens.

Dorsal Spine Fractures

Fractures of the dorsal spine may also result from significant trauma. However, underlying bone diseases can weaken the vertebrae and pathologic fractures may occur with little or no trauma. A few of the underlying diseases that may cause pathologic fractures are primary and secondary bone tumors, Paget's disease, osteopetrosis, osteoporosis, and osteomalacia (Fig. 12-27).

Lumbar Spine Fractures

Fractures commonly occur in the lumbar spine and are usually diagnosed by radiography (Fig. 12-28A, B). MRI may be helpful in assessing the effect of the fracture fragments on the thecal sac (Fig. 12-28C). As in other areas of the spine, CT imaging is helpful to evaluate the extent of the fractures and to precisely locate the fracture fragments within the neural canal and their relationship relative to the thecal sac (Fig. 12-28D).

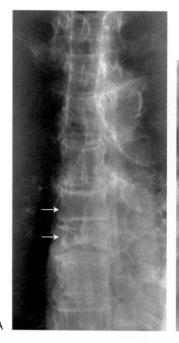

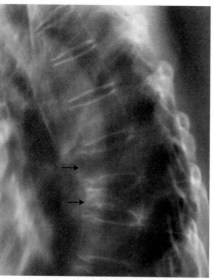

FIG. 12-27. Dorsal spine AP **(A)** and lateral **(B)** radiographs. Osteopenia due to senile osteoporosis with secondary pathologic compression fractures of the T7 and T8 vertebral bodies. The compression fractures *(straight arrows)* are manifest by a decrease in the vertical height of the T7 and T8 vertebral bodies when compared to the other dorsal vertebral bodies. Notice the overall decreased density (osteopenia) of all the osseous structures due to osteoporosis.

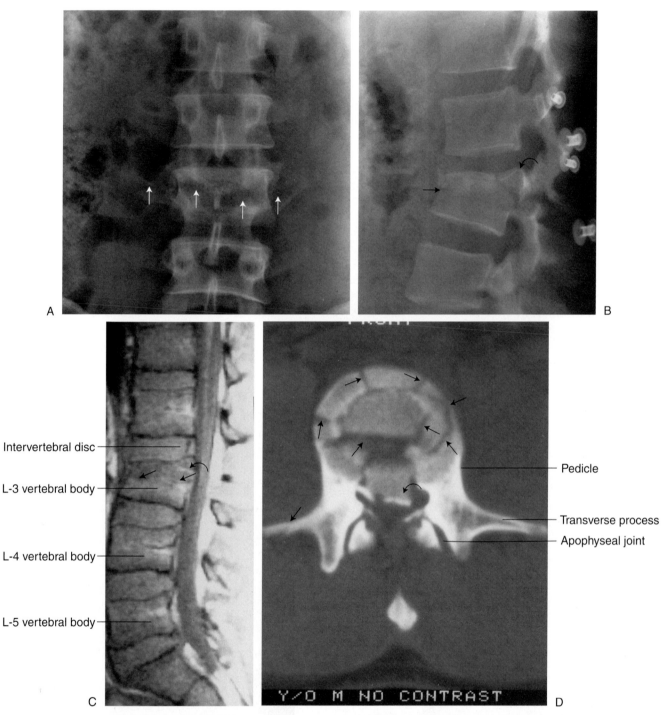

FIG. 12-28. Lumbar spine AP **(A)** and lateral **(B)** radiographs. Seat belt fracture of the L3 vertebrae. This 30-year-old was wearing a lap seat belt when involved in a motor vehicle accident, and this is a flexion injury caused by the mobile upper body flexing on the lower body that is fixed by the lap seat belt. There is a transverse fracture through the L3 vertebra involving the vertebral body and the transverse processes (straight arrows in A and B). A large fracture fragment arising posteriorly from the vertebral body is displaced into the neural canal *(curved arrow in B)*. The L3 vertebral body height is less than normal secondary to compression or collapse caused by the fracture. There is mild dorsal angulation of the spine at the level of the L3 fracture. These fractures may be either stable or unstable. The remainder of the lumbar spine is normal. Note the clothing snaps. **C:** Lumbar spine sagittal proton-dense MR image. A lap seat belt L3 displaced fracture in another 30-year-old patient. The L3 vertebral body is mildly compressed secondary to a fracture *(straight arrows)*, and a posterior fracture fragment resides in the neural canal compressing the neural canal *(curved arrow)*. **D:** Lumbar spine axial CT image. L3 vertebra displaced burst-type fracture in a 23-year-old involved in a motor vehicle accident. The mechanism of injury is axial compression with or without flexion and/or rotation. The straight arrows indicate the severe comminuted fracture of the L3 vertebral body. Typically, there is displacement of a posterior vertebral body fracture fragment *(curved arrow)* into the neural canal resulting in neural canal compromise and neural sac compression.

Spondylolysis and Spondylolisthesis

Spondylolysis and spondylolisthesis are difficult and confusing terms for the beginner. However, an understanding of these conditions and their clinical significance is necessary as they will commonly be encountered in clinical practice. *Spondylolysis* refers to a defect in the pars interarticularis that lies between the superior and inferior articular processes of a vertebra. In other words, the neck of the scotty dog is missing (see Fig. 12-9A). The defect is usually bilateral but can be unilateral, and when present the defect can potentially be seen on all lumbar spine radiographs, especially the oblique views (Fig. 12-29). It is widely believed that spondylolysis results from a chronic strain (stress fracture) or, on occasion, from an acute fracture. Some believe that on rare occasions the condition may be congenital (2). *Spondylolisthesis* is the forward movement of a vertebra relative to the more stable vertebra below. Usually, the forward movement is made possible by a bilateral spondylolysis defect in the vertebra (Figs.

12-29 and 12-30). Actually, it is the vertebral body, pedicles, and superior articular processes that move forward or ventrally, whereas the laminae, inferior articular processes, and the spinous process remain in their normal positions (see Fig. 12-30). The majority of the spondylolysis with spondylolisthesis cases occur in the lumbar spine, especially at L5–S1 levels, and it is uncommon in the dorsal and cervical spine. Spondylolisthesis may be asymptomatic, and the most frequent symptom is low back pain probably due to muscle spasm and instability. Symptoms, when they occur, are not necessarily related to the severity of the disease (1). Spondylolisthesis secondary to spondylolysis must be differentiated from the spondylolisthesis secondary to degenerative or osteoarthritis without spondylolysis. Degenerative spondylolisthesis is best imaged on a lateral radiograph of the lumbar spine (Fig. 12-31), and it most commonly occurs at the L4–5 level. There are usually degenerative changes in the disc space and the apophyseal joints *without a defect in the pars interarticularis.*

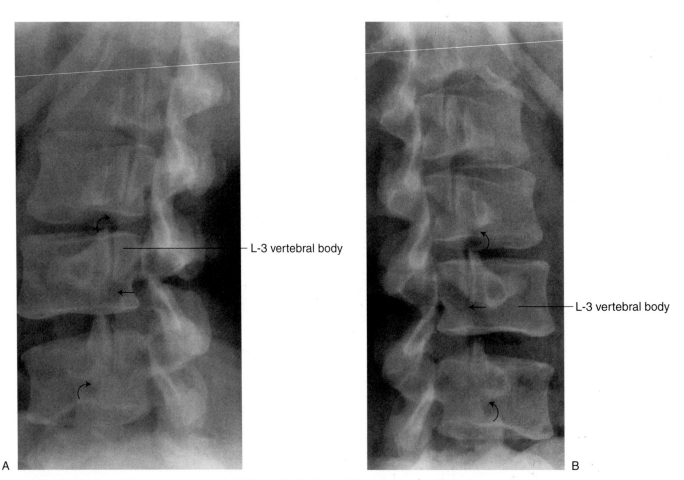

A   L-3 vertebral body   L-3 vertebral body   B

FIG. 12-29. A and B: Lumbar spine right **(A)** and left oblique **(B)** radiographs. Bilateral spondylolysis of L3 *(straight arrows)*. The pars interarticularis or the scotty-dog neck is absent bilaterally in the L3 vertebra. Normal scotty-dog necks or pars interarticulares are present in the L2 and L4 vertebrae bilaterally *(curved arrows)*.

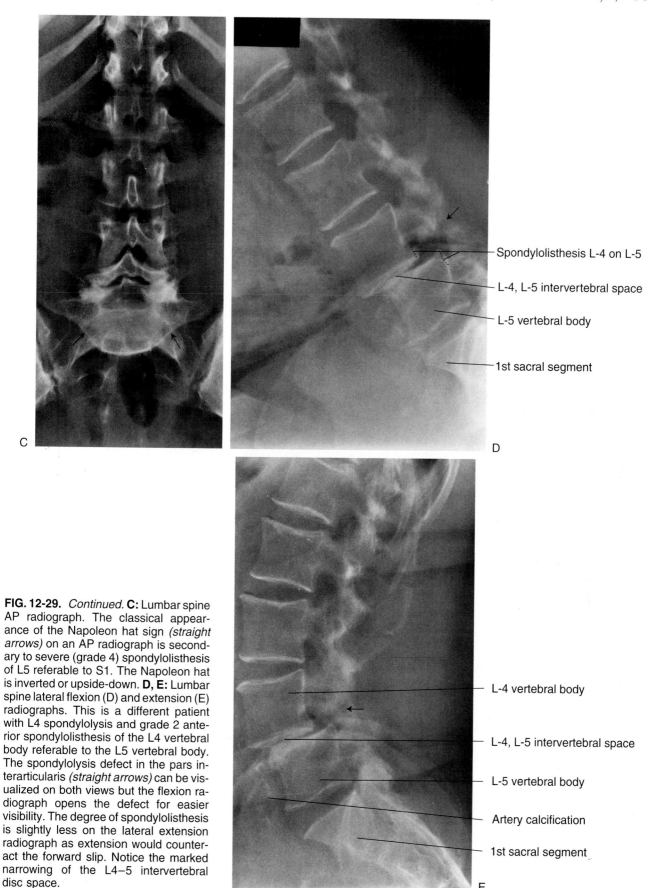

C

D

— Spondylolisthesis L-4 on L-5

— L-4, L-5 intervertebral space

— L-5 vertebral body

— 1st sacral segment

— L-4 vertebral body

— L-4, L-5 intervertebral space

— L-5 vertebral body

— Artery calcification

— 1st sacral segment

E

FIG. 12-29. *Continued.* **C:** Lumbar spine AP radiograph. The classical appearance of the Napoleon hat sign *(straight arrows)* on an AP radiograph is secondary to severe (grade 4) spondylolisthesis of L5 referable to S1. The Napoleon hat is inverted or upside-down. **D, E:** Lumbar spine lateral flexion (D) and extension (E) radiographs. This is a different patient with L4 spondylolysis and grade 2 anterior spondylolisthesis of the L4 vertebral body referable to the L5 vertebral body. The spondylolysis defect in the pars interarticularis *(straight arrows)* can be visualized on both views but the flexion radiograph opens the defect for easier visibility. The degree of spondylolisthesis is slightly less on the lateral extension radiograph as extension would counteract the forward slip. Notice the marked narrowing of the L4–5 intervertebral disc space.

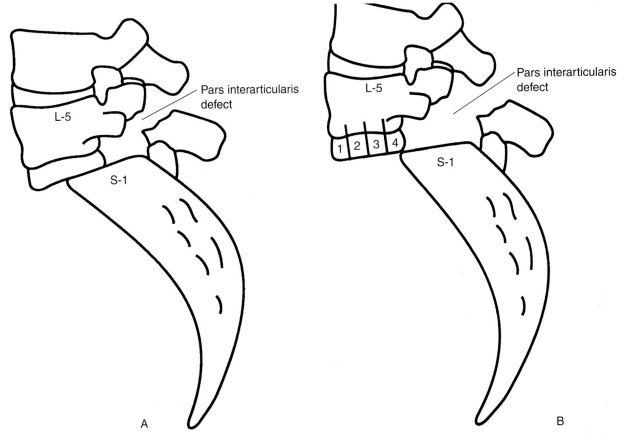

FIG. 12-30. A: Illustration of spondylolysis and spondylolisthesis on a lateral radiograph. The L5 vertebral body, pedicles, and superior articular processes have moved forward or ventral relative to the sacrum. However the L5 inferior articular processes, laminae, and the spinous process remain in their normal position. **B:** Illustration of spondylolisthesis classification or grading system. The sacrum is divided into fourths and the forward movement of L5 is simply given a grade of 1–4.

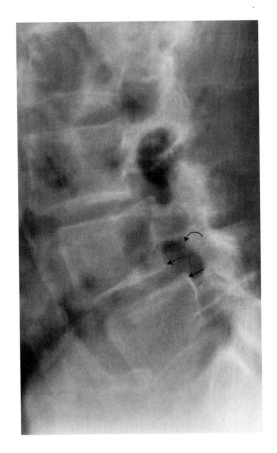

FIG. 12-31. Lumbar spine lateral radiograph. Degenerative grade 1 spondylolisthesis of L4 referable to L5 *(straight arrows)*. This is a common complication of degenerative spine changes. The pars interarticularis is intact *(curved arrow)*. The spondylolisthesis is secondary to the degenerative changes in the intervertebral space and the apophyseal joints that allow L4 to move forward relative to L5.

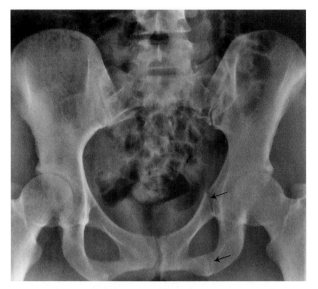

FIG. 12-32. Pelvis AP radiograph. Fractures of the left superior and inferior pubis rami *(straight arrows)*. Sacral fractures are present but are obscured by the overlying intestinal gas.

Pelvic Fractures

Fractures of the pelvis are common and result from a variety of injuries (Fig. 12-32). They are usually multiple rather than single. The major problem with pelvic fractures is that the bladder, urethra, and other pelvis soft tissues may be damaged by fracture fragments as was demonstrated in Chapter 10.

TABLE 12-7. *Intervertebral disc herniation nomenclature*

Bulge—entire width of disc displaced posteriorly
Protruding—only a portion extends beyond disc space
Extruded—a fragment of disc displayed away from the disc space
Limbus vertebra
Schmorl's node

A variety of opaque foreign bodies encountered on pelvis radiographs are demonstrated in Fig. 12-33.

Herniated Intervertebral Disc Disease

Intervertebral disc herniations occur at all levels in the spine including the dorsal spine. Although intervertebral discs cannot be visualized on radiographs, disc disease should be suspected whenever there is intervertebral disc space narrowing on radiographs. Noninvasive CT and MRI are increasingly being used in conjunction with or in place of the myelogram as they are more accurate and have a lower complication rate than myelography.

Some confusing terms have developed in the classification of herniated intervertebral discs, but the following is a simple approach to this terminology problem. *Herniation* is a general umbrella term, and it can be divided into three main categories, i.e., bulging, protruding, and extruded discs (Table 12-7). A *bulging disc* means that the entire width of disc has moved or is mildly displaced dorsal to the posterior aspect of the

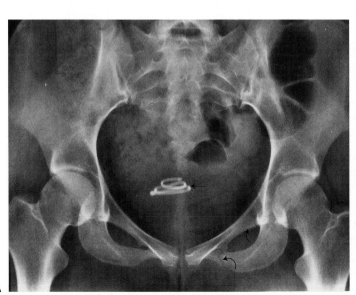

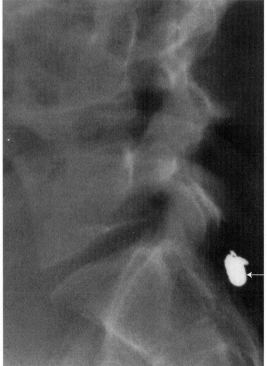

A   B

FIG. 12-33. A: Pelvis AP radiograph. Intrauterine contraceptive device *(straight arrow)* and left superior and inferior pubis fractures *(curved arrows)*. **B:** Lumbar spine lateral radiograph. Metallic bullet or slug foreign body *(straight arrow)* in soft tissues posterior to the sacrum.

vertebral body. A *protruding disc* refers to only a portion of the disc extending lateral and/or posterior beyond the disc space. The protruding disc fragment remains attached to the main disc body. An *extruded disc* means that a fragment of the disc is displaced from the disc space.

Herniated lumbar intervertebral disc disease is common especially at the L4–5 and L5–S1 levels (Fig. 12-34). Usually, disc herniations are lateral and/or posterior. However, when the disc herniates anteriorly, this results in a vertebral defect with a classical appearance called a limbus vertebra (Figs. 12-35 and 12-36). When the disc herniates into the vertebral endplate, the resulting defect is called a Schmorl's node (Figs. 12-35 and 12-36). There are some people who feel that a Schmorl's node is congenital.

Scheuermann's disease (Fig. 12-36) is osteochondrosis of the epiphyseal plates in teenagers who often complain of back pain. The diagnosis of Scheuermann's disease usually can be made on lateral spine radiographs. The radiographic features include fragmented and sclerotic epiphyseal plates of the vertebrae, wedge-shaped vertebral bodies with increased AP diameter, and narrowed disc spaces. Limbus vertebrae and Schmorl's nodes may be present.

TABLE 12-8. *Arthritides*

Osteoarthritis
Diffuse idiopathic disseminated hyperplasia
Inflammatory arthritis (rheumatoid arthritis and ankylosing spondylitis)
Neuropathic joint (Charcot's joint)
Infectious arthritis

ARTHRITIDES

Because the spine has multiple joints, it is not surprising that most of the arthritides involve the spine (Table 12-8).

Osteoarthritis

Osteoarthritis or degenerative arthritis (Fig. 12-37) is the most common arthritis, and the spine is frequently involved. Patients with osteoarthritis will usually complain of pain and/or limited motion in the involved spine. As in the extremities, the typical radiologic features include irregular joint narrowing, sclerosis, and osteophyte formation (Fig. 12-37). The differential diagnosis of degenerative or osteoarthritis must include neuropathic joints and diffuse idiopathic skeletal hy-

text continues on page 338

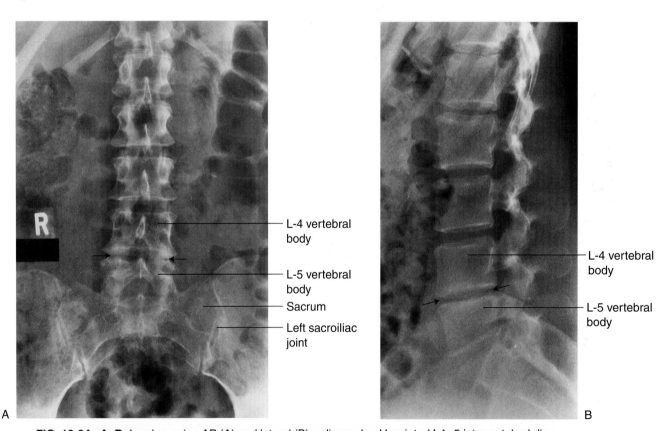

L-4 vertebral body
L-5 vertebral body
Sacrum
Left sacroiliac joint

L-4 vertebral body
L-5 vertebral body

FIG. 12-34. A, B: Lumbar spine AP (A) and lateral (B) radiographs. Herniated L4–5 intervertebral disc. The patient is a 30-year-old woman with bilateral leg weakness greater on the right than the left. There is significant narrowing of the L4–5 intervertebral disc space *(straight arrows)* suggesting disc disease at this level. Again, the disc is not visible on the radiograph. The disc space narrowing is more apparent when you compare the L4–5 disc space to the other lumbar disc spaces. Normally the L4–5 disc space height is greater than the other lumbar spine disc spaces.

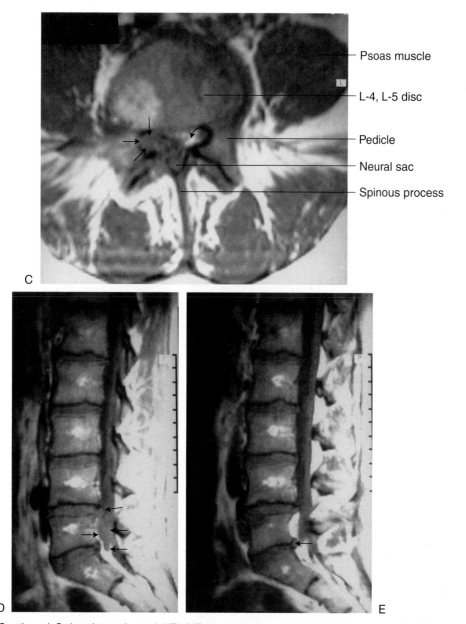

Psoas muscle

L-4, L-5 disc

Pedicle

Neural sac

Spinous process

C

D   E

FIG. 12-34. *Continued.* **C:** Lumbar spine axial T1 MR image in the same patient. Large extruded L4–5 intervertebral disc. The disc is extruded posterolaterally to the right *(straight arrows)*, and it is creating extrinsic pressure on the neural sac and obliterating the epidural fat on the right side. Normal epidural fat is present on the left *(curved arrow)*. **D, E:** Lumbar spine sagittal T1 MR images in the same patient. Caudally extruded L4–5 intervertebral disc (D) and a protruding L5–S1 intervertebral disc (E). Notice in image (D) that the extruded L4–5 disc *(arrows)* has migrated inferiorly to the level of the L5–S1 disc space posteriorly and is severely compressing the neural sac. In image (E) there is a bulging disc at the L5–S1 level *(straight arrow)*.

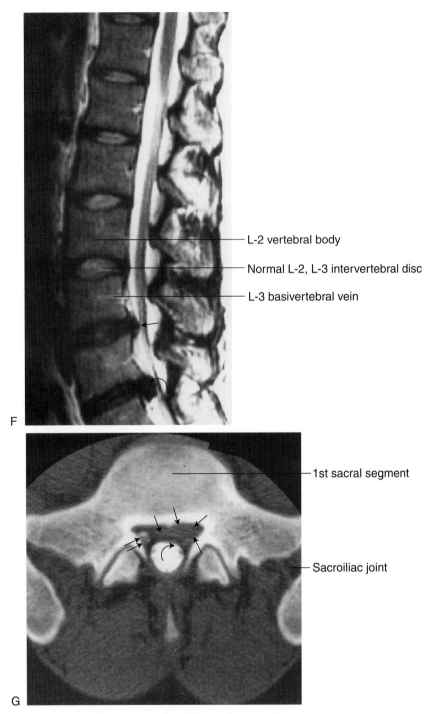

F

G

FIG. 12-34. *Continued.* **F:** Lumbar spine sagittal T2 MR image. Herniated lumbar discs at multiple levels in a 29-year-old man. There is a bulging L3–4 disc *(straight arrow)* and an extruded L4–5 lumbar disc *(curved arrow).* **G:** Lumbar spine axial CT image. Protruded L5–S1 intervertebral disc. The straight arrows outline the protruded disc at the L5–S1 level. The disc is causing mild extrinsic pressure on the thecal sac *(curved arrow).* The double arrows indicate the right nerve root, whereas the left nerve root is displaced and not visible.

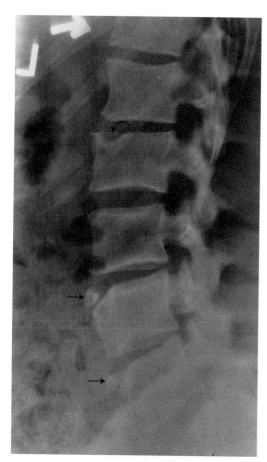

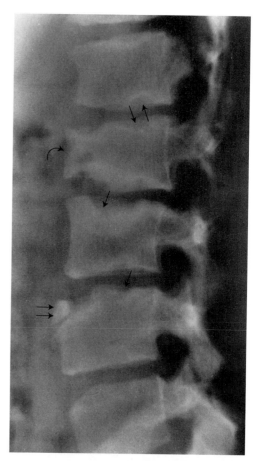

FIG. 12-35. Lumbar spine lateral radiograph. Limbus vertebrae and a Schmorl node. A limbus vertebra *(straight arrows)* should not be confused with a fracture or a secondary ossification center. The Schmorl node defect *(curved arrow)* is the scooped-out area in the vertebral endplate.

FIG. 12-36. Lumbar spine lateral radiograph. Scheuermann's disease. The involvement of three or more vertebrae by Schmorl's nodes *(straight arrows)* is called Scheuermann's disease. Anterior wedging and increased AP diameter of the vertebral bodies *(curved arrow)* may result from this process. There is a limbus vertebra *(double straight arrows)*. Note the wavy appearance of the endplates.

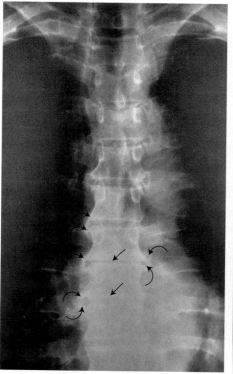

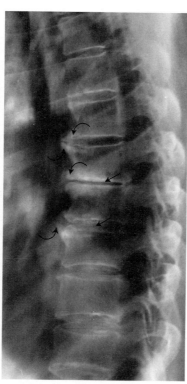

FIG. 12-37. Dorsal spine AP **(A)** and lateral **(B)** radiographs. Osteoarthritis or degenerative arthritis. Multiple osteophytes *(curved arrows)* are present and multiple disc spaces are narrowed *(straight arrows)* secondary to degenerative disc disease.

A

B

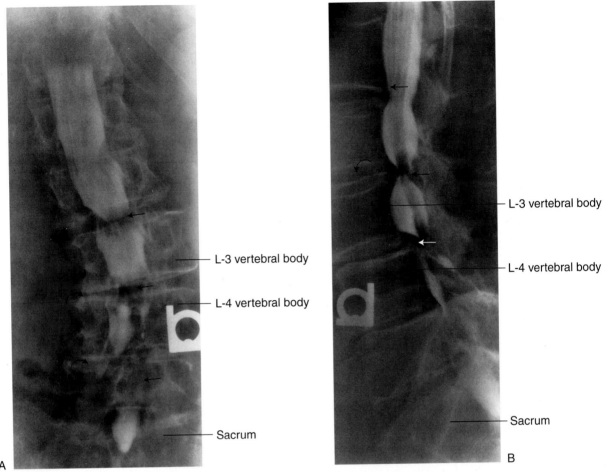

FIG. 12-38. Lumbar myelogram PA **(A)** and lateral **(B)** radiographs. Spinal stenosis. The straight arrows indicate multiple levels of neural sac compression secondary to spinal canal narrowing that is in turn secondary to degenerative changes in and around the neural canal. There is also scoliosis of the lumbar spine and the L3–4 and L4–5 intervertebral disc spaces are markedly narrowed *(curved arrows).*

perplasia. Common complications of osteoarthritis are spinal stenosis (Fig. 12-38) and spondylolisthesis.

Spinal stenosis describes a vertebral or neural canal that is too narrow, and the multiple etiologies can be classified as congenital, developmental, and idiopathic (3). Although myelography dramatically demonstrates this abnormality, CT enjoys excellent patient acceptance, and in general is a good way to make the diagnosis (Fig. 12-39).

Diffuse Idiopathic Skeletal Hyperplasia

Diffuse idiopathic skeletal hyperplasia (DISH) or Forestier's disease is best demonstrated on a lateral spine radiograph (Fig. 12-40) and is characterized by ossification involving the anterior aspect of the disc spaces and vertebral bodies. It is characteristically accompanied by exuberant osteophytes. The overall ap-

pearance is similar to the bamboo spine of ankylosing spondylitis, however, ankylosing spondylitis is usually accompanied by obliteration of the sacroiliac joints and advanced osteoporosis. Spinal stenosis is a significant complication of DISH (Fig. 12-41).

Neuropathic Joints

Charcot's joints or neuropathic or neurotrophic joints can occur in the spine as well as the extremities (Fig. 12-42). The joint changes are secondary to lost pain sensation and/or unstable joints found in a variety of neurologic conditions including diabetes mellitus, syringomyelia, and spina bifida with meningocele. The radiographic findings are disc space narrowing, bone destruction and fragmentation, sclerotic subchondral bone, subluxation and dislocation, and marginal bone mass formation. Many of these findings can be found in osteoarthritis.

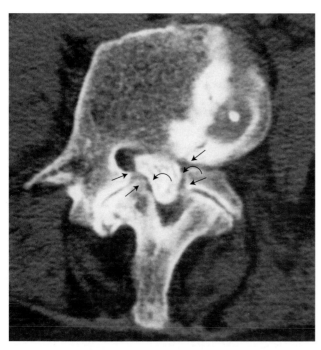

FIG. 12-39. Lumbar spine axial CT image with contrast. Spinal stenosis at the L3–4 level secondary to hypertrophic facet changes in this 71-year-old man. The straight arrows outline the marked narrowing of the spinal canal, and the curved arrows indicate the deformity of the thecal sac secondary to the spinal stenosis.

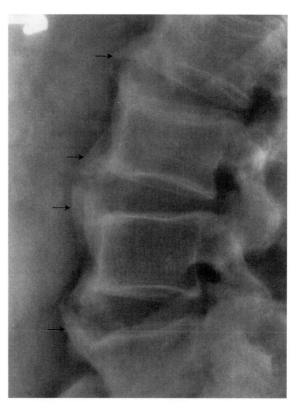

FIG. 12-40. Lumbar spine lateral radiograph. Diffuse idiopathic skeletal hyperostosis, or DISH. Note the large osteophytes *(straight arrows)* along the anterior vertebral bodies that extend anteriorly across the disc spaces. The intervertebral disc spaces are normal in height.

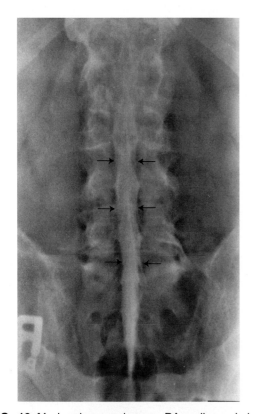

FIG. 12-41. Lumbar myelogram PA radiograph in a different patient. Spinal stenosis secondary to diffuse idiopathic skeletal hyperostosis (DISH). The straight arrows indicate multiple levels of spinal stenosis and neural sac compression due to DISH changes in the spinal canal. The overall appearance of the spine is somewhat similar to the bamboo spine of ankylosing spondylitis.

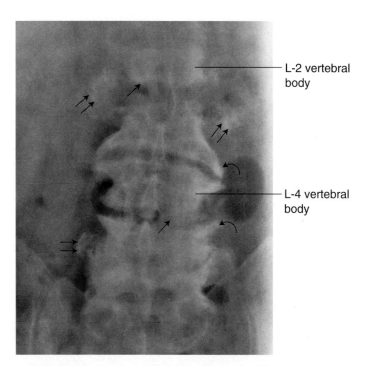

L-2 vertebral body

L-4 vertebral body

FIG. 12-42. Lumbar spine AP radiograph. Diabetic neuropathic arthropathy. The characteristic changes of neuropathic arthropathy are present including sclerotic and destructive changes *(single straight arrows)*, fragmentation and marginal bone mass formation *(double straight arrows)*, and osteophyte formation *(curved arrow)*.

TABLE 12-9. *Some primary spine bone tumors (3)*

Benign:
    Hemangioma
    Osteoid osteoma
    Osteoblastoma
    Aneurysmal bone cyst
    Osteochondroma
    Giant cell tumor
Malignant
    Multiple myeloma (most common)
    Condrosarcoma
    Osteosarcoma
    Ewing's sarcoma

Rheumatoid Arthritis

There are many synovial joints in the spine, thus rheumatoid arthritis often involves the spine. The severity of rheumatoid arthritis of the spine ranges from mild to severe. There may only be mild narrowing of cervical disc spaces. However, when rheumatoid arthritis involves the odontoid and the atlantoaxial joint, the result can be weakening of the transverse atlantal ligament that holds the odontoid close to the anterior arch of C1. When this ligament becomes involved, subluxation or even dislocation of the atlantoaxial joint may occur (Fig. 12-43). These patients can experience cervical pain either at rest or with head movement. On a lateral radiograph, the normal distance between the anterior border of the odontoid and posterior aspect of the C1 anterior arch is usually less than 2.5 mm in adults. When there is subluxation or dislocation of this joint, the distance becomes greater than 2.5 mm, especially when the cervical spine is flexed.

Flexion and extension lateral cervical spine radiographs are indicated in rheumatoid arthritis patients when they experience pain with head movement, and before undergoing general anesthesia or any other procedure wherein their head might be hyperflexed or hyperextended. These precautions help to prevent spinal cord injury. As elsewhere, rheumatoid arthritis often is associated with osteopenia and secondary pathologic fractures. The differential diagnosis for osteopenia and vertebral fracture includes osteoporosis, metastatic disease, primary bone tumor, infection, and trauma.

Ankylosing Spondylitis

Ankylosing spondylitis, or Marie-Strumpell disease (Fig. 12-44; see Fig. 11-78) is an inflammatory arthritis that usually involves young men who often present with back pain. The disease can result in obliteration of the sacroiliac joints and squaring of the vertebral bodies, creating the bamboo spine appearance.

TUMORS

Benign

Benign tumors may involve the spine (Table 12-9). One such tumor is the hemangioma. These are usually asymptomatic and an incidental finding in the spine. Hemangiomas in the spine require no therapy unless they become symptomatic. Symptoms may develop when the tumor causes a pathologic fracture or the lesion extends outside the vertebrae and compresses the spinal cord. Hemangiomas can develop in other bones, but in the spine they have a classic appearance with prominent or thickened vertical trabeculae that simulate

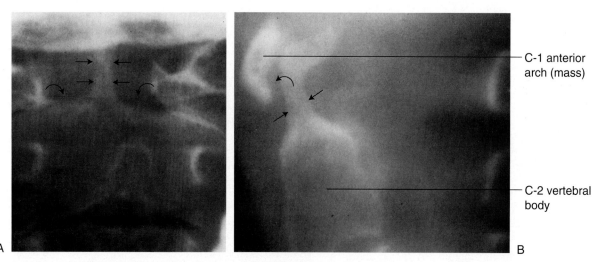

FIG. 12-43. A: Cervical spine AP open mouth radiograph. Rheumatoid arthritis. The odontoid process *(straight arrows)* is narrowed, osteopenic, and poorly marginated. Note the increased distances between the odontoid process of C2 and the inferior articular processes of C1 *(curved arrows)* due to partial loss of odontoid bone. **B:** Cervical spine lateral tomograph in the same patient. Rheumatoid arthritis. The odontoid *(straight arrows)* is markedly narrowed. The space between the anterior odontoid and the anterior arch of C1 *(curved arrow)* is greater than the normal 2.5 mm or less. This can also occur in ankylosing spondylitis.

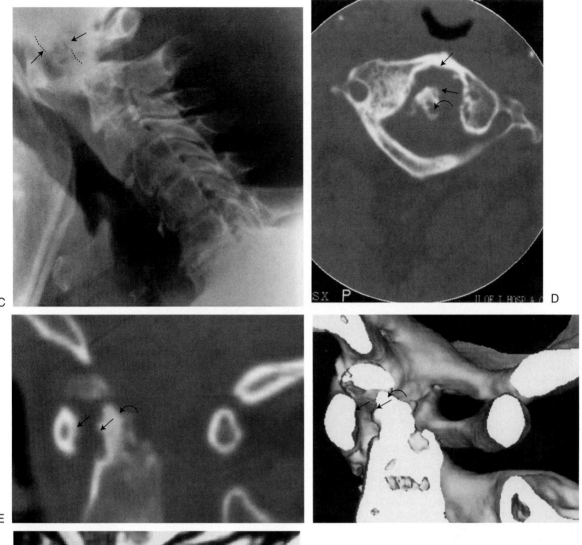

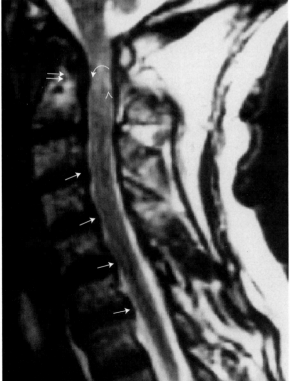

FIG. 12-43. *Continued.* **C:** Cervical spine lateral flexion radiograph in a different patient than shown in B. Rheumatoid arthritis. When the cervical spine is flexed, the space *(straight arrows)* between the anterior surface of the odontoid and the posterior aspect of the anterior arch of C1 *(dotted lines)* is dramatically widened. This widening represents an unstable dislocation of C1 relative to C2. There is grade 1 anterior spondylolisthesis of C2 relative to C3. Note the narrowing of all the cervical disc spaces and the generalized osteopenia. **D:** Cervical spine axial CT image. Rheumatoid arthritis with spinal stenosis in a 55-year-old man. The C1–2 joint is abnormal with 8 mm distance between the anterior arch of C1 and the odontoid *(between the straight arrows)*. There are advanced erosive changes in the odontoid *(curved arrow)*. **E, F:** Cervical spine CT sagittal reconstruction (E) and sagittal CT three-dimensional reconstruction (F) in the same patient as shown in D. The odontoid is involved with erosive changes and has a distal penciled appearance *(curved arrows)*. There is redemonstration of the abnormal C1–2 joint *(between the straight arrows)*. **G:** Cervical spine sagittal T2 MR image in the same patient as shown in D–F. The odontoid *(double arrows)* is displaced posterior resulting in spinal stenosis and cervical cord compression *(curved arrow)*. The increased signal in the compressed cord *(arrowhead)* probably represents edema and/or chronic reaction to the compression. The single straight arrows indicate multiple levels of mild spinal stenosis.

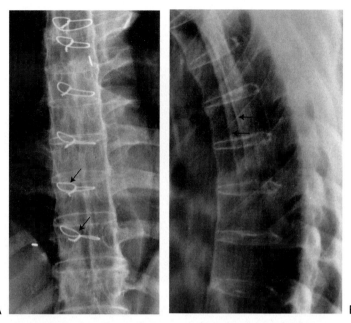

FIG. 12-44. Dorsal spine AP **(A)** and lateral **(B)** radiographs. Ankylosing spondylitis. There is an overall bamboo appearance to the spine and generalized osteopenia. The straight arrows on the AP radiograph indicate opaque wire sutures. On the lateral radiograph the scapulae *(straight arrows)* are nicely visualized.

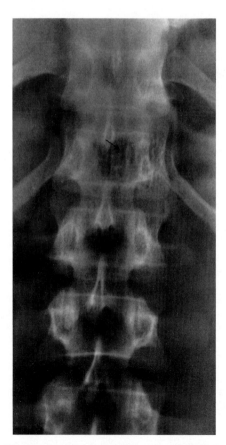

FIG. 12-45. Dorsolumbar spine AP radiograph. T12 vertebral body hemangioma. The prominent vertical trabecular pattern is characteristic of bone hemangioma *(straight arrow)*. Compare the appearance of the T12 vertebral body to those above and below that level.

jail bars (Fig. 12-45). The differential diagnosis should include severe osteoporosis, osteolytic metastatic disease, primary bone tumors, and Paget's disease. However, in Paget's disease the vertebrae tend to have a picture frame appearance. Osteoporosis tends to be osteopenic or hypolucent with prominent vertebral endplates, whereas metastatic osteolytic disease in the spine is usually radiolucent and destructive.

Aneurysmal bone cysts (ABCs) are benign and generally occur in young people. Some believe that they are not primary bone lesions but exist secondary to other processes such as infection, other tumors, or trauma. They occur in the posterior portions of the vertebrae, ends of long bones, and in flat bones. Pain is usually the presenting symptom. On radiographs (Fig. 12-46) they appear multicystic, expansile or ballooning, and may have a fracture or a blowout point associated. In general, these lesions are lytic in appearance, and they must be differentiated from osteoblastoma, giant cell tumor, and tuberculosis (4). It should be remembered that an ABC can arise from a primary bone tumor, but the primary bone tumor could be overlooked because the ABC appearance is dominant.

Osteoblastoma (Fig. 12-47) is a rare bone tumor that is usually considered benign, but a small percentage of them recur or invade locally. Thus, they are considered to be at least potentially malignant. The patients generally present with local pain, and occasionally a mass is palpable. The most frequent sites of involvement are the pedicles, lamina, and spinous processes. When the tumor mass invades the neural canal, a variety of secondary neural symptoms may be present. The appearance of this lesion is so variable that the differential

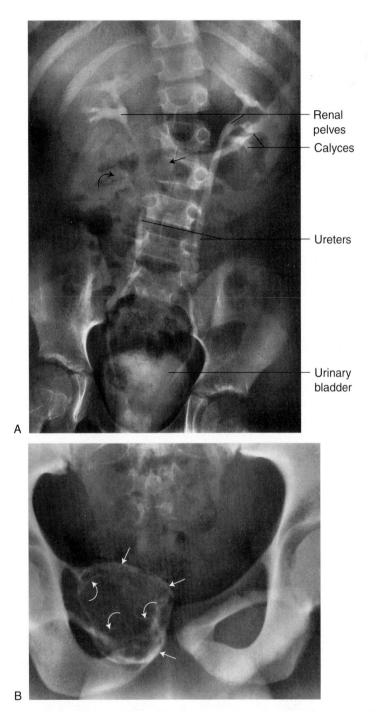

Renal
pelves

Calyces

Ureters

Urinary
bladder

A

B

FIG. 12-46. A: Abdomen AP radiograph selected from an excretory urogram. Aneurysmal bone cyst of the L3 lumbar vertebra. This 11-year-old girl complained of back pain. The right pedicle of L3 vertebra is missing *(straight arrow)* and there is scoliosis of the lumbar spine. Further workup revealed a partially calcified, large, and contiguous soft tissue mass lesion to the right of L3. The approximate location of this lesion's soft tissue component is indicated by the curved arrow. This is difficult to see on this image. However, it was the missing L3 pedicle that led to a more thorough workup and the correct diagnosis. This is a good example of how a missing pedicle can be the principal clue to the presence of an abnormality. **B:** Pelvis AP radiograph. Aneurysmal bone cyst of the right superior pubis ramus *(straight arrows)*. The lesion has the classic ballooned and thinned cortex *(straight arrows)* as well as a multicystic appearance. The curved arrows indicate bony septa that traverse the lesion.

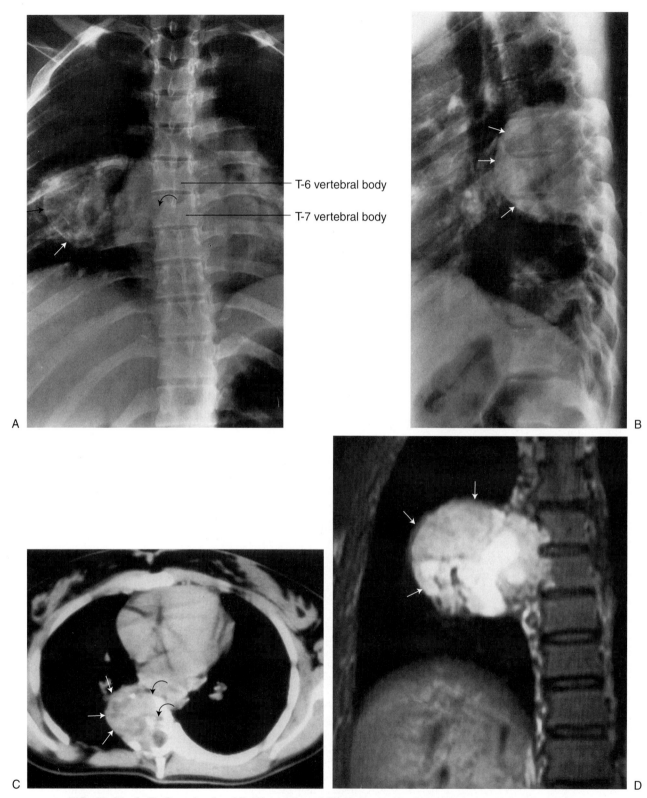

T-6 vertebral body

T-7 vertebral body

A

B

C

D

FIG. 12-47. A, B: Dorsal spine AP (A) and lateral (B) radiographs. Osteoblastoma of the T7 vertebra. This 22-year-old had back pain, and a mass lesion was discovered on a chest radiograph. A large dense lesion projects to the right of dorsal spine *(straight arrows)*. The right pedicle of T7 is missing *(curved arrow).* **C, D:** Dorsal spine axial CT image (C) and coronal T2 MR image (D) in the same patient. The osteoblastoma *(straight arrows)* is clearly demonstrated on both CT and MRI. The extensive destruction of the vertebral body *(curved arrows)* is evident on the CT image.

diagnosis must include a wide variety of benign and malignant bone tumors. Thus osteoblastoma should be included in the differential diagnosis of any bone lesion in the spine. Figures 12-47C and D illustrates the important role that CT and MRI play in the workup of bone tumors.

Malignant

As previously discussed in Chapter 11, *metastatic disease is the most common neoplasm in bone and this includes the spine.* As in other bones, metastatic disease involving the spine can be osteolytic (Fig. 12-48) with and without destruction and/or osteoblastic activity (Fig. 12-49). The primary neoplasms causing osteolytic and osteoblastic bone lesions are listed in Table 12-10.

The importance of visualizing the vertebral pedicles is emphasized in Fig. 12-50. When one or both pedicles are missing in patients with known or suspected cancer, the first diagnosis that must come to mind is metastatic disease. MRI is very useful to confirm the presence of metastatic disease in a vertebra with a missing pedicle

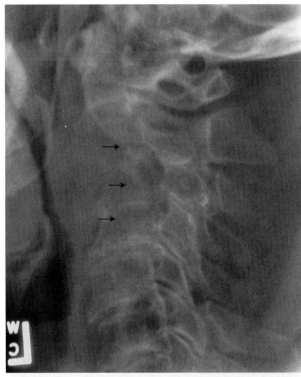

A

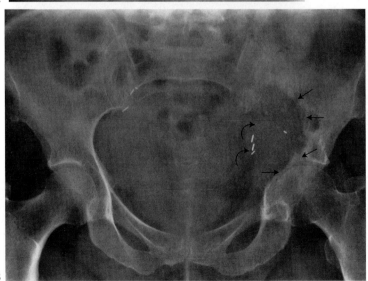

B

FIG. 12-48. A: Cervical spine lateral radiograph. Osteolytic metastatic disease of multiple cervical vertebrae. The C2, C3, and C4 vertebral bodies are involved by destructive (lytic) metastatic disease from the lung *(straight arrows).* **B:** Pelvis AP radiograph. Osteolytic metastatic carcinoma of the cervix involving the left ilium and ischium *(straight arrows).* The extensive involvement of the left ischium has resulted in left acetabular protrusio. There is a large soft tissue metastatic mass in the left pelvis *(curved arrows).*

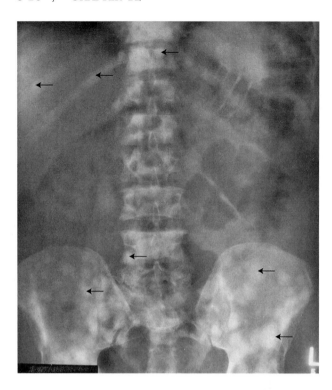

FIG. 12-49. Abdomen AP radiograph. Osteoblastic metastatic carcinoma of the prostate. The multiple areas of increased density *(straight arrows)* represent the metastases that involve the pelvis, lumbar spine, dorsal spine, and ribs.

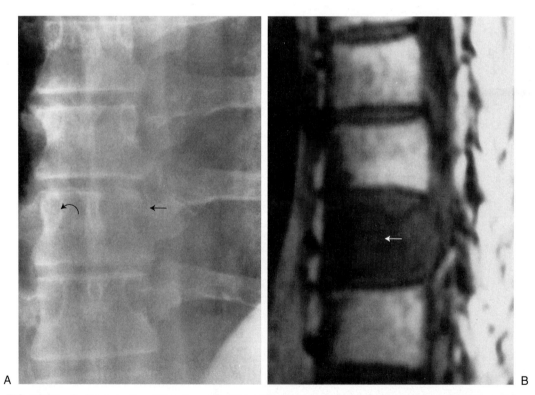

A

B

FIG. 12-50. A: Dorsal spine AP radiograph. Osteolytic metastatic lesion of the left T9 vertebral pedicle. The missing left T9 pedicle *(straight arrow)* was destroyed by metastatic disease while the uninvolved normal right T9 pedicle *(curved arrow)* remains clearly visible. This finding prompted further investigation by MRI that proved the missing pedicle was destroyed by a metastatic lesion. **B:** Dorsal spine sagittal T1 MR image in the same patient. Metastatic disease of the T9 vertebra. The metastatic disease involving the T9 vertebral body *(straight arrow)* has replaced almost all of the bone marrow fat, resulting in a low-intensity signal. This abnormality of T9 is quite obvious when compared to the high-intensity signals from the normal bone marrow of the uninvolved vertebral bodies above and below T9.

TABLE 12-10. *Characteristics of metastases*

Osteoblastic:
  Prostate
  Breast
  Lymphoma
  Carcinoid
  Neuroblastoma (occasional)
Osteolytic:
  Breast
  Lung
  Almost all other metastatic tumors

(see Fig. 12-50B) and to assess the extent and location of the metastases (Fig. 12-51).

Malignant primary bone lesions of the spine occur in an older age group and are more likely to involve the vertebral body than benign lesions (3). All primary bone tumors can occur in the spine including multiple myeloma (most common), chondrosarcoma, osteosarcoma,

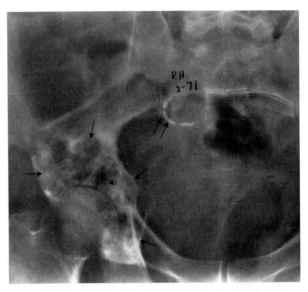

FIG. 12-52. Pelvis AP radiograph. Chondrosarcoma of the right ischium and ilium *(straight arrows)* in a 69-year-old. Note the classic popcorn calcification within the tumor *(curved arrows)*. There is residual barium in the appendix *(double straight arrows)* following a gastrointestinal barium study.

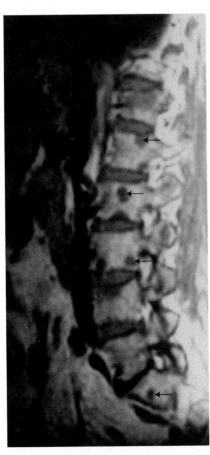

FIG. 12-51. Lumbosacral spine sagittal T1 MR image. Metastatic carcinoma of the breast. The patient complained of severe back pain, but the radiographs were negative. The straight arrows indicate some of the many metastatic lesions present in the lumbar and sacral spine. The metastatic lesions appear black on the T1 MR image but white or gray on T2 images.

Ewing's sarcoma, and lymphoma (3). Multiple myeloma and all primary bone tumors must be differentiated from metastatic disease, and this is sometimes very difficult. Chondrosarcomas (Fig. 12-52) tend to be slow growing and produce cartilage. They often involve the pelvis as well as the long bones, and the lesions tend to be expansile with popcorn-like calcifications.

Primary tumors of the thecal sac and the spinal cord can mimic bone tumors of the spine. Thus tumors arising from these structures should be considered in the differential diagnosis when dealing with back pain and abnormal radiographs and myelograms.

METABOLIC DISEASES

Paget's disease is due to an imbalance of osteoclastic and osteoblastic activity that may be metabolic in origin (4), and this has been discussed in Chapter 11. It often involves the spine and, more frequently, the pelvis (Fig. 12-53). The classic spine appearance is the picture frame vertebra caused by increased peripheral vertebra density and central lucency.

Osteopenia, osteoporosis, and osteomalacia have been discussed in the metabolic disease section of Chapter 11. The typical patient with osteoporosis (Fig. 12-54) is elderly and complains of back pain, especially if secondary compression fractures are present. Vertebral fractures not only cause back pain, but will often result in loss of height and kyphosis. The typical

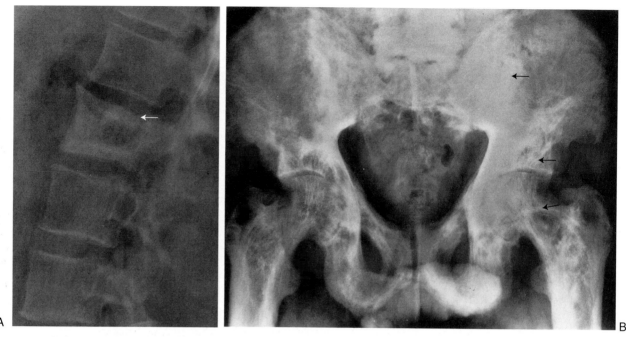

FIG. 12-53. A: Lumbar spine lateral radiograph. Paget's disease L2 vertebra *(straight arrow)*. The L2 vertebra has the classic picture frame appearance secondary to the increased trabecular density in the periphery of the vertebral body. There is mild loss of the L2 vertebral body height compared to the vertical heights of L1 and L3, and this is compatible with a mild compression fracture. The remainder of the lumbar spine is not involved by the Paget's disease. **B:** Pelvis AP radiograph. Paget's disease. The bone trabeculae are coarse *(straight arrows)* with an overall increased density and widening or expansion of the bones.

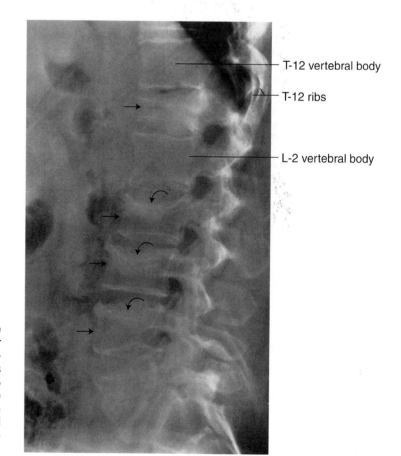

FIG. 12-54. Lumbar spine lateral radiograph. Senile osteoporosis. Note the overall decreased density or osteopenia of the spine. There are multiple compression pathologic fractures secondary to osteoporosis *(straight arrows)*. The fractures of L1, 3, 4, and 5 are manifest by a loss of the vertical heights of the involved vertebral bodies. Compare the fractured vertebrae to the normal vertical heights of the T12 and L2 vertebral bodies. Note the multiple fish-mouth deformities *(curved arrows)*.

radiographic appearance of osteoporosis in the spine is decreased overall density of the vertebral bodies, and as a result the vertebral endplates appear prominent. As the vertebra become softer than the disc, the endplates can sag (4), resulting in fish-mouth deformities of the vertebrae.

Sickle cell anemia is a Mendelian dominant hereditary trait. The disease is variable in severity and characterized by crises that include anemia, fever, severe abdominal and bone pain, and bone infarction. Radiographs may show osteoporosis, bone infarcts, aseptic necrosis, and fish-mouth vertebrae (Fig. 12-55).

INFECTION

Osteomyelitis or bone infection is common and has been discussed in Chapter 11. Spine infections are caused by a wide range of organisms, but staphylococcal infections are the most common. Vertebral osteomyelitis is becoming more prevalent because of drug addiction. As with osteomyelitis, elsewhere, patients with spinal osteomyelitis usually have fever and localized pain. The radiographic findings are nonspecific, and there often is some degree of destruction of the vertebral body and/or disc spaces (Fig. 12-56). Osteomyelitis should be in the differential diagnosis of all lytic bone lesions. Radionuclide scanning is often helpful to detect osteomyelitis, especially when the radiographs are negative. MRI is sensitive to detect osteomyelitis (Fig. 12-57). On T1 MR images, the infections have a decreased signal intensity (they appear black), whereas on T2 images the infections have an increased signal intensity (they appear white). CT scanning may detect bone and joint destruction that is not visible on radiographs.

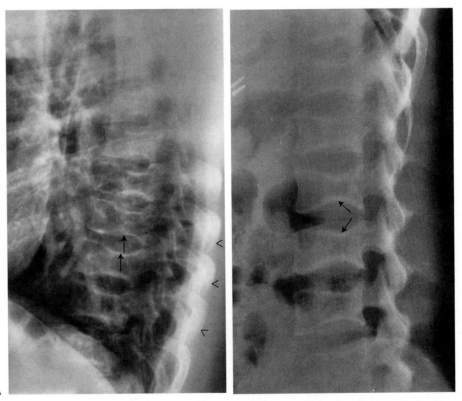

FIG. 12-55. Dorsal spine **(A)** and lumbar **(B)** spine lateral radiographs. Sickle cell anemia. There is overall osteopenia and the fish-mouth deformities of the vertebral bodies *(straight arrows)* are similar to those in senile osteoporosis (Fig. 12-54). Note the ribs in A *(arrowheads)*.

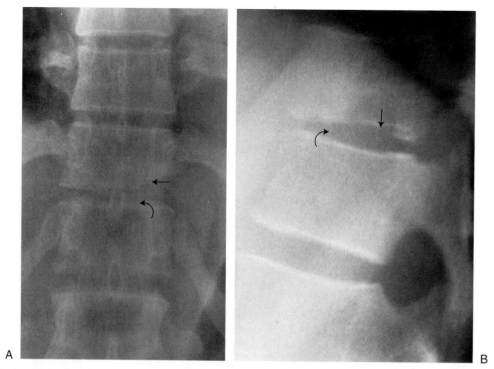

FIG. 12-56. Lower dorsal and upper lumbar spine AP **(A)** and lateral **(B)** radiographs. Osteomyelitis of T11 vertebral body. This 41-year-old patient had back pain and a low-grade fever. There is destruction of the posterior portion of the T11 inferior endplate *(straight arrows)*, and the marked narrowing of the T11–12 intervertebral disc space *(curved arrows)* suggests disc and joint destruction.

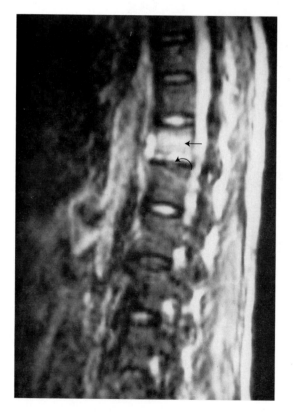

FIG. 12-57. Thoracic and lumbar spine T2 sagittal MR image. Osteomyelitis of the T11 vertebral body and infectious destruction of the T11–12 intervertebral disc space. The white appearance of the T11 vertebral body confirms the clinical impression of osteomyelitis *(straight arrow)*. Compare the abnormal density of T11 vertebral body to the normal density of the uninvolved vertebral bodies above and below the T11 vertebra. Notice that a large portion of the T11–12 intervertebral disc is missing *(curved arrow)* compatible with probable disc destruction. Compare the involved abnormal disc space at T11–12 to the normal-appearing discs above and below.

Key Points

- Basic observations on spine radiographs should include spinal alignment, the vertical heights of the vertebral bodies and the intervertebral disc spaces, osseous density, presence of the pars interarticularis in the lumbar spine, and presence of the pedicles on each vertebra. An absent pedicle is abnormal and should make you suspicious of a destructive process such as primary and secondary bone neoplasm.
- Spine CT is good for bone detail, localization of fracture fragments and their relationship to the spinal canal and cord, and diagnosis of herniated intervertebral disc disease.
- Spine MRI is good for imaging disease processes that involve the bone marrow fat such as tumor and infection. MRI is also valuable for diagnosis and staging of herniated intervertebral disc disease and evaluating the spinal cord.
- Most congenital anomalies of the spine are asymptomatic.
- Hyperflexion injuries include tear-drop fractures, posterior ligament injury, and facet locking. Locked facets commonly have associated spinal cord injury.
- Odontoid process fractures are unstable and result from hyperflexion and hyperextension injuries. Open mouth AP radiographs, CT, and tomography are useful tools to diagnose odontoid fractures.

REFERENCES

1. Edeiken J. *Roentgen Diagnosis of Diseases of Bone*, 4th ed. Baltimore: Williams and Wilkins, 1990.
2. Greenspan A. *Orthopedic Radiology*, 2nd ed. Philadelphia: JB Lippincott, 1992.
3. Weinstein J. *The Lumbar Spine.* Philadelphia: WB Saunders, 1990.
4. Griffiths H. *Basic Bone Radiology*, 2nd ed. Norwalk, CT: Appleton and Lange, 1987.

CHAPTER 13

Brain

Wilbur L. Smith

BRAIN IMAGING

Neuroradiology was a relatively unsophisticated branch of imaging prior to 1970. Plain radiographs of the skull were insensitive for predicting neurologic disorders, and obtaining more useful diagnostic imaging information about the brain and spinal cord was cumbersome, painful, and yielded images that were difficult to interpret without advanced knowledge of neuroanatomy. The early brain imaging techniques were all at least minimally invasive and many involved such gruesome activities such as injecting air into the spinal canal and rolling the patient about in a specially devised torture chair. Few patients willingly returned for another one of those exams! The highest level of comfort that the poor patient who needed brain imaging could anticipate was a direct puncture carotid arteriogram or a spinal tap.

The invention and widespread utilization of the technique of computerized axial tomography (CAT), or computed tomography (CT), allowed relatively painless access to the processes inside the skull and allowed the field of neuroradiology to become a premier subspecialty within radiology. The old scans were slow, lacking in detail, and hard to manage (Fig. 13-1), but they were such a marvelous advance that they were embraced as a revolution in medical imaging. Indeed, Sir Godfrey Hounsfield, the pioneer of CT imaging, won many international awards and was knighted for his work. Despite advances in developing many other imaging modalities to date, CT still forms the basis for most diagnostic studies of the brain and spine and is the most common

neuroimaging study performed in the United States. CT scans are routinely performed either with or without intravenous contrast enhancement and certain indications are generally predictive of the need for contrast, although there are many variations. Table 13-1 gives the usual indications for contrast use, however, if in doubt, radiologists are always available for consultation on individual cases.

In CT scanning, images of the brain are acquired in axial (horizontal) planes and then viewed at different digital levels, so that one can see the bones of the face and skull as well as the tissues of the brain itself. Two image acquisitions are not required to get this data, but rather two different levels of viewing the same digital data. The sections that result from the CT scans depict the anatomy at predetermined intervals depending on the parameter of slice thickness. Generally, the thicker the slices the fewer the sections needed to get through the brain, but as the slices are thickened, anatomy is depicted in less detail. In the standard brain CT scan, there are several key landmarks to observe for proper orientation. Figure 13-2 illustrates some of the highlights for which you should look in orienting yourself to the anatomy depicted by the slices.

Let's begin with the caudal sections and work cephalad. The fourth ventricle, a cerebrospinal fluid space located dorsal to the brain stem and in the midline of the posterior fossa, is a good marker for identifying the level of the pons, cerebellar vermis, and the base of the anterior cranial fossa (Fig. 13-2A). On the same section lying ventral to the brain stem is the suprasellar cistern and the dorsum sellae. Note that the figures depict the

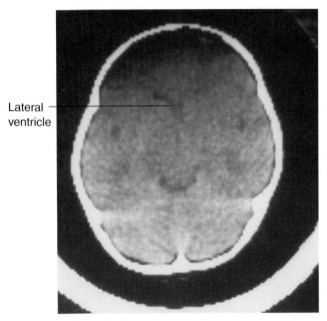

Lateral ventricle

FIG. 13-1. A scan of the brain performed in 1976 on an EMI device. This single section took about 1 minute to acquire. The coarse pixels make anything but the larger brain structures such as the ventricles difficult to appreciate. This was, however, a huge improvement over the pneumoencephalogram.

TABLE 13-1. *A brief listing of common indications for CAT scanning emphasizing those needing intravenous contrast enhancement*

Indications for CAT scan	IV contrast
Trauma	No
Infection	No
Congenital anomalies	No
Tumor	Yes
Metabolic disorder	No
Multiple sclerosis	Yes
Hydrocephalus	No

cle, one encounters the ambient cistern and cephalad portion of the suprasellar cistern (Fig. 13-2B). The former is an important landmark for the point where the cerebral peduncles (an extension of the brain stem) pass through the tentorium cerebri. Ventral to this landmark and slightly cephalad are located the third ventricle and the anterior horns of the lateral ventricles. At the lateral margins of the anterior horns of the ventricles are the basal ganglia, identifiable as masses of gray matter bordering the lateral and third ventricles (Fig. 13-2C). The caudate nuclei protrude into the anterior horns of the lateral ventricles. Further cephalad the scans depict the brain cortex and the orderly interfaces between the gray and white matter (Fig. 13-2D). Note that each section of gray matter has an accompanying area of white matter arranged in a predictable pattern. Symmetry is everything in looking at CT scans of the brain, providing that the patient is properly positioned, structures should match up from side to side.

Despite its immense success, CT has limitations that inhibit its value. CT is inherently limited in its ability to display high degrees of tissue contrast. If two tissues absorb roughly the same number of photons, CT cannot

anatomy of the posterior fossa less sharply than some of the more cephalad sections of brain. CT scans in the posterior fossa are somewhat degraded owing to the absorption of x-rays by the large amount of dense surrounding bone, therefore, detail of the cerebellar hemispheres may be obscured. This technique limitation is mitigated to some degree by faster and better scanners, but bone artifact is a limitation of CT scanning. Proceeding to sections cephalad from the fourth ventri-

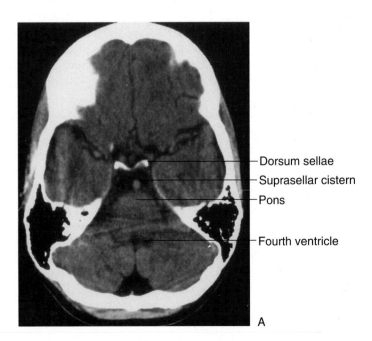

Dorsum sellae
Suprasellar cistern
Pons
Fourth ventricle

A

FIG. 13-2. A: CT scan of a normal adult at the level of the 4th ventricle. The brain stem structure ventral to the fourth ventricle is the pons. Further anterior lies the five-pointed star representing the suprasellar cistern. Lying within the suprasellar cistern are the vessels of the circle of Willis and the dorsum sella or back of the sella turcica.

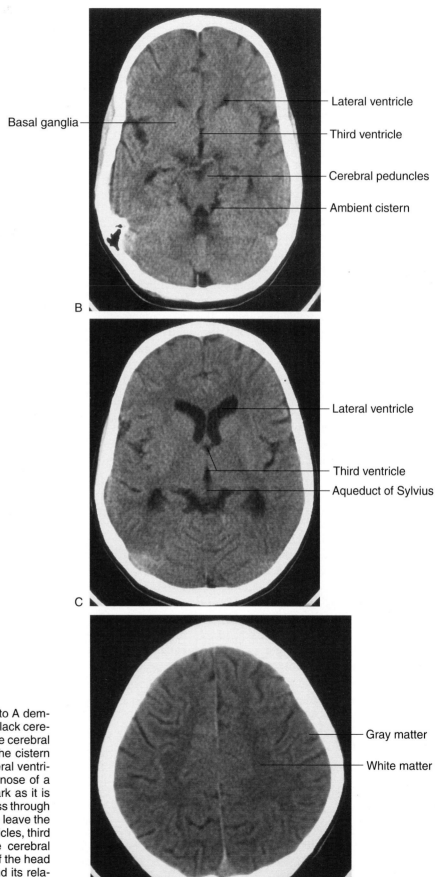

FIG. 13-2. *Continued.* **B:** A cut cephalad to A demonstrates the ambient cisterns as curved black cerebrospinal fluid densities just posterior to the cerebral peduncles. If you use your imagination, the cistern is the mouth, the anterior horns of the lateral ventricles the eyes, and the third ventricle the nose of a smiling man! This is an important landmark as it is the point where the cerebral peduncles pass through the tentorium. **C:** Proceeding cephalad we leave the posterior fossa and image the lateral ventricles, third ventricles, aqueduct of Sylvius, and the cerebral hemispheres. **D:** A scan near the vertex of the head depicts the white matter (black on CT) and its relationship to gray matter. Note that each area of gray matter has an associated column of white matter.

TABLE 13-2. *A comparison of indications and factors affecting the choice of CT or MRI*

Factor	CT	MRI
Cost	++	+++
Availability	+++	++
Tissue differentiation	+	+++
Multiplanar sequences	+	+++
Speed of exam	+++	++
Bone reconstruction	+++	+

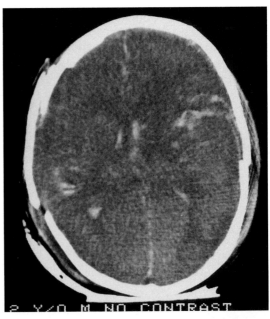

FIG. 13-3. A child injured in a severe auto accident shows multiple white areas in the brain as well as disruption of the skull. The white areas are intraparenchymal hemorrhage. Note also the disruption of the normal brain architecture (compare to Fig. 2D, which shows a section at roughly the same level) reflecting the severe cerebral edema.

discriminate between them. Bone or other high-density items such as aneurysm clips degrade the CT image. While the time needed to obtain a section by CT has declined substantially in recent years, there are physical limitations to CT scanning in moving and positioning uncooperative or disabled patients.

The newest technique in the imaging of the brain and spinal cord is magnetic resonance imaging (MRI). This technique also had humble beginnings; the first scanners were used to quantify fat in livestock coming to market. MR images are wonderfully detailed, but the studies require more time and are more expensive to carry out than CT scans. Despite the great potential of MRI and its proliferation from a research device in the early 1980s to a staple of most imaging departments in the United States, CT scans still provide the bulk of diagnostic brain images. Table 13-2 compares the strengths and limitations of CT and MRI.

TRAUMA

Perhaps the most common indication for brain imaging is trauma. Human heads are extremely vulnerable to injury; consequently, the trauma CT scanner rarely lacks sufficient business. In assessing a CT performed for trauma, one has a finite number of search parameters for major findings that represent conditions likely to demand immediate intervention.

The presence of blood in the head, but outside the vascular system is often a key to the correct diagnosis. Fortunately, when blood is loose in the head, it usually appears as a conspicuous white blob on the CT scan. Therefore the first rule of looking at trauma CT scans is to "look for the white collections inside the skull" (Fig. 13-3). Your diagnosis often can be even more specific because the white (or blood) tends to align in certain predictable ways according to its anatomic location. As an overview, the locations of intracranial bleeding are first separated into intraaxial, meaning within the brain tissues themselves, or extraaxial. The extraaxial hemorrhages occur in spaces with characteristic shapes that can assist in localizing the hemorrhage. Fluid in the epidural space, between skull and dura, usually presents as a crescentic mass, convex to the brain (Fig. 13-4).

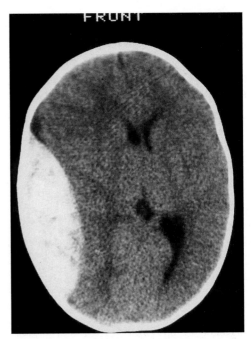

FIG. 13-4. A large mass of white (blood) density convex toward the brain is characteristic of an epidural hemorrhage. Most of these occur due to traumatic tear of an artery and are surgical emergencies. The brain is shifted by the hematoma as evidenced by the shift of midline.

The subdural space between dura and arachnoid membranes, however, is usually concave paralleling the surface of the skull, therefore subdural hematomas are differentiated from epidural bleeding by their shape (Fig. 13-5). Subarachnoid blood diffuses over the surface of the gyri and fills the CSF cisterns around the brain (Fig. 13-6). Intraaxial bleeding is often confined to the area of the ruptured vessel and is entirely enclosed within the substance of the brain. By first finding the "white" blood, then looking at its shape and anatomic location, one can be pretty precise about the diagnosis and the location of the blood. As the hematoma ages, the blood assumes different image characteristics. Table 13-3 is a description of the differing appearances of blood in the head with age of the bleed.

After looking for bleeding in trauma patients, the next step is to look for mass effect, a clue that there is pressure impinging on an area of the brain. For most injuries, the best way to find significant mass effects is to look for asymmetry with displacement of the midline structures, the most prominent of which are the falx cerebri, lateral ventricles, and interhemispheric fissure (Figs. 13-4 and 13-7). A midline shift away from a lesion, e.g., an epidural blood collection, is usually an emergent situation, particularly in the context of trauma. However, a word of caution is advisable: Midline shift does not always signal a need to take out your pocket knife to perform emergent, kitchen-table-type neurosurgery. Diffuse edema of one hemisphere of the brain (Fig.

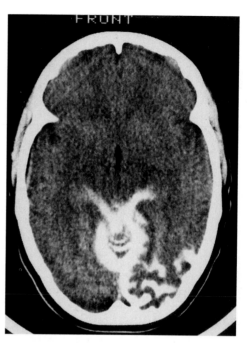

FIG. 13-6. A CT scan at the level of the ambient cistern showing the cistern as white (blood) instead of black (cerebrospinal fluid) (compare to Fig. 2B). Note that the white density also surrounds the brain stem and has an irregular pattern outlining the gyri of the occipital lobe. When blood mimics cerebrospinal fluid distribution it is usually extraaxial and in the subarachnoid space flowing around and over the brain tissues.

13-7) or even atrophy of the contralateral hemisphere can cause apparent (or real) shift. The important concept is midline shift. When the brain structures are shifted away from the side of the evident abnormality, such as a hematoma, increase your level of suspicion and urgency in evaluating your patient.

After searching for blood and mass effects on the brain CT scan, the next important step is to assess the densities of the brain tissues themselves. Earlier we described how the gray and white matter components of the brain should be visible on the CT scan (see Fig. 13-2D). The lateral ventricles and CSF spaces are black and should be easily distinguished as separate from the tissues of the brain. Variations on this theme are generally bad news. The most prominent and dangerous sign

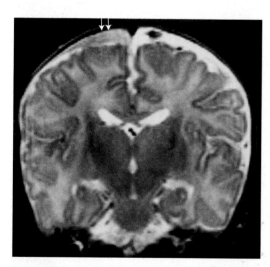

FIG. 13-5. MRI of the brain, shown to illustrate that MRI is also effective in showing trauma. This is an abused child who has a subdural space hematoma *(arrows)*. Note that the surface is concave, reflecting the contour of the cerebral cortex, but not extending among the gyri. This configuration is typical for a subdural hematoma. Note also that the signal densities are different on MRI. Imaging of bleeding is more complex on MRI than by CAT.

TABLE 13-3. Characteristics of intracranial blood by imaging

| Time of bleed | CT | MRI | |
		T1-weighted	T2-weighted
Immediate	White	Black	Black
Acute	White	White	Black
Subacute	White	White	White

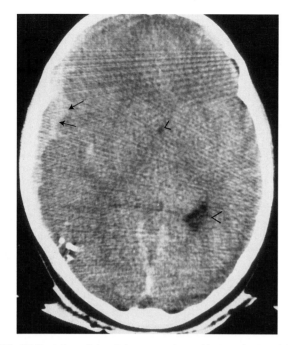

FIG. 13-7. Intraaxial or intraparenchymal hemorrhage of the brain in a trauma patient. The white densities (blood) do not conform to any definable space and are actually within and between the tissues of the brain. A subdural hematoma *(arrows)* is also present in this patient. Note that the lateral ventricle and its temporal horn *(arrowheads)* are displaced by the mass effect.

is the obliteration of the distinction between the gray and white matter, which indicates profound edema in the area. If this is a universal pattern, there is a special name for the profound edema that occurs obliterating all brain landmarks; "the bad black brain" (Fig. 13-8). This finding usually portends a poor outcome, representing diffuse breakdown of tissue integrity with ensuing cerebral edema. The cause of this catastrophic chain of events is almost always a limitation of the oxygen supply to the brain tissues, owing to either a compromise of the blood supply or a loss of oxygen to the brain cells. In the latter instance, as the brain swells, cerebral blood supply is compromised by loss of the arterial perfusion gradient and ultimately there is no circulation to the brain. Owing to different tissue densities and less vulnerable perfusion, the basal ganglia and brain stem are often particularly conspicuous against the uniform density of the "bad black brain" and their conspicuity results in the so-called reversal sign (Fig. 13-9).

Please note the intentional lack of a detailed discussion of skull fractures in this section on trauma. That is because in general skull fractures aren't very important in the immediate outcome of a patient. It is the effect of the trauma on the brain that does your patient harm, not the crack in the bone (Fig. 13-10). A significant big exception is the depressed skull fracture, a situation where the bone is driven directly back into the menin-

geal coverings and the brain itself. CT imaging and bone windows are of great importance in documenting the depth and extent of this type of injury, as well as documenting any intracranial air leaks owing to tears of the dura or meninges (Fig. 13-11). In this type of trauma, surgery is usually needed and the identification of the fracture, depth of the fragment(s), surface brain injury, and pneumocephalus (air inside the skull) are the key observations.

MRI is not to be totally omitted in any discussion of trauma, but its role is usually secondary. Owing to the limitations of patient access (ventilator limitations, difficulty in patient observation, etc.) and the longer examination times, MRI is rarely the first imaging modality employed for acute trauma. After the acute, life-threatening emergencies have been handled, MRI is extremely sensitive for assessing the extent of parenchymal injury to the brain or defining more precisely the compartment of localized extraaxial fluid. In each of these instances the prognosis and etiology of the injury is better defined after MRI. MRI spectroscopy, a study of brain metabolism, holds great promise for predicting the outcome of some injuries. The utility of MRI for finding subarachnoid blood is debatable, but MRI is unparalleled in defining precisely which gyrus was smashed in a previous auto accident (Fig. 13-12). The instances where MRI is critical in deciding the urgent management of a trauma patient are few, but it is an invaluable secondary tool in selected patients.

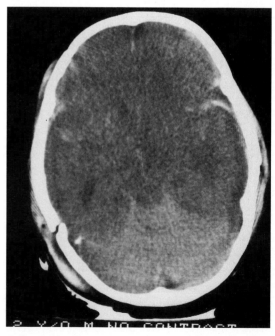

FIG. 13-8. This severely brain-injured child has neither recognizable ventricles nor gray/white matter differentiation (compare with Fig. 13-2D). In fact, the whole neocortex, except for the areas of hemorrhage, is a uniform shade of black. This severe brain edema portends a poor prognosis.

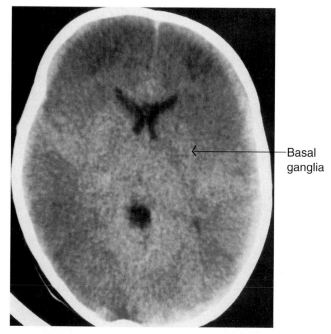

FIG. 13-9. A child with diffuse hypoxic injury of the brain demonstrates the reversal sign. Note that the basal ganglia are gray and the neocortex black, particularly in the frontal and parietal regions.

Basal ganglia

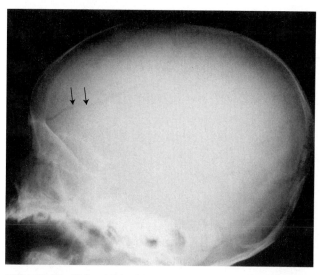

FIG. 13-10. This child with a linear skull fracture *(arrows)* was completely asymptomatic (except for a palpable bump on his skull) because the brain underlying the skull was not affected. The presence of the skull fracture documents trauma but is of little importance in patient management.

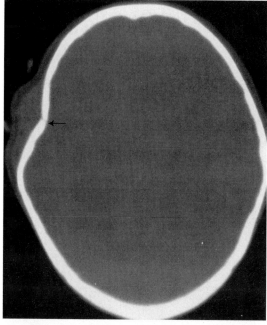

FIG. 13-11. Bone windows of a CT scan demonstrate the depth of injury in a depressed skull fracture *(arrow)* after this teenager was struck with a hammer.

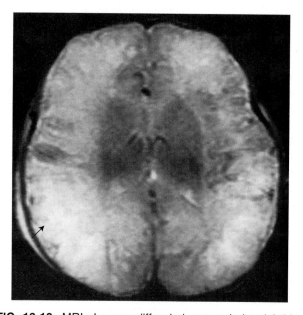

FIG. 13-12. MRI shows a diffusely increased signal (white indicated by arrow) in the posterior parietal lobes of a blunt head trauma victim. This is owing to a cortical contusion that was subtle on the CT scan. Although the finding explained the patient's symptoms and documented the severity of injury, the lesion did not require urgent intervention.

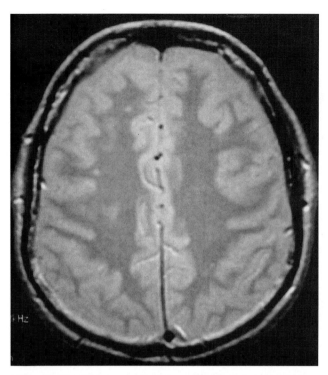

FIG. 13-13. Widely scattered unidentified bright objects (UBOs) in the white matter of this octogenarian are not of significance. These UBOs are common near the basal ganglia but can be seen anywhere and are assumed to represent small artery disease with lacunar infarctions.

In summary, a CT scan of an acute trauma patient should be evaluated for the following findings: (a) white densities defining bleeding, including the shape and distribution of the blood collection(s); (b) mass effect, particularly with shift of the midline structures; and (c) loss of normal contrast characteristics (or asymmetry) of the normal tissue and CSF interfaces. These rules won't get you every answer on every trauma patient, but they will help you in almost 95% of the cases you see. For the other 5%, you may have to do a radiology or neurosurgery residency!

VASCULAR DISEASE

Just after trauma as an indication for brain imaging is vascular disease, and the most prevalent form is stroke. Stroke results from occlusion of the vascular supply (usually arterial but occasionally venous as well) to a focal area of the brain causing tissue ischemia. Many "strokes" are small and not even detected clinically. Most people in their fifth or sixth decade have small areas of abnormal signal called UBOs (unidentified bright objects) on MRI of the brain (Fig. 13-13), and there are some who ascribe the origin of UBOs to silent strokes. We have a lot of brain tissue that we don't fully use, so that loss of these small areas isn't necessarily perceived as a clinical problem.

Only when either a large or a particularly critical area of brain becomes ischemic do emergent symptoms appear and neuroimaging come into play. CT scans are often the first examination, however, their use is problematic as there is a significant incidence of falsely negative CT scans in the first 24–48 hours after a stroke. The size, severity, and presence of hemorrhage clearly affect the CT picture of stroke, so that some strokes appear almost immediately, however, the sensitivity of CT scan for the diagnosis is considerably higher after the first 24–48 hours (Fig. 13-14).

The most reliable finding in stroke on CT scan is the loss of normal architecture of brain substance. The area of the stroke is depicted as a dark (edematous) blotch obliterating the normal tissue density. Occasional strokes will have associated bleeding, particularly in patients with hypertension, and the blood will show up on CT as a white density within the darker area of infarct (Fig. 13-15). A stroke may also change in nature as the tissue is destroyed and revascularization takes place. Bleeding may ensue such that initially nonhemorrhagic strokes can develop high signal characteristic of internal bleeding. This change often portends a poor prognosis.

There is a developing body of knowledge suggesting that early treatment of stroke may restore circulation and limit brain tissue damage. This has led to a change

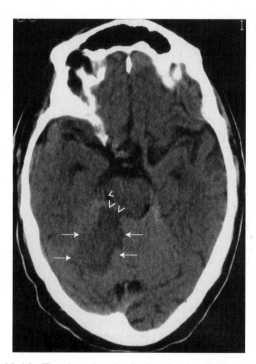

FIG. 13-14. The low-density lesion in the right cerebellar hemisphere represents an acute stroke owing to arterial occlusion. Note that there is swelling of tissues involved in the stroke as evidenced by effacement of the ambient cistern on the right *(arrowheads)*. The lesion does not contain blood because there is no white signal on CT.

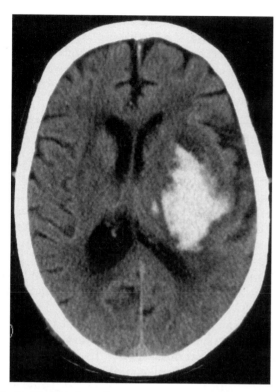

FIG. 13-15. This huge hematoma in the left side of the brain has an irregular margin and edema surrounding the white area of fresh hemorrhage. This is a 53-year-old hypertensive executive who suffered a fatal acute hemorrhagic stroke.

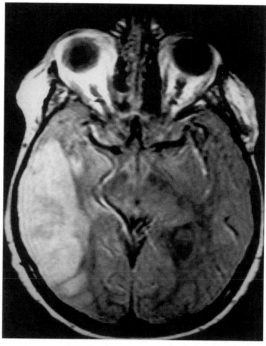

FIG. 13-16. The white area in the right temporal lobe on this patient is a newly symptomatic stroke as depicted by gadolinium-enhanced MRI.

in imaging to emphasize early diagnosis. MRI is more sensitive to the early changes and has assumed a larger role in the imaging of acute stroke. On MRI the damaged tissues are white (on T2) owing to the large amount of free water leaked by the ischemic cells. The use of MRI contrast (gadolinium) has improved detection even further and MRI may soon be the standard for stroke imaging (Fig. 13-16).

So far we've discussed acute strokes. Chronic strokes result in atrophy of the brain tissue (Fig. 13-17) manifested by either focal or diffuse shrinkage of the brain owing to cell death. Of special note is diffuse multi-infarct dementia, a condition that is difficult to differentiate from Alzheimer's disease. Here the strokes are small and confined to the areas near the ventricles, so that the ventricles enlarge at the expense of the dead tissue (Fig. 13-18). The patient's CT scan looks like the ventricles are dilated, with the gyri and sulci appearing unusually prominent—a condition sometimes referred to as *hydrocephalus ex vacuo.* These cases are truly a conundrum because Alzheimer's disease, normal pressure hydrocephalus of the elderly, and diffuse brain atrophy from any cause all look the same. Functional brain imaging with spectroscopy, blood perfusion analy-

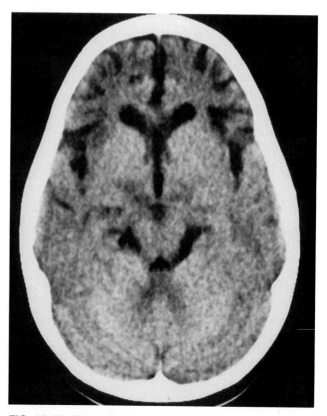

FIG. 13-17. This elderly man has diffusely dilated ventricles as well as deep sulci over the brain surface because of atrophy presumably associated with multiple prior infarcts.

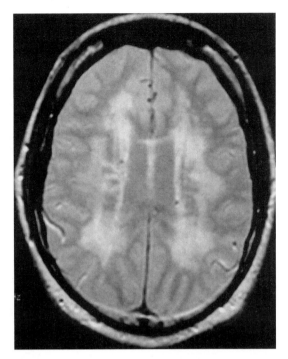

FIG. 13-18. T2-weighted scan at the level of the lateral ventricles demonstrates multiple high-signal periventricular infarcts owing to lack of perfusion of the deep layers of the brain. These patients present with dementia and movement disorders that may mimic a number of degenerative neurologic conditions.

sis, and/or metabolic measurement is of future consideration for this diagnosis. There is no easy imaging answer and at present there is no specific treatment with good efficacy for any of these conditions, however, this is a rapidly developing area of medicine and exciting imaging developments are to be anticipated.

TUMOR

The third common application of brain imaging is tumor evaluation. In adults, metastases (Fig. 13-19) constitute the most common tumors, with primary benign or malignant tumors being somewhat less common. The converse is true in children owing to the lower frequency of primary malignancies that metastasize to brain. The location of the tumors also differs with age. A greater proportion of adult tumors are in the cerebral cortex, whereas in children the proportion of tumors originating below the tentorium is much greater (Fig. 13-20).

CT scanning for tumor follows the same general principles as for trauma, with the major exception that most tumor scans are performed after the administration of intravenous contrast. The theory, which works most of the time, is that the abnormal tumor circulation allows contrast to penetrate the blood–brain barrier and enhance the tumor. Because contrast enhancement is white on a CT scan the tumor becomes conspicuous. However, tumors can bleed, and the white of the contrast may obscure the white of the bleeding. Because the appearance of blood is an important issue in tumor patients, we often have to study them both with and

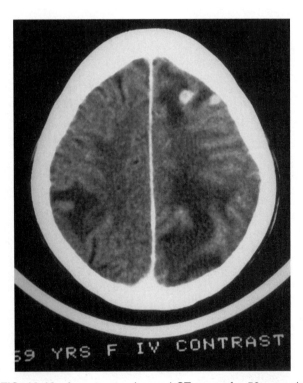

FIG. 13-19. A contrast-enhanced CT scan of a 59-year-old woman with known lung cancer shows multiple high- and mixed-density lesions. These were metastases from the lung tumor.

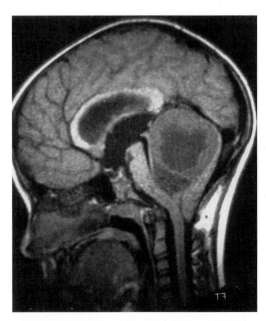

FIG. 13-20. T1-weighted MRI documents a huge tumor that arises from the cerebellar vermis and pushes the brain stem forward. This is typical behavior of a medulloblastoma.

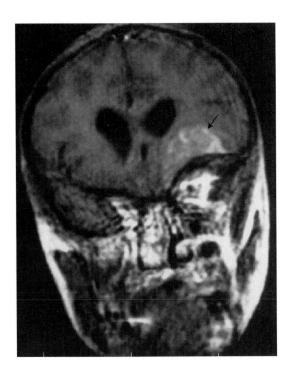

FIG. 13-21. This large tumor *(arrow)* has a broad base along the roof of the orbit and displaces the frontal lobe of the brain superiorly. This growth is typical of an extraaxial tumor, in this case a meningioma.

without intravenous enhancement. In defining tumor and normal anatomy imaging MRI equals or surpasses CT in efficacy, however, CT is cheaper and more widely available, and therefore it remains the most common initial examination for the diagnosis of brain tumor.

Just as with trauma, it is important to differentiate intraaxial masses (within the brain tissues) from extraaxial masses, as the differential diagnosis and approach are different. Determining tumor origin is one of the most difficult diagnostic tasks. In general, an extraaxial tumor will display its widest base at the brain surface and will smoothly indent the brain from without (Fig. 13-21). Extraaxial tumors tend to be related to the meninges or the bones of the skull. Occasionally, a parenchymal brain tumor originates at the brain surface and differentiation is impossible. Conversely, extraaxial tumors sometimes grow from slips of tissues insinuated into the brain, giving the appearance of parenchymal masses.

Tumors that are entirely enveloped within the brain tissues are usually of glial cell origin, with astrocytoma being the most common primary tumor (Fig. 13-22) and metastasis being the most common. When the distinction of intraaxial from extraaxial is difficult and critical, using another modality with multiplanar imaging capability, such as MRI, is invaluable. MRI also offers different tissue contrast parameters, and contrast-enhanced MRI adds yet another dimension.

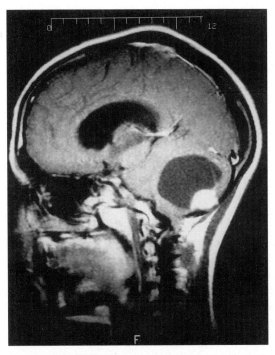

FIG. 13-22. On gadolinium-enhanced MRI this cerebellar tumor contains a very bright nidus of tissue within a cystic mass. This is characteristic of a pilocytic astrocytoma.

Once the tumor is diagnosed and localized to the proper anatomic location, the next job is to look at the mass effect caused by the tumor and to assess the likelihood of damage to critical centers of the brain which may require emergent action. Here, the same principles applied in trauma are useful. Does the tumor cause displacement of the normal structures, such that they are sufficiently compressed to cause compromise of the blood supply or direct pressure damage to the cells of the normal brain tissue? If so, you have to move quickly. Once again, shift away from the tumor and alteration of the normal differentiation of the brain tissues are key to the proper determination.

CONGENITAL ANOMALIES

Although CT is often employed for the diagnosis of congenital anomalies of the brain, MRI, with its superior tissue contrast, is invaluable in this area. Congenital anomalies usually present in childhood, either with abnormal physical findings or with seizures. Physical abnormalities most often associated with congenital brain abnormalities include macrocephaly (big head), abnormal appearance of the face (particularly with midline abnormalities such as cleft palate), and meningocele. Each of these findings should tip you off to pursue a specific type of abnormality.

In the case of macrocranium (a big head), the likely diagnosis is hydrocephalus or dilatation of the ventricles because of abnormal cerebrospinal fluid (CSF) circulation. The lateral ventricles stand out so well owing to their CSF content that CT is well adapted to the initial diagnosis and monitoring of treatment for hydrocephalus (Fig. 13-23). The most critical factor is determining the cause of the hydrocephalus so that you can predict whether or not surgical shunting will be of value for the patient. In most instances the method is straightforward: One looks for the most caudal dilated ventricle and assumes that the obstruction is between that site and the most cephalad normal ventricle. For example, if the lateral and third ventricles are dilated but the fourth ventricle is normal, the obstruction is likely at the outflow area of the third ventricle or the aqueduct of Sylvius (Fig. 13-24).

Often obstructive hydrocephalus can become static owing to equilibration of the CSF dynamics of production and absorption. In this case, it may not be necessary to place a shunt to drain the CSF. Once the dilated ventricles are detected, the need to shunt can be determined by following the ventricular size over time. This should, of course, be coupled with close observation of the patient's clinical status. Don't ever let the imaging hold you back if your patient is deteriorating. CT scans provide sufficient detail for monitoring progression of hydrocephalus. MRI is often of value in the initial evalu-

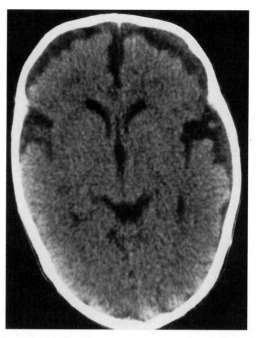

FIG. 13-23. This child presented with a large head. Family history documented macrocranium in several other family members including the father. The head CT scan shows the ventricles to be slightly enlarged and the subarachnoid spaces to be prominent. This constellation of findings is diagnostic for benign familial macrocranium. In this instance, the child needed no treatment and the CT scan was sufficient to exclude a major problem.

ation of hydrocephalus, but follow-up monitoring is the domain of CT. Hydrocephalus can occur on other than a congenital basis, but the rules outlined here for evaluation hold for most instances.

MRI is the best method for initial evaluation of most babies with complex defects of the face and brain because of its multidimensional imaging capability. Holoprosencephaly, or failure of division of the embryonic forebrain, is always associated with facial anomalies and is a good prototype for illustrating the value of MRI. This complex series of anomalies ranges all the way from a totally malformed brain, a condition not compatible with life, to agenesis of the septum pellucidum and optic abnormalities (septooptical dysplasia), conditions compatible with long life (Fig. 13-25). Whereas CT scans are sufficient for the gross defects of holoprosencephaly, MRI can show sufficient detail to define the absence of the septum pellucidum as well as showing the midline defects of the optic tracts. If you have one test to do in these children, MRI is the best.

Meningocele is a common condition caused by failure of closure of the embryonic neural tube. This condition is almost invariably associated with a complex series of abnormalities called the Arnold–Chiari malformation. The reason all of these brain anomalies are associated

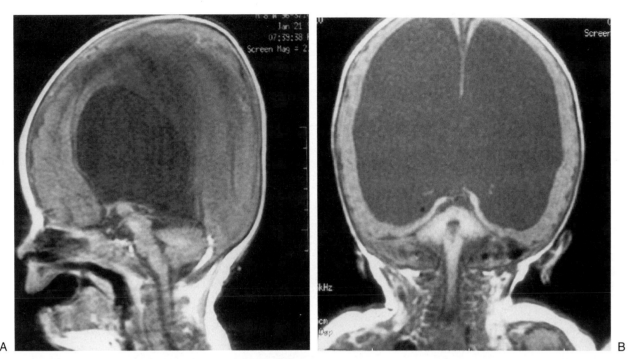

FIG. 13-24. A sagittal **(A)** and coronal **(B)** MRI of an infant with a huge head at birth. The child has severe hydrocephalus involving the lateral and third ventricles but a normal fourth ventricle. This is suggestive of an aqueductal obstruction.

with what commonly is a spinal abnormality is complex, but the findings are reproducible and best demonstrated by MRI (Fig. 13-26). The tethering of the spinal cord that occurs with meningocele is associated

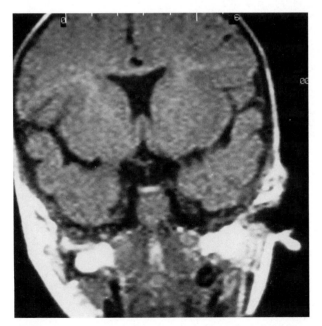

FIG. 13-25. MRI of an infant with septooptical dysplasia documents the minimal abnormality of incomplete septation of the lateral ventricles by showing a deficiency of the septum pellucidum.

with protrusion of the cerebellar tonsils below the foramen magnum. As with our other examples, the complex anatomy in developmental brain anomalies is best shown by MRI.

The finding of seizures in a child suggests a congenital defect, either structural or owing to a metabolic problem. In either case, MRI is more likely to yield the correct answers. Structural abnormalities include errors of neuronal migration where the brain tissues are arrested in their normal growth, leaving focal islands of tissue in abnormal locations throughout the brain (Fig. 13-27). Other structural abnormalities result from abnormal rests of tissues proliferating and disrupting the normal brain tissue. A good prototype condition here is tuberous sclerosis (Fig. 13-28), although any of the other phakomatosis can give similar problems. Metabolic abnormalities causing seizures usually cause demyelination, thereby affecting the white matter either diffusely or as focal lesions (Fig. 13-29). MRI is clearly superior to CT here, although the findings are not specific for one disease process, focal infection or demyelinating disorders such as multiple sclerosis can look the same as metabolic defects.

There are many other potential uses for CT scanning in neurologic disease. However, if you retain the general principals elucidated here, you can make most of the diagnoses needed for patient care, whether or not you completely master all of the nuances of the differential diagnosis.

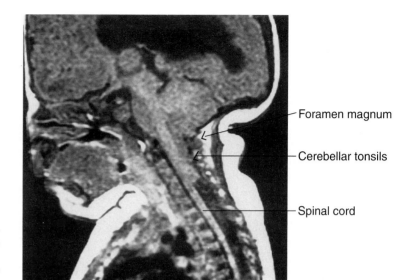

Foramen magnum

Cerebellar tonsils

Spinal cord

FIG. 13-26. MRI from a baby with lumbar myelo-meningocele. The posterior fossa is small and the cerebellar tonsil protrudes far below the foramen magnum. This is a constant component of the Arnold-Chiari malformation.

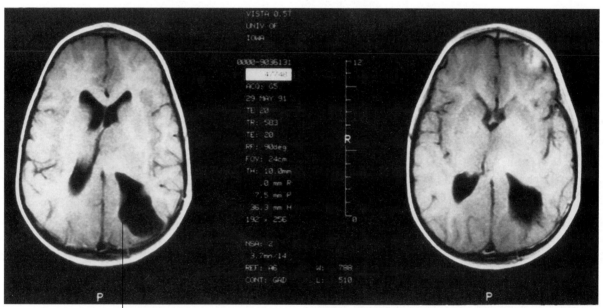

Schizencephalic cleft

FIG. 13-27. A child with seizures. MRI shows a cleft from the posterior portion of the left lateral ventricle all the way to the brain surface. This condition, caused by a failure of proper migration of neurons as the brain is formed, is called *schizencephaly*.

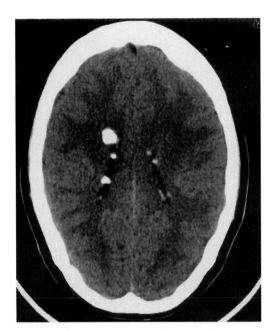

FIG. 13-28. CT scan of the brain demonstrates calcification in the roof of each lateral ventricle. These calcifications are within the hemartomas or tubers. MRI would also demonstrate the hemartomas as well as showing the lesions that are not calcified.

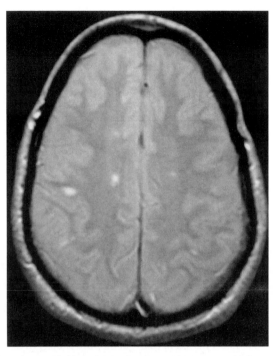

FIG. 13-29. Multiple high-density white matter lesions are consistent with a myelodegenerative phenomenon, in this case multiple sclerosis. These findings are not specific and must be combined with the clinical and laboratory results in order to be diagnostic.

Key Points

- Computerized axial tomography (CAT), or computed tomography (CT), is the most commonly performed neuroimaging study in the United States. CT scans can depict the brain in horizontal planes that can be viewed at different levels.
- When assessing a CT scan for potential trauma, begin by looking for blood in the head outside the vascular system. Blood appears on CT initially as a white blob.
- Mass effect is a clue that pressure is impinging on an area of the brain. The best way to find significant mass effect is to look for asymmetry with displacement of the midline structures.
- Obliteration of the distinction between gray and white matter in the brain represents profound edema. If the edema is universal, you are witnessing a "bad black brain," which portends a poor outcome and is almost always caused by a limitation of oxygen in the brain.
- On CT, acute strokes often initially appear as a dark edematous blotch obliterating the normal tissue density. On MRI, the damaged tissues are white due to water leaked by the ischemic cells.
- Tumors that are entirely enveloped in the brain tissues are usually of glial cell origin, with astrocytoma being the most common primary tumor.
- Complex anatomy in developmental brain anomalies is best shown with MRI.
- Physical abnormalities most often associated with congenital brain abnormalities include macrocephaly (big head), abnormal appearance of the face (particularly with midline abnormalities such as cleft palate), and meningocele.

SUGGESTED READING

Osborn A. *Diagnostic Neuroradiology.* St. Louis: CV Mosby, 1994.

CHAPTER 14

Head and Neck Radiology

Wilbur L. Smith

HEAD AND NECK IMAGING

Head and neck radiology in many practices is considered an offshoot of neuroradiology. The structures are in close proximity and share many common functions, however, for this text we will emphasize the differing approaches to imaging and the different indications that make head and neck radiology unique. This field, unlike neuroradiology, still has a great reliance on plain radiographs for initial diagnosis, particularly for common conditions such as paranasal sinusitis and trauma imaging. Computed tomography (CT) and magnetic resonance imaging (MRI) are liberally used for complex cases and surgical planning, especially if tumor is suspected or to amplify the findings on the screening radiographs. This is a pattern seen with increasing frequency, and in the future the reliance on plain radiographs may dwindle as the cost of CT and MRI declines and access to these devices becomes universal.

The plain films of the facial series, like all other plain film studies, illustrate three-dimensional anatomy in two planes, therefore, it is necessary to have two views of the structures (e.g. an anterior view and a lateral view) in order to infer the third plane. The most commonly employed plain radiograph of the face is the Waters' view (Fig. 14-1). An easy way to visualize the Waters' is to think of yourself (with x-ray eyes) facing the patient, then having the patient tilt his or her head back about 30 degrees from the horizontal plane. You could then in theory look right up the middle of the patient's maxilla and nasal cavity! The anterior structures of the midface are optimally demonstrated by the Waters' view.

Because most facial trauma originates from anterior and the maxillary sinuses are most commonly suspect for infection, the Waters' is the most widely used facial radiograph. Obviously, some things will be distorted in this view, e.g., the mandible is not optimally seen, the ethmoid sinuses are inconspicuous, and only the anterior orbital rim is evident. Other standard views are clearly necessary and a number of specialized views exist. The Caldwell view is used predominately to see the orbits and ethmoid sinuses (Fig. 14-2). To visualize this projection, picture the patient looking straight into your x-ray eyes. You get a great view of the orbit, although the middle ear structures are superimposed. The ethmoid and frontal sinuses are clearly delineated as is the upper portion of the nose and the frontal bone of the skull. The maxillary sinuses are partially overlapped by the orbits making this view less valuable for seeing the maxilla. The final commonly obtained projection is a lateral (Fig. 14-3), the third dimension to complete the dimensional prospective. Because the Caldwell and Waters' views are posterior-to-anterior projections, you cannot see the posterior walls of structures or the angle of the mandible without the lateral view. The sphenoid sinus, a deep skull base structure, is only clearly visible on the lateral projection. Table 14-1 outlines the structures optimally visualized by different projections of the facial bones on radiographs.

INFECTION

Sinusitis, implying an infection of the mucosa of one or more of the four major paranasal sinuses, is probably

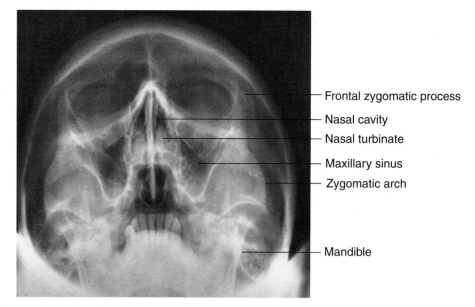

Frontal zygomatic process
— Nasal cavity
— Nasal turbinate
— Maxillary sinus
— Zygomatic arch

— Mandible

FIG. 14-1. Normal Waters' view of the face showing the good delineation of the maxilla. The maxillary sinuses are optimally displayed and the anterior portions of the orbit and the nasal cavity are clearly outlined.

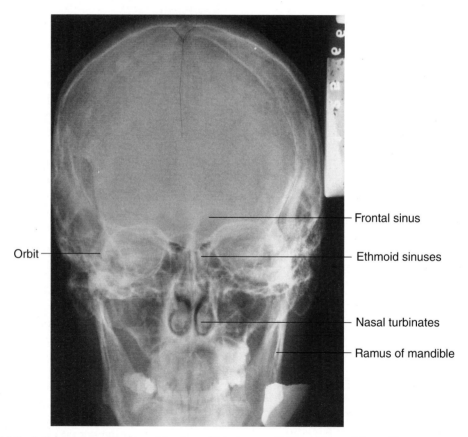

Orbit

— Frontal sinus

— Ethmoid sinuses

— Nasal turbinates

— Ramus of mandible

FIG. 14-2. A Caldwell, or PA view of the face. Note how well the orbits and frontal bone are seen. The maxilla is superimposed on the skull base to some degree. The structures of the internal auditory canals are visible through the orbits.

TABLE 14-1. *Structures optimally visualized by different projections in radiographs*

Projection	Anatomic structures visualized
Waters'	Maxilla, maxillary sinus, anterior orbit
Caldwell	Orbit, ethmoid sinus, frontal sinus
Lateral	Maxillary sinus, airway, sphenoid sinus

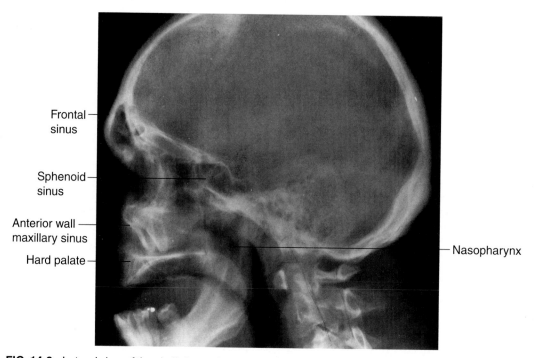

Frontal
sinus

Sphenoid
sinus

Anterior wall
maxillary sinus

Hard palate

Nasopharynx

FIG. 14-3. Lateral view of the skull shows the posteriorly located sphenoid sinus and the nasopharyngeal airway. This view complements the others adding the third dimension to the structures of the head and neck.

the most common indication for head and neck radiographic imaging. The clinical picture of pain, swelling over the sinuses, and leukocytosis may be convincing no matter what the radiograph shows, and in patients with that triad, there is litle to be gained by imaging except perhaps to stage disease. In most instances, however, the patient's symptoms are nonspecific and the diagnosis is assumed based upon either an air–fluid level, a fluid-filled sinus, or thickening of the mucosal lining of the sinus. The cardinal assumption is that the radiographically opacified sinus is indeed infected. Fluid can come from many causes, and the diagnosis is rarely documented by bacteriologic means, therefore, despite a positive radiograph, a healthy degree of skepticism is warranted. Some authorities recommend that a CT scan of the sinuses be performed in equivocal cases where the plain radiographs are negative, and the clinical suspicion is high (Fig. 14-4). While the CT scan is a better anatomic definition of the opacified sinus, the assumption is the same, i.e., that fluid means infection. Secondary evidence such as bone destruction from osteomyelitis or erosion and expansion of the sinus by an organized inflammatory polyp, will add credibility to the surety of the imaging diagnosis of inflammatory sinusitis.

Children under age 5 merit special skepticism when a diagnosis of sinusitis is based on radiographs. Studies

have shown that children who are in mid-tantrum can fill their maxillary sinuses with tears which they clear by simply blowing their noses! That is pretty thin evidence on which to base a diagnosis of sinusitis! The sinuses develop at different ages in children, so that it is futile, for example, to look for frontal sinusitis in a 2-year-old as the sinus has not aerated at that age. Table 14-2 outlines sinus development by age. Sinusitis is an example of a diagnosis for which strong clinical correlation is desirable before accepting a diagnosis based solely on images.

In studying children's sinuses, it is important to note a unique relationship between ethmoid sinusitis and periorbital cellulitis of the child. The same antibiotics that treat the cellulitis will fix the sinusitis in most instances, so that it is often a moot point as to whether there is sinus disease present, however, it is also true that the periorbital cellulitis cases associated with sinus-

TABLE 14-2. *Sinus development by age*

Sinus	Age of aeration
Ethmoid	Birth
Maxillary	2 years
Sphenoid	6–7 years
Frontal	10–12 years

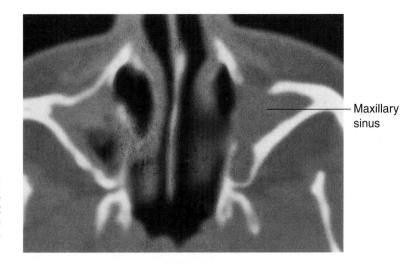

FIG. 14-4. CT scan of the maxillary sinuses in this 7-year-old child with fever and leukocytosis documents complete opacification of the left maxillary sinus and partial opacification of the right. Based on this clinical picture, this child almost certainly has sinusitis.

itis tend to be the more severe ones (Fig. 14-5). Recognizing the ethmoid cellulitis can be the tip off to deeper layers of orbital involvement including occasionally an intraorbital abscess (Fig. 14-6). Once the screening studies are completed by plain radiographs, CT scanning is the best technique for diagnosing the extent of sinus disease. MRI has a minimal role in the diagnosis of inflammatory disease of the sinuses. Many patients with severe periorbital cellulitis will require CT scanning.

TRAUMA

When accompanied by a good clinical examination, simple facial fractures can usually be adequately diagnosed from appropriate radiographs. Whenever complex trauma of an extensive nature is suspected, or when the plain radiographs show less injury than suspected on the basis of physical examination, then supplementary CT scans should be used and are invalu-

able. Any facial bone may be injured after trauma, but two types of fracture complex are both distinctive and frequent, warranting a detailed description; the "blowout" orbital floor fracture and the "tripod" fracture of the maxilla. Other bones may be broken and these fractures are frequently a component of more complex deep structure fractures. Whatever you do once you find one type of fracture, don't stop! Particularly in the face, the structures are small and close together, so that multiple fractures are the norm rather than the exception.

The blowout fracture occurs when an object strikes the eye straight on. The force is transmitted through the fluid-filled eyeball, rupturing the bone of the floor of the orbit and forcing the inferior rectus muscle through the fracture defect, and into the superior portion of the maxillary sinus. The eye muscle entrapment is manifested by limited range of motion of the eyeball, particularly for upward gaze. The characteristic radio-

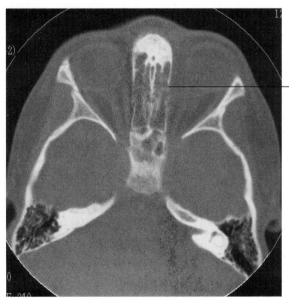

FIG. 14-5. CT scan of the orbit in a child with periorbital cellulitis shows extensive opacification of the ethmoid sinuses. A substantial portion of children with periorbital cellulitis have ethmoid involvement.

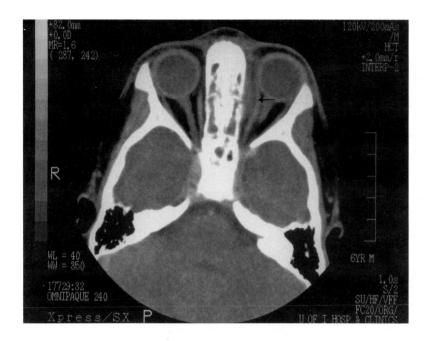

FIG. 14-6. CT scan with soft tissue windows of the child shown in Fig. 14-5 documents a soft tissue mass just medial to the medial rectus muscle of the orbit. This mass is an abscess *(arrows)* from the ethmoid sinusitis and osteomyelitis.

graph shows a mass within the roof of the maxillary sinus and disruption of the floor of the orbit (Fig. 14-7). This diagnosis is not hard clinically once muscle entrapment has occurred, however, occasionally the blowout is part of another complex series of fractures and the examination and plain radiographs are equivocal. In this situation, a CT in the coronal plane is definitive. Remember that a conventional CT scan plane will be parallel to the fracture and the fragment, making the diagnosis difficult, so that you need to look at a coronal plane or at coronal reconstructions to be sure. This injury requires prompt corrective surgery before vascular and nerve damage to the muscle ensue, therefore, you must suspect it and act promptly to confirm your diagnosis.

The tripod fracture is a close relative of the blowout except the site of the impact is a little lateral, missing the eyeball and striking the upper cheek just below the eye in a vulnerable spot where the frontal bone, zygomatic arch, and maxilla come together forming the eminence of the cheek. A blow in this area disrupts these three bones and their articulations, usually fracturing the zygoma and lateral wall of the maxillary sinus and disrupting the frontal zygomatic articulation to complete the tripod effect (Fig. 14-8). Tripod fractures can be diagnosed by plain film, but a CT scan is often valuable for assessing possible associated deeper injuries and planning any needed surgical repairs. If injuries go deeper into the face, they can disrupt the fixation of the facial bones to

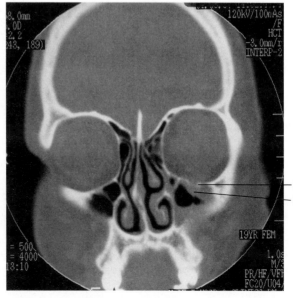

Blowout fracture
Entrapped muscle

FIG. 14-7. A blowout fracture of the orbit caused by a fist to the eye. Note the soft tissue mass protruding into the maxillary sinus. This woman had no gaze abnormality upon presentation for care but developed one shortly thereafter. The fracture required surgical reconstruction but the patient now has a normally functioning eye.

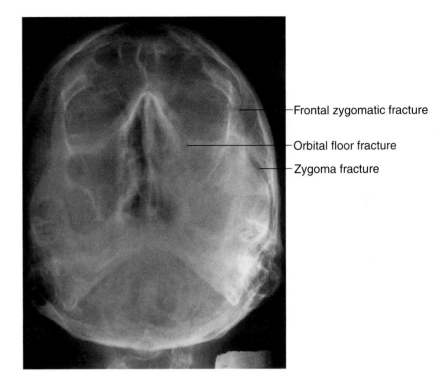

Frontal zygomatic fracture

Orbital floor fracture

Zygoma fracture

FIG. 14-8. After a fist fight this adult had severe facial swelling. The Waters view shows three components of the left tripod fracture; however, there are other fractures as well. This person needs a CT scan!

the skull base, the so-called LaForte fractures (Fig. 14-9). These need CT scanning for precise diagnosis and surgical planning, but the trauma necessary to cause such a fracture is so severe that the need for complex imaging is evident from the clinical examination.

Penetrating trauma in the face is also a major opportunity for imaging. Generally, plain radiographs are good for locating the foreign body (providing it is radiopaque), however, sectional imaging is almost always necessary for definition of the effects (Figs. 14-10 and 11).

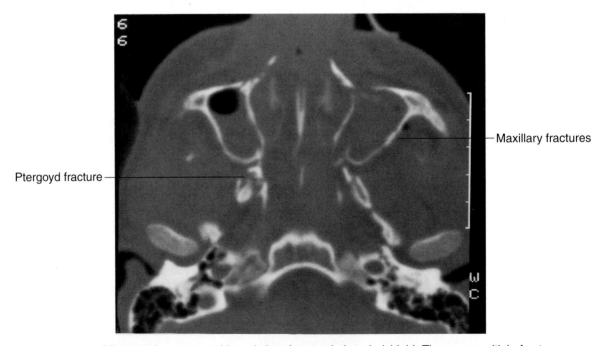

Ptergoyd fracture

Maxillary fractures

FIG. 14-9. CT scan of an auto accident victim who struck the windshield. There are multiple fractures including disruption of the deeper structures of the face (ptergoyd plates illustrated). This is a complex fracture pattern of the LaForte type and can only be defined well with CT.

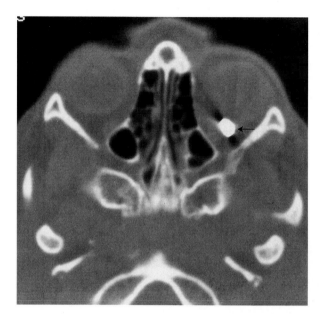

FIG. 14-10. Metallic BB *(arrow)* in the eye of a child. CT gives superior definition of the location and affected structures.

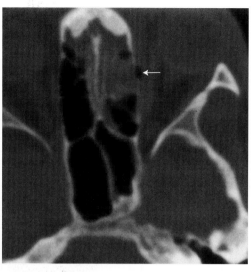

FIG. 14-11. This child was running with a pencil in hand. She fell impaling her eye on the pencil. The CT shows the disruption of the bones of the medial wall of the orbit and the air pushed in along the track of the pencil.

TUMORS

Head and neck tumor imaging is dependent on multiple complex interrelationships of tumor and normal structures, therefore, films are usually not definitive. Most cancers center about the nasopharynx, larynx, and mouth, requiring some type of sectional imaging for a definitive diagnosis of the extent of the lesion. The choice as to CT or MRI is frequently not an easy one and often both are needed, particularly if curative surgery is possible. The structures of the pharynx and face are small, complex, and closely interrelated, therefore, a tumor tends to creep along the paths of least resistance, spreading through tissue planes or bony canals to involve a number of important structures in a relatively small space (Fig. 14-12). Distant metastasis and ability to excise the tumor without removing vital normal tissues are key. These tumors tend to spread via the lymphatics, and it is wise to ensure that you carefully inspect lymph nodes in the area of the tumor prior to selecting

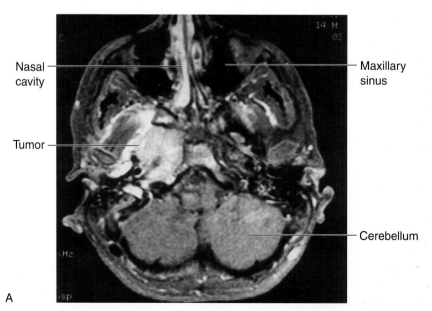

Nasal cavity

Maxillary sinus

Tumor

Cerebellum

A

FIG. 14-12. A: Axial MRI of the nasopharynx shows a large malignant squamous cell carcinoma infiltrating the soft tissue planes of the face and growing along the skull base. The tumor is white owing to enhancement with gadolinium. A tumor this extensive carries a poor prognosis.

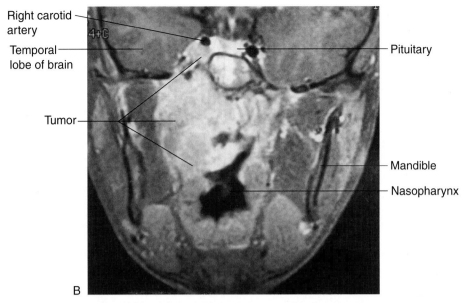

Right carotid artery

Temporal lobe of brain

Tumor

Pituitary

Mandible

Nasopharynx

B

FIG. 14-12. *Continued.* **B:** A coronal view of the face demonstrates the value of being able to visualize structures in multiple planes by MRI. Here we see the tumor distorting the lateral wall of the nasopharynx and invading the skull base lifting the right carotid artery and abutting the pituitary gland.

a course of action (Fig. 14-13). A monograph on facial and laryngeal diagnosis is beyond the scope of this chapter. The important message is that sectional imaging and help from the radiologist are key for diagnosis and staging.

Benign tumors and congenital anomalies of the head and neck abound. While plain radiographs are helpful, particularly for bony lesions, sectional imaging and ultrasound are the usual methods for definition of the abnormality. The reason that ultrasound is valuable in

children is that many of the tumors are cystic and the differentiation of cyst from solid alters the diagnostic probabilities.

In summary, head and neck radiology employs plain radiographs for the diagnosis of trauma and sinusitis. Tumors almost always need more complex sectional imaging. The definition of the normal tissue plains is key to understanding tumor spread and the possibility for curative surgery. Usually these data can only come from CT or MRI.

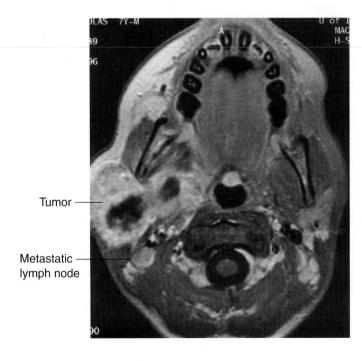

Tumor

Metastatic lymph node

FIG. 14-13. Gadolinium-enhanced scan of a 40-year-old with a necrotic cancer of the parotid gland. The metastasis to a regional lymph node is evident on the scan. Imaging not only defines the tumor, but confirms the presence of metastasis.

Key Points

- The most commonly employed radiograph of the face is the Waters view, in which the structures of the midface are optimally demonstrated by filming the patient with his or her head tilted back at around a 30-degree angle from the horizontal plane.
- Sinusitis is among the most common indications for head and neck imaging. The diagnosis is often based on an air–fluid level, a fluid-filled sinus, or thickening of the mucosal lining of the sinus. In most cases it is assumed that a radiographically opacified sinus is indeed infected.
- Because structures in the face are small and in close proximity to one another, multiple fractures are the norm rather than the exception. Two of the most distinctive and frequent of the fracture complexes in the face are the blowout orbital floor fracture and the tripod fracture of the maxilla.
- Tumors of the pharynx and the face tend to creep along the path of least resistance to involve a number of important structures in a relatively small space. Usually, either CT or MRI is necessary for a definitive diagnosis in these cases.

SUGGESTED READINGS

Harnsberger RH. *Handbook of Head and Neck Imaging,* 2nd ed. St. Louis: CV Mosby, 1995.

Peters S, Curten H. *Head and Neck Imaging,* 3rd ed. St. Louis: CV Mosby, 1996.

Subject Index

Note: An f after a page number denotes a figure; a t after a page number denotes a table.